Contemporary Perspectives in Wound Healing

Contemporary Perspectives in Wound Healing

Edited by Connie Freeman

hayle
medical

New York

Hayle Medical,
750 Third Avenue, 9ᵗʰ Floor,
New York, NY 10017, USA

Visit us on the World Wide Web at:
www.haylemedical.com

ISBN: 978-1-63241-573-8

Cataloging-in-Publication Data

Contemporary perspectives in wound healing / edited by Connie Freeman.
    p. cm.
Includes bibliographical references and index.
ISBN 978-1-63241-573-8
1. Wound healing. 2. Wounds and injuries. 3. Wounds and injuries--Treatment.
4. Dermatology. I. Freeman, Connie.
RD94 .C66 2019
617.1--dc23

Table of Contents

Preface

Wound healing is a complex process of repair where the skin and the tissues in an injured area repair themselves. In undamaged skin, the dermis and the epidermis constitute a protective barrier against the external environment. When this barrier is ruptured, a sequence of hemostasis, inflammation, proliferation or tissue growth and tissue remodeling occurs to repair the damage. This process of healing can be interrupted by factors, such as diabetes, infection, venous or arterial disease or metabolic deficiencies of old age, leading to the formation of non-healing chronic wounds. The major complications of wound healing include deficient and excessive scar formation, deficient contraction, exuberant granulation, dystrophic calcification, Marjolin's ulcer, etc. Various skin substitutes, biologics, biomembranes and scaffolds are used to facilitate wound healing. This book is a valuable compilation of topics, ranging from the traditional to the contemporary clinical perspectives in the domain of wound healing. It aims to present researches that have advanced the understanding of wound healing. This book, with its detailed analyses and data, will prove immensely beneficial to professionals and students involved in this area at various levels.

This book unites the global concepts and researches in an organized manner for a comprehensive understanding of the subject. It is a ripe text for all researchers, students, scientists or anyone else who is interested in acquiring a better knowledge of this dynamic field.

I extend my sincere thanks to the contributors for such eloquent research chapters. Finally, I thank my family for being a source of support and help.

Editor

Alternative Approaches to Wound Healing

Anuradha Majumdar and Prajakta Sangole

Abstract

The history of wound healing across the globe abounds with usage of various herbs for treating simple cuts and bruises to serious burns. Wound healing is a complex and dynamic process and, moreover, depends a lot on the wound bearing person's immunity and mental status. Synthetic medicine may give rise to side effects of allergy and resistance with usually higher cost of treatment. Whereas the alternative and complementary medicine such as Ayurveda, Siddha, Unani, Chinese medicine, and ozone therapy can lessen these side effects considerably and offer treatment at lower costs, thus elevating the overall quality of life of the patient. In today's times the patient is more demanding and has the ability to partake in treatment decisions. It is then the moral responsibility of the scientists to apply modern up-to-date scientific acumen to provide evidenced-based concept to alternative therapies of wound healing to ensure that these practices are safe and efficacious.

Keywords: wound healing, alternative therapies, Ayurveda, Siddha, Unani, Traditional Chinese Medicine, ozone therapy

1. Introduction

Wound healing continues to pose a challenging clinical problem despite scientific developments in the field. A correct and efficient wound management is essential. Emphasis is required on new and alternative therapeutic approaches and development of technologies for acute and chronic wound management. A wound can be defined as a damage or a disruption to the normal anatomical structure and function [1]. This can range from a simple break in the epithelial integrity of the skin or it can be deeper, extending into subcutaneous tissue with damage to other structures such as tendons, muscles, vessels, nerves, parenchymal organs, and even bones [2]. Depending on the time of repair, wounds can be divided as acute, chronic, and complicated. Wound healing is a natural, complex, dynamic yet continuous process, and is initiated as any injury occurs and continues till the entire repair of the wound and tissue remodelling is complete. The process can be randomly divided into (i) coagulation and haemostasis, (ii) inflammation, (iii) proliferation, and (iv) wound remodelling with scar tissue formation. If the wound healing is interrupted by any infection, tissue hypoxia, edema, growth factor imbalance or nutritional, and metabolic status of the host, then the wound may take extended time for repair. Normal wound healing is a dynamic and complex process involving a series of coordinated events including bleeding, coagulation, initiation of an acute inflammatory response to the initial injury, regeneration, migration, and proliferation of connective tissue and parenchyma cells, as well as synthesis of extracellular matrix proteins, remodelling of new parenchyma, connective tissue, and collagen deposition [3–7]. Modern synthetic allopathy-based medicines have their share of limitations of allergy, resistance, cost, etc., which has prompted the scientists and wound care professionals to consider alternative approaches to wound healing and validating their use using modern technology. The perception toward alternative medicine such as Ayurveda, Siddha, Unani, and Chinese has changed. The World Health Organisation (WHO) defines traditional medicine as "the sum total of the knowledge, skills, ands practices based on the theories, beliefs, and experiences indigenous to different cultures, whether explicable or not, used in the maintenance of health as well as in the prevention, diagnosis, improvement or treatment of physical and mental illness" [8]. Each of the above-mentioned systems of medical practice offers a variety of medicines for wound management and has been traditionally practiced since ancient times in few parts of the world and is fast getting acceptance in rest of the globe. Ayurveda or Indian traditional and Chinese medicine have rich abundance of knowledge and have been well known as ethnopharmacological and folklore-based systems. Siddha also has origin in south of India, Tamilnadu, which aims in providing ultimate cure to both mind and body systems. "Food as medicine" is the principle behind Siddha treatment. Unani system of medicine has its origin in Iran and also has documented evidences of antimicrobial herbs possessing wound healing properties. Ozone therapy has been in use since World War I times and offers remarkable bactericidal action. The abovementioned alternative therapies offer an economical approach to wound healing. Besides this benefit, they have significant lesser side effects thus increasing patient compatibility as compared to modern medicine.

2. Alternative approaches in wound healing

2.1. Ayurvedic products

A rich heritage of knowledge on preventive and curative medicines is available in ancient scholastic work included in the Atharvaveda (an Indian religious book), Ayurveda (Indian traditional system of medicine), etc. Many Ayurvedic plants have a very important role in the process of healing of wounds (*vrana*). Plants are more potent healers because they promote the repair mechanisms in the natural way. Plant-based therapy not only accelerate healing process, moreover, also maintain the esthetics. More than 70% of wound healing Ayurveda-based pharma products are plant-based, 20% are mineral-based, and remaining contain animal products as their base material. The plant-based materials are used as first aid — antiseptic coagulants and wound wash [9]. Different Ayurvedic preparations are made and used topically for healing of wounds. Ghee is used in many Ayurvedic traditional preparations and also finds use as an ointment base. It is rich source of essential fatty acids (EFAs), which regulate prostaglandin synthesis and hence induce wound healing. Cow ghee (*Goghrita*) specifically possesses regenerative properties promoting the growth of healthy cells and is clinically proven. *Bhasma* is a calcined preparation in which the gem or metal is converted into ash. *Grithas*, also called as *neyyu*, are medicated clarified butter. *Taila* or medicated oil is manufactured by steeping powdered medicinal substances, water, vegetable drugs in paste form and fragrance-producing materials such as cardamon, saffron, sandalwood, camphor. *Malam* (Cream) too is applied topically and has been documented in ancient ayurvedic texts for its helpfulness in wound healing. Some of the herbal drugs that are mentioned in Ayurvedic texts which have been specifically studied for their wound healing properties (*vranaropaka*) are mentioned below.

2.1.1. Aloe vera

A. vera finds a mention in Ayurvedic practice since centuries regarding its wound healing property. A study carried out by Yadav *et al.* [10] in 2012 provides the scientific rationale for the traditional use of *A. vera* gel for management of wound using wound excision model in experimental rats. The effect produced by *A. vera* gel with reference to wound contraction, wound closure, decrease in surface area of wound, tissue regeneration at the wound site, and histopathological characteristics were significant in treated rats. The effect of *A. vera* gel on biochemical studies revealed significant increase in collagen and decreased hexosamine content and malondialdehyde levels when compared with control. The authors concluded that *A. vera* gel is very effective on open wounds and a promising herbal drug. It also had a marked influence on the collagen level which is the precursor protein for wound healing mechanism. *A. vera* gel reportedly accelerated epithelialization, neovascularization, and increased wound contraction in the later stage of the wound healing process.

2.1.2. Cleome rutidosperma DC.

A study [11] justifies the use of folklore plant *C. rutidosperma* for the treatment of wounds. Petroleum ether, chloroform, methanol, and aqueous extracts of *C. rutidosperma* (Family: Capparidaceae) roots were evaluated for their wound healing activities in rats using excision and incision wound models, respectively. The effects of wound healing were assessed by the rate of wound closure, period of epithelialization, and wound breaking strength. Nitrofurazone (0.2% w/w) in simple ointment IP was used as reference standard for the activity comparison. The authors concluded that the animals treated with methanol and aqueous extracts of *C. rutidosperma* showed faster rate of wound healing compared with other extracts under study. The wound healing property of the roots can be attributed to the presence of flavonoids, triterpenoids, and tannins which possess the antimicrobial and astringent properties which seem to be responsible for wound contraction and increased rate of epithelialization.

2.1.3. Kshatantak Malam

It is a combination of *Acyranthes aspera*, *Allium cepa*, and *Cannabis sativa* also known as *Baharer nani* has been traditionally reported by Bengal School of Ayurvedic Physicians as external healer for open cuts, complicated wounds and burns but still a scientific document proving its quality was not available. Gangopadhyay *et al.* [12] reported its pharmacological evaluation and chemical standardization for its wound healing activity in rats. The test drug was applied topically on a 8 mm diameter full thickness punch in Wistar rats. Framycetin and povidone-iodine ointment were used as standard comparators. Parameters such as wound contraction size (mm^2), wound index, healing period (days), tensile strength (g), DNA (mg/g), RNA (mg/g), total protein (mg/g), hydroxyproline (mg/g), PAGE study, and histological analysis were carried out for analysing the effects of the malam. Out of the three constituents, *A. aspera* specifically possesses potent wound healing activity, *A. cepa* owns antimicrobial activity, and *C. sativa* is capable of tissue repair by virtue of its anti-inflammatory property.

2.1.4. Katupila (Securinega leucopyrus) (Willd.)

Another plant used since ancient times in Saurashtra region of India and Srilanka is known as *Katupila* in Srilanka and *Humari* in India. It is mentioned as one of the 60 measures for wound healing by *Acharya Sushruta* (Ancient spiritual Hindu teacher). *Katupila* leaves act as antiseptic, and the paste is capable of removing extraneous material from the wounds without the need of surgery [13].

2.1.5. Ayurvedic polyherbal formulation

Rawat and Gupta [14] reported wound healing activity of a prepared ayurvedic formulation containing *Jasad Bhasma*, *Gandhak*, *Tankankhar*, and *Ras Kapoor*. *J.* (*Yashad*) *Bhasma* is ash containing zinc. *Gandhak or Gandhaka Rasayan* is an ayurvedic mineral-based medicine, which contains detoxified sulfur processed with herbal juice as a main ingredient. *Gandhak Rasayan* is a great antibacterial, antiviral, and antimicrobial ayurvedic medicine. *Tankankhar* is borax applied topically for its analgesic property. Ras Kapoor are pills made out of camphor (*karpoora/ kapoor*), mercury compound (*Shuddha Hingula*), purified opium (*Papaver somniferum*), nutgrass (*Musta/ Cypeus rotundus*), Connessi seed (*Indrayava/ Holarrhena antidysenterica*), and Nutmeg (*Jatiphala/ Myristica fragrans*). The preparation was studied on excision and incision wound models in rats. The preparation exhibited remarkable wound healing in rats and the authors suggest further mechanism-based probing to prove the effectiveness of the constituents to be utilised in humans.

Few more folklore plants which were validated by means of preclinical wound healing studies are mentioned below in **Table 1**. Almost all the plants are shown to be wound healers by applying their extracts topically on wounds created by punches on rats. Their subsequent effect on wound healing models such as excision, incision, and dead space wound models in rats corroborate their wound healing properties. These plants ultimately are reported to stimulate wound contraction, increase hydroxyproline and eventually collagen content thus strengthening the wound area, increase the wound closure rate, reduce scar area, and epithelialization period. Few plants such as *A. cepa, Ageratum conyzoides,* and *Heliotropium indicum* are known to specifically heal the wounds by benefit of their antioxidant property. Dexamethasone is a potent anti-inflammatory glucocorticoid which is used in skin allografts but is known to delay wound healing. Plants such as *Ocimum sanctum, Gossypium herbaceum, Ficus hispida, Pyrus communis,* and *Tetrapleura tetraptera* have been specifically shown to promote dexamethasone suppressed wound healing tested in wound healing models (**Table 1**). *Alafia multiflora* is found to be one of the plants which contains retinoids and have shown marked interaction with steroids like dexamethasone and was reported to further delay the healing of dexamethasone-suppressed wounds. Thus, vitamin A even if known to hasten the process of wound healing is shown to interact with steroids and thus concomitant application should be avoided in dexamethasone suppressed wounds. Few plants such as *Echinacea* species, Vitamins such as A and E found in plants, Bromelain, and Grape seed extract have demonstrated few interactions with conventional therapies used for wound healing (**Table 1**).

No.	Name	Wound healing activity
Plants effective on acute wounds in rats		
1.	*Mimusops Elengi (Linn.)* (Sapotaceae)	The methanolic extract ointment of *M. elengi* in rats effectively stimulated wound contraction; increased tensile strength of incision and dead space wounds as compared to control group [15]
2.	*Carica papaya* (Caricaceae)	Contains a mixture of cysteine endopeptidases such as papain. Chympopapain A and B, papaya endopeptidase-II, papaya endopeptidase-IV, omega endopeptidase, chinitase, protease-inhibitors, and proteins. Papaya fruits possess wound healing properties; papaya latex was applied to the burn wound using hydrogel as a vehicle system [16]
3.	*Tephrosia purpurea (Linn.)* (Leguminosea)	Contains glycosides, rotenoids, isoflavones, flavones, chalcones, flavonoids and sterols. It is used in the treatment leprous wound and the juice is used for the eruption on skin [17]
4.	*Adhatoda vasica (Linn.)* (Acanthaceae)	Leaves and stems of the plant have been reported to contain an alkaloid mimosine, leaves also contain mucilage and root contains tannins. The methanolic, chloroform and Diethyl ether extract ointment (10% w/w) of *A. vasica* has significant wound healing activity. In both extract ointment, the methanolic extract ointment (10% w/w) showed significant effect when compare to standard drug and other two extract in excision wound model [18]
5.	*Piper betle* (Piperaceae)	In Indian folkloric medicine, betel leaf is popular as an antiseptic and is commonly applied on wounds and lesions for its healing effects. This particular property has paved way for further experimental studies, which have established pan extract to have antimicrobial and anti-leshmian properties. Fresh juice of betel leaves is also used in many Ayurvedic preparations [19]
6.	*Moringa oleifera (Linn.)* (Moringaceae)	It has anti-inflammatory, antibacterial and counter irritant action, which helps in wound healing. The aqueous extract was studied and it was found that there was

No.	Name	Wound healing activity
		significant increase in wound closure rate, skin-breaking strength, granuloma breaking strength, hydroxyproline content, granuloma dry weight and decrease in scar area was observed [20]
7.	*Eucalyptus globules* (Myrtaceae)	It is used for cuts, wounds and to boost the immune system [21]
8.	*Terminalia Chebula* (Combretaceae)	Traditionally, fruit pulp is used to stop bleeding. Recent studies showed that various aqueous and organic extracts increased cell proliferation and reduced free radical production thus promoting wound healing. Significant utility of the plant is in cases where ammonia accumulation is a limiting factor [22]
9.	*Aegel marmelos* (Bael) (Rutaceae)	Methanolic extract was found to heal wounds faster when tested in wound healing models in rats. *A. marmelos* treated wounds were reported to epithelialize faster and rate of wound contraction was higher as compared to control group of rats [23]
10.	*Alternanthera sessilis* (*Linn.*) (Amaranthaceae)	Consist of chemical constituents like α and β-spinosterols lupeal isolated from roots. The leaves are used for cuts and wounds. The wound healing property of *A. sessilis* (*Linn.*) attributed to sterols present in the plant [24]
11.	*Mussaenda frondosa.* (*Linn.*) (Rubiaceae)	The leaves extract was tested on wound healing models in rats. *M. frondosa* treated rats displayed Increased wound concentration and tensile strength, augmented hydroxyproline content along with antibacterial activity [25]
12.	*Aristolochia bracteata* (Aristolochiaceae) and *Cassia tora* (Leguminosae)	Wound contracting ability of the extracts was significantly greater than that of the control, which was comparable to that of the reference standard 0.02%w/w nitrofurazone ointment [26]
13.	*Mimosa pudica* (Mimosaceae)	Used in folklore medicine for arresting bleeding and in skin diseases. *M. pudica* has been reported to contain mimosine (an alkaloid), free amino acids, sitosterol, linoleic acid and oleic acid. The wound healing studies on roots indicated that phenols constituents/tannins play an important role in wound healing process. The result of excision wound model is indicating that significant increase in wound contraction compared with standard group, revealing that the extract has ability to induce cellular proliferation. The increase in tensile strength of wounded skin indicates the promotion of collagen fibers [27]
14.	*Anthocephalus Cadamba* (Rubiaceae)	The potent wound healing capacity was shown from the wound contraction and increased tensile strength has thus validated the ethno therapeutic claim [28]
15.	*Lantana camara* (*Linn.*) (Verbenaceae)	Showed considerable signs of dermal healing and significantly decrease mean wound healing time and reduced scarring at the wound enclosure [29]
16.	*Carapa guianensis* (Meliaceae)	The ethanolic leaf extract of *C. guianensis* showed increase in the rate of wound contraction, skin breaking strength, the rate of epithelialization [30]
17.	*Curcuma longa* (*Linn.*) (Zingiberaceae)	Curcumin has potent anti-inflammatory and analgesic activities. Volatile oil isolated from *C. longa* also exhibits antibacterial and potent anti-inflammatory activity. *C. longa* also contains protein, fats, vitamins (A, B, C, etc) all of which have an important role

No.	Name	Wound healing activity
		in would healing and regeneration. Turmeric has been used for treating the wounds in the rats. The presence of vitamin A and proteins in turmeric result in the early synthesis of collagen fibers by mimicking fibroblastic activity. Juice of the fresh rhizome is commonly applied to recent wounds, bruises and leech bites [31]
18.	*Tecomaria capensis* (Bignoniaceae)	*T. capensis* significantly stimulated wound contraction. The breaking strength of the treated incision wounds increased in *T. capensis* extract when treated groups compared with the control group [32]
19.	*Hyptis suaveolens* (*Linn.*) (Lamiaceae)	Aqueous, alcoholic and petroleum ether extracts were tested in rats in wound healing models. Petroleum ether extract was found to show enhanced wound healing activity compared to other extracts. Period of epithelialization, granulation strength, hydroxyproline content was found to be increased in petroleum ether extract as compared to other extracts. Histopathological study of this extract too revealed more collagen and macrophages as compared to other extracts [33]
20.	*Arnebia densiflora* (*Ledeb.*) (Boraginaceae)	Rats treated with *A. densiflora* showed rapid healing than the control group. Wound closure and collagen production were faster and healing occurred on the 14th day after wounding [34]

Plants possessing anti-oxidant property contributing to wound healing activity

No.	Name	Wound healing activity
21.	*Allium cepa* (Liliaceae)	It contains kampferol, β-sitosterol, ferulic acid, myritic acid, prostaglandins. Flavonoids have been documented which is believed to be one of the most important components of wound healing. The enhanced wound healing in rats when *A. cepa* was administered orally may be due to free radical scavenging action and the antibacterial property of the phytoconstituents present in it [35]
22.	*Ageratum conyzoides* (Asteraceae)	The leaves are applied to the wounds act as septic and heel them quickly. Several Phytoconstituents like alkaloids and saponins are known to promote wound healing process due to their antioxidant anti-microbial activities. The wound healing property of *A. conyzoides* appears to be due to the presence of its active principles, which accelerate the healing process and confers breaking strength to the healed wound [36]
23.	*Heliotropium Indicum* (Boraginaceace)	Various extracts of *H. indicum* were tested in wound healing models in rats. The methanolic and aqueous extracts were shown to be working better than petroleum ether extract. Increase in the granulation tissue weight, hydroxyproline content, and increased activity of superoxide dismutase and catalase level was reported to be contributing factors for better wound healing of *H. indicum* as compared to 0.2% w/w nitrofurazone ointment [37]

Plants reported to improve dexamethasone suppressed wound healing

No.	Name	Wound healing activity
24.	*Ocimum sanctum* (*Linn.*) (Labiaceae)	Ethanolic extract of *O. sanctum* significantly decreased the anti-healing effect of dexamethasone in all wound models like incision, excision and dead space wound model. It was reported that the plant has various actions like free radical scavenging effect, metal chelation and immune modulation [38]

No.	Name	Wound healing activity
25.	*Gossypium herbaceum* (*Linn.*) (Malvaceae)	Ethanol and ethyl ether fractions of *G. herbaceum* were tested in wound models to test the effect of the plant on diabetes and dexamethasone delayed wounds. The plant displayed significant increased wound contraction, breaking strength and decreased epithelization period. Hydroxyproline and collagen content was increased [39]
26.	*Ficus hispida* (*Linn.*) (Moraceae)	Ethanolic extract of roots of *F. hispida* was investigated in normal and dexamethasone depressed healing conditions, using incision, excision and dead space wound models in albino rats. Collagen and hydroxyproline content was increased thus proving the pro-healing effect of the plant [40]
27.	*Pyrus communis* (Rosaceae)	Ethanol and ethyl acetate extracts of *P. communis* were tested in dexamethasone delayed wound healing model in rats. The study reported that plant treated wounds displayed fast healing of infectious wound, in immunosuppressed and disease condition like diabetes [41]
28.	*Tetrapleura tetraptera* (Mimosaceae)	The stem bark aqueous extract was studied for effect on dexamethasone delayed wounds in excision and incision wound models in rats. The authors reported excellent potential of the plant related to epithelialization, contraction and tensile strength improvement [42]
Plant reported to display interaction with dexamethasone and further delay wound healing (drug–herb interaction)		
29.	*Alafia multiflora* (*Stapf.*) (*Apocynaceae*)	The study on *A. multiflora* highlights the drug-herb interaction. Aqueous extract of the plant was studied for its effect on normal and dexamethasone delayed wounds in rats utilizing excision and incision wound models. It showed beneficial effects in normal rats. But in dexamethasone delayed wounds, the plant extract further deteriorated the wound healing. This proved the known interaction between retinoids occurring in the plant and the steroid but also indicated at involvement of some other constituent contributing to the delayed wound healing [43]
Plants with interactions with conventional therapies and reported side effects		
30.	*Echinacea* species (*Echinacea purpurea, Echinacea pallida, Echinacea angustifolia*) (Asteraceae)	Risk of poor wound healing in chronic users [44]
31.	Vitamin A (Retinoic acid)	Interaction with steroids to further delay wound healing [45]
32.	Bromelain (Protein extract from pineapple, *Ananas sativus*)	Can improve wound healing but carries risk of bleeding. Recommended to stop its usage 2 weeks before surgery [46]
33.	Vitamin E	Can improve wound healing owing to its antioxidant property but carries risk of bleeding. Recommended to stop its usage 2 weeks before surgery [47]
34.	Grape seed extract	Possesses antioxidant activity owing to the presence of active proanthocyanidin content. Proanthocyanidin is a bioflavonoid that acts as a strong antioxidant, protecting DNA from harmful free radicals. Additionally, grape seed extract has been

No.	Name	Wound healing activity
		reported to reduce inflammation, stabilize collagen and elastin, act as a natural antihistamine, and protect and heal connective tissue. It seems safe overall with no studies pertaining to its interactions were found to be reported. Seems safe overall [48]

Table 1. Ayurvedic plants with reported wound healing activity.

2.2. Siddha medicines

Siddha is the traditional system of medicine practiced in Tamilnadu, South India, and Tamil speaking areas of the world. The Siddhars' (founders of Siddha medicine) used lots of herbs to treat cardiac and respiratory conditions, heal wounds, treat snake and scorpion bites, dreaded diseases like cancer, and documented them in the form of palm leaf manuscripts, stone, and copper scriptures, etc. The claim of the Siddha physicians is that the medicinal plants are commonly identifiable, easily available throughout the year, cost effective, and with lesser adverse effects [49]. The Siddha system of medicine aims at offering complete cure to mind and body. It follows the principle of "Food as medicine" [50]. The Siddhars have documented many oils (*Tailam*) and ointments (*Kalimbu*) effective in wound healing. There are few plants mentioned in Siddha system of traditional medicine which have been evaluated preclinically for their wound healing activity.

Few noteworthy studies using Siddha medicines are mentioned below.

2.2.1. Siddha polyherbal oils

Siddha medicine has used *Kayathirumeniennai, punguthailam, and mathanthailam* as polyherbal (medicated oils) since centuries, but recently, Sabarianandh *et al.* in 2014 made efforts to scientifically validate the use of these oils on experimentally induced burn wounds in Wistar rats. The study showed wound contraction was significantly decreased; epithelialization was increased as compared to the vehicle treated group. This was even confirmed by the histopathological analysis [51].

2.2.2. Heritage Sanjeevi

Pugalendhi *et al.* demonstrated the effect of Heritage *Sanjeevi* (a Siddha combination drug) on wound healing in Wistar rats. "Heritage *Sanjeevi*" is a medication made up of *Curcuma Aromatia, Psoralea Corylifolia, Vernonia Anthemintica (Willd.), Hydnicarpus Laurifolia, Elettaria Cadamomum*, coconut milk, mercury, sulphur, hydrogyrum schloride calomel, "Sulphie" of lead, copper sulphate, zinc sulphate, and camphor. The mixtures of these compounds were processed in the manner that all the inorganic material is detoxified using an ancient detoxin called *Pooneer*. The extracted oil is filtered and stored in glassware. It is used for external application only, and its shelf life is six years, and it has been claimed to have excellent healing property against burns, scalds, chemical burns, acid burns, and radiation burns. The medication was tested on Wistar rats by external application till the time the wound which was created using a punch was completely healed. The study results demonstrated significant reduction in the size of the wound. The authors claimed that wound healing can be credited to one or few constituents of the medication causing collagen production and thus helping in faster wound correction [52].

2.2.3. Siddha Kalimbu

Another study revealed the wound healing ability of a polyherbal Siddha formulation, *Siddha kalimbu* consisting of 10 gm each of *Ficus spp* (*Itthi*), *Adenanthera Pavonina* (*Manjeti*), sandalwood (*Santhanam*), jasmine (*malligai*), *Symplocos racemosa* (*Roxb.*) (*Vellilothram*), *Ficus hispida* (*Atthi*), *Alstonia scholaris* (*Satvin*), and dried roots of 12.5 gm of *Curcuma longa* (*Manjal*) when mixed with 60 ml of Eal oil (muscle relaxant drug), 10 ml neem oil (*Azadirachta indica*), 20 ml of coconut oil, and 10 ml *Millettia pinnata* (*Pungai*) oil. The formulation was tested on excision and incision wound models in rats, and it was reported that the Siddha treatment significantly healed the wound by synthesizing collagen and influencing the growth hormone. The topical application of the formulation increased the wound breaking strength, wound contraction, and period of epithelialization [53].

2.2.4. Polyherbal formulation

Krishnamoorty *et al.* in 2012 reported an *in vitro* study of a polyherbal formulation comprising of extracts of *Wrightia tinctoria*, *Aloe vera*, *Curcuma longa*, and *Terminalia chebula*. They studied the impact of the formulation on fibroblast cell migration and proliferation using scratch wound assay technique. Fibroblast cell migration and proliferation were studied employing cell migration assay. Carbomer-based gel with beeswax made for a novel delivery system and the formulation proved significantly effective in management of superficial wounds and first degree burns [54].

2.2.5. Kungiliya vennai and Kalchunna thailam

Vennai (*Butter*) *and thailam* (*Balm*) are mentioned and used in Siddha medicine as wound healing bases. *Kungiliya vennai* is herbal formulation containing *Shorea robusta*, *Sesamum indicum*, and *Cocos nucifera*. It is traditionally recommended by Siddha practitioners for wound healing. *Kalchunna thailam* finds a mention in Siddha medicine for wound healing and is a preparation of limestone and coconut oil mixed in equal proportions. In an excision wound model in Sprague Dawley rats, the *Kungiliya vennai and Kalchunna thailam* treated rats showed positive outcome in the wound healing process. The preparations were comparable with the standard 2% Mupirocin ointment. The authors reported *Kungiliya vennai* has additional property of regenerating adnexal structures such as hair follicles, sweat, and sebaceous glands [55].

Few more Siddha plants which were preclinically evaluated for wound healing activity are mentioned below (**Table 2**).

No.	Plant name	Wound healing activity
1.	Banyan tree (*Ficus benghalensis*)	Ethanolic and aqueous extracts of *F. benghalensis* were evaluated in excision and incision wound models. Both extracts exhibited significant wound-healing activity, which was proven by decrease in the period of epithelialization, an increase in the rate of wound contraction and skin-breaking strength. Proteoglycans and glucosaminoglycans have been shown to play important roles in wound healing [56]
2.	Common wireweed (*Sida acuta*)	Was studied respectively on two types of wound models in rats, (i) the excision and (ii) the incision wound model. Wound contracting ability of the *S. acuta* ointment (5% w/w) significantly greater than that of the control nitrofurazone ointment (0.2% w/w) which was employed as standard comparator drug [57]
3.	Barmuda grass (*Cynodon dactylon*)	Flavanoid fraction of *C. dactylon* in Swiss albino mice demonstarted the wound healing activity, when it was applied externally daily on excised wound area for 8 days [58]
4.	Country fig (*Ficus racemosa*)	Aqueous and ethanolic extract of roots of *F. racemosa* in Wistar albino rats showed significant increase in percentage closure by enhanced epithelialization. The effect can be linked to enhanced collagen synthesis. Results showed the herb hastened the wound healing process by decreasing the surface area of the wound [59]
5.	Purging nut (*Jatropha curcas*)	Bark extract showed significant wound healing activity in albino rats. It accelerated the healing process by increasing the skin breaking strength, wound contraction, dry granulation tissue weight, and hydroxyproline levels. Epithelization period was also significantly decreased [60]
6.	Maasikkai (*Quercus infectoria*)	Ethanol extract of the shade-dried leaves of was studied in rats and it showed a positive effect on wound healing, with a significant increase in the levels of the antioxidant enzymes, superoxide dismutase and catalase, in the granuloma tissue [61]
7.	Pomegranate (*Punica granatum*)	Ethanolic extract on Wistar rat showed significant the wound healing activity. It significantly increased the rate of wound contraction and collagen turnover [62]
8.	Red silk cotton (*Bombax malabaricum*)	Alcoholic Bark extract resulted in a significant decline in the wound in rats. When compared with standard drug, nitrofurazone, it was found superior in terms of wound contracting ability, wound closure time, and tensile strength [63]
9.	Rhus olina (*Lannea coromandelica*)	Ethanol and acetone extracts of barks were applied to male Wistar rats in the form of simple ointments exhibited wound healing activity in excision and incision methods. Framycetin sulphate was taken as standard control. It displayed potent wound healing activity in terms of significant wound contraction and increased tensile strength [64]
10.	Plantain tree (*Musa paradisiaca*)	The extract of *M. Paradisiaca* holds substantial wound healing activity in rat models [65]
11.	Kino tree (*Pterocarpus marsupium*)	The effect of heart wood extract of *P. marsupium* on wound healing has been studied in diabetic and normal animals. The effect has also been compared with standard (mupirocin ointment) application. The results show that application of heart wood extract significantly increased wound healing in both normal and diabetic animals [66]

Table 2. Siddha herbs with reported wound healing activity.

2.3. Unani medicines

Unani system of medicine has its origin in Iran and also has documented evidences of anti-microbial herbs possessing wound healing properties. Like Siddha, Unani system too has a mention of cow's ghee (*Roghan-e-gao*), *Shorea robusta*, etc. Following are examples of wound healing plants or medicines (*marham*) according to Unani system of medicine.

2.3.1. Iranian wound healing plants

Pirbalouti *et al.* reported the wound healing properties of five traditional Iranian plants on alloxan-induced diabetic wounds in rats. Wound area, epithelialization time, and histopathological characteristics were studied upon treatment with *Malva sylvestris*, *Punica granatum*, *Amygdalus communis*, *Arnebia euchroma*, and *Scrophularia deserti*. The results corroborated the traditional wound healing use of the above plants [67].

2.3.2. Marham-e-Ral

Similarly, a study described the wound healing effect of a Unani formulation *Marham-e-Ral* in rats. Ingredients of this formulation are *Shorea robusta Gaertn* (*Ral*), Camphor (*Kafoor*), Catechu (*Katha*), *Roghan-e-Gao*, and Beeswax. *Marham-e-Ral* was administered topically once a day till complete epithelialization occurred. Wound contraction and epithelialization were measured. Both excision and incision wound models were developed. Rate of wound contraction was significantly enhanced so was the epithelialization period. The plant extracts have revealed presence of flavonoids, triterpenoids, and tannins which are known to contribute to wound healing. They also possess astringent, antimicrobial and antiinflammatory effects. Based on their study, the authors claimed the prohealing stroke *Marham-e-Ral* possesses [68].

2.3.3. Aloe (Elva)

Aloe is one of the oldest plants documented across the globe and also features in Unani system of medicine where it is called as '*Elva*'. Oryan *et al.* [69] reported the detailed account of wound healing activity of *A. vera* in rats. They demonstrated that the wound healing was 50% faster with aqueous extract of *A. vera* as compared to silver sulfadiazine in case of open wounds.

2.3.4. Golnar-e-farsi

Punica granatum (*Linn.*), known as *Golnar-e-farsi* in Iran, popularly known as pomegranate flowers and *Achillea kellalensis* (*Bioss.*) and *Hausskn* a well known traditional herb used in tribal medicine of Iran is locally known as *Golberrenjas or Bumadaran-e-Sabzekoh* were studied scientifically by Pirbalouti *et al.* in 2010. The authors reported their significant wound healing properties in rat excision wound model owing to their increased wound contraction ability and collagen turnover [70].

2.3.5. Shorea robusta

Shorea robusta finds a mention in both Siddha and Unani systems of medicine. A study carried out by Wani *et al.* in 2011 reported the wound healing property of *S. robusta* Gaertn. f. in excisional and incisional wound models in rats. The ethanolic extract was found to accelerate wound contraction, increased tensile strength, and hydroxyproline content thus acting as a wound healer [71].

2.4. Chinese herbs

As are Ayurveda and Siddha to India and Unani to Iran, traditional Chinese system of medicine has been practiced for ages in China. Traditional Chinese Medicine (TCM) focuses on the concept of Yin and Yang which describes two opposing yet complementary aspects of any one phenomenon. Yin is associated with poor circulation and healing and stagnation, while Yang is related with being overheated and excess of scar tissue. Thus for optimum wound healing, an ideal balance needs to be struck between Yin and Yang. Raw Chinese formulas are created specific to each patient. A raw formula means simply that the herbs in the formula are in their natural state without modification. Traditionally, raw Chinese formulas are given in their organic form, cooked for several hours, and then ingested, but it tends to have an undesirable taste. However, with wound healing, a topical application is convenient, effective, and has no or less side effects. Herbs can be utilized in their natural state and with their maximum potency. Few of the examples of wound healer herbs of TCM are as follows:

1. Tam *et al.* [72] were the first to report a combination of *Radix astragali* and *Radix rehmanniae* in the ratio of 2:1 for the treatment of diabetic foot wounds. The herb combination showed its effectiveness in treating diabetic wound healing through the actions of tissue regeneration, angiogenesis and anti-inflammation.

2. *Angelica sinensis* (AS) called as *Dang-Gui* in Chinese, was analysed in detail by Hsiao *et al.* [73] using proteomics to demonstrate range of pharmacological effects associated with AS which will prove fruitful in developing it as a wound healing herb. The authors concluded that AS extract and its active component ferulic acid (FA) participate in the modulation of wound healing process associated with fibroblasts. FA specifically acts as a ROS scavenger. Additionally, FA is also able to trigger proteins like heme oxygenase-1 (HO-1), heat shock protein 70 (HSP70), Extracellular signal-regulated kinases (ERK ½), and Protein kinase B (Akt), which help cells to respond to environmental stress thus contributing to its enhanced wound healing ability.

3. Hou *et al.* [74] recently demonstrated the wound healing property of a four-herb Chinese medicine ANBP which is a pulverized mixture of four herbs including *Agrimonia eupatoria* (A), *Nelumbo nucifera Gaertn* (N), *Boswellia carteri* (B), and *Pollen Typhae Angustifoliae* (P) explored the effect of four-herb Chinese medicine ANBP. The herb was evaluated on the basis of wound healing and scar formation in rabbit ear hypertrophic scar models of full-thickness skin defect. Compared with the control group, local ANBP treatment not only significantly improved wound healing, but also reduced scar formation. The study results demonstrated that ANBP treatment along with reducing collagen synthesis, blocked

excessive deposition of collagen and also promoted collagen maturity, thus obstructing the formation of scar. The mechanism of the effect of ANBP on collagen expression is different in the early and late stages of wound healing, which is favourable for wound closure and scar contraction. Using proteomics approach, the authors suggested that ANBP promoted wound healing and condensed scarring by bidirectional regulation of the Transforming Growth Factor β (TGF- β)-/Smad-dependent pathway.

4. Chinese medicine book, Compendium of Materia Medica proclaims *Lucilia sericata* known as *'WuGuChong'* in Chinese for treating superficial purulent diseases like carbuncle. Zhang *et al.* reported that fatty acid extracts of *Lucilia sericata* can promote murine cutaneous wound healing by virtue of its remarkable angiogenic activity. Wound excision model in rats followed by Vascular Endothelial Growth factor (VEGF) expression analysis by western blotting, RT-PCR and immunohistochemistry strongly suggested the mechanism involved in wound healing property of the herb [75].

5. Chak *et al.* [76] demonstrated the effect of another Chinese medicine *Shiunko* consisting of sesame oil, *Lithospermi radix, (LR; Lithospermum erythrorhizon Sieb. et Zucc.)*, *A. sinensis*, lard, and beeswax. The authors reported that *Shiunko*-treated fibroblasts induced range of biochemical events engaged in the wound healing process, including cell proliferation and anti-apoptosis, anti-oxidant activity, secretion of collagen, and cell mobility. It was also noted that Stathmin, a differentiation marker was greatly induced by *Shiunko*, which is a sign of good healing process. Proteomics suggested peroxiredoxin and glutathione S-transferase were involved in antioxidantion offered by *Shiunko*. Also, superoxide dismu-tase was enhanced after *Shiunko* treatment which again contributed to its wound healing property. TGF-β was upregulated on *Shiunko* treatment which happens to be upstream regulator of collagen expression and an indispensable factor for wound healing.

6. *Terminalia chebula* is mentioned in other systems of medicine like Ayurveda for its wound healing ability. Likewise, it was proven by Li *et al.* [77] that tannin extracts from immature *Terminalia chebula* fruits helps in cutaneous wound healing in rats. The immunohisto-chemical, transcriptional and translational levels of VEGF analysed in the study helped the authors conclude that the wound healing property was by the virtue of anti-angiogenic effects. Also, the proliferation of bacteria like *Staphylococcus aureaus* and *Klebsiella pneu-monia* were inhibited by the extract thus conferring the much needed antibacterial effect beneficial for faster wound healing. Thus the study concluded that tannin extracts from immature fruits of *Terminalia chebula Fructus (Retz.)* stimulated cutaneous wound healing in rats.

2.5. Ozone therapy

Ozone therapy dates back to the year 1914 when it was used during World War I for the treatment of gas gangrene. Ozone has multiple therapeutic effects in wound healing due to the property of releasing nascent oxygen, which has been shown to have bactericidal capabil-ities and to stimulate antioxidant enzymes. There are few randomized clinical trials to verify the use of ozone therapy in the early stages of wound healing. To verify the same, Zhang *et al.* [78] recently carried out a study assessing the use of ozone therapy in the early stages of diabetic foot ulcer by estimating the expression of VEGF, TGF-β, and Platelet derived growth factor (PDGF). The authors claimed that the oxygen-ozone therapy increased the levels of all the above three endogenous growth factors which contributed to its enhanced wound healing ability. Similarly, Wainstain et al. [79] demonstarted that oxygen–ozone therapy along with conventional therapy for 24 weeks hastened the healing of diabetic foot ulcer. The theory that ozonated oil has wound healing property was investigated at our laboratory in an excision wound model using Sprague Dawley rats. The animals were divided into four groups, which were treated with sesame oil (vehicle), framycetin (standard), or two doses of ozonated sesame oil (peroxide values 500 and 700 mEq/1000 g, respectively). The formulations were topically applied on the excision wounds once daily for 11 consecutive days, and the animals were euthanized on the 12th day. Ozonated oil treated wounds had significantly higher tensile strength, collagen content, and superoxide dismutase activity than that of the vehicle treated wounds. Histopathological analysis of skin of the excised wound area treated with ozonated oil revealed better healing activity in comparison with the vehicle-treated wounds. Thus it was concluded that ozonated oil can be of potential remedial use for healing wounds [80]. Another animal study was carried out by Kim et al. [81] to evaluate the therapeutic effects of ozonated olive oil in guinea pigs in acute cutaneous wound healing model. Full thickness punch wound was created on the back of guinea pigs and ozonated olive oil treatment was compared with pure olive oil and no treatment control group. The immunohistopathological results demonstrated that topical application of ozonated olive oil increased the levels of VEGF, TGF-β, and PDGF thus accelerating acute cutaneous wound healing. A study conducted by Travagli et al. [82] reported a deleterious effect of ozone treatment on aged mice. The authors claimed that ozone therapy in 8-week mice enhanced wound healing, while when administered to 18-week mice, the full thickness excisional wound displayed delayed healing. This may also be attributed to reduced bacterial infection and/or increased O_2 tension by O_3 contact in wound area in younger population.

3. Clinical studies supporting the folklore use of alternative therapies

Scientists advocate more clinical studies to be conducted to provide robust proof-of-concept of folklore wound healing property of the herbs mentioned in alternative therapies. Few of the clinical studies carried out are documented subsequently.

3.1. Ayurveda-based clinical studies

3.1.1. Katupila study

A case study of diabetic wound of a 55-year-old female patient wherein Katupila paste [(Securinega leucopyrus) (Willd.)] was applied daily and after a month the wound was reported to have healed completely leaving a minimal scar. The healing properties of Katupila were attributed to its antimicrobial, antiseptic, and wormicidal qualities. Also it was shown to possess abundant quantities of flavonoids and tannins which offer the antioxidant effects [13].

3.1.2. Manjishthadi Gritha

A clinical study employing *Manjishthadi Gritha* was carried out by Baria *et al*. The *Gritha* was prepared using seven herbs namely, *Manjishtha* (*R. cordifolia Linn.*), *Daruharidra* (*B. aristata DC.*), *Mocharasa* (*Salmalia malabaricum*), *Dhatakipushpa* (*Woodfordia fruticosa (Linn.) Kurz.*), *madhuka* (*Madhuca indica J. F. Gmel*), *Lodhra* (*Symplocos racemosa Roxb.*) and *Rasanjana* (*Extractum berberis*). The *Gritha* was applied topically on wounds mostly from anorectal cases twice a day for 21 days. The observation period of 1 month recorded the results of the study. Out of 45 patients, 24 were treated with the *Gritha* and 21 with povidone iodine ointment. The *Gritha*-treated patients showed better wound healing, no left-over scar, no excess pigmentation, and absence of adverse effects. The authors reported *Manjishthadi Gritha* as an economical and effective wound healing combination [83].

3.1.3. Honey: A pilot study

Vijaya *et al*. [84] reported a pilot study using honey for healing the cutaneous wounds of 10 randomly selected patients of both sexes. Honey collected locally was applied daily for 20 days and the size of the wound was measured on day 7, 15, 20, and after complete wound healing. The authors concluded that honey was remarkable in healing the wounds and can be very effectively used as first aid dressing material. A case study [85] was reported employing honey for the cure of a chronic infected wound on the right lower limb of a 70-year-old female. Every morning the wound was cleaned with neem bark decoction, and Dabur® honey was applied on the wound. Along with the local application, following drugs were administered orally every 12 hours: *Glycerrhiza glabra* (*Linn.*), *Asparagus racemosus* (*Willd.*), *Tribulus terrestris*, *Tinispora cordifolia* (*Willd*). At the end of fifth week, the authors reported a complete healing of the wound leaving a minimal scar. Sushruta Samhita has mentioned *honey* (*madhu*) as a wound healer centuries ago. The above case study practically proved the effectiveness of honey. It is hyperosmolar so confers antibacterial effect. It has high viscosity so acts as physical barrier. Presence of enzyme catalase in honey gives it antioxidant properties. The four drugs given orally possess antioxidant, adaptogenic, and immunomodulatory activities. Clinical studies employing honey with bigger population although would yield more authentic conclusions.

3.2. Unani medicine-based study

3.2.1. Dragon's blood cream

Namjoyan *et al*. [86] reported a clinical study using Dragon's blood cream, a deep red resin obtained from four different sources, *Croton spp.*, *Dracaena spp.*, *Daemonorops spp.*, and *Pterocarpus spp.* 60 patients referred to remove their skin tags were included in this randomized clinical trial to receive either Dragon's blood cream or placebo cream. Wound measurement and process of healing was checked on 3rd, 5th, 7th, 10th, 14th, and 20th day of the trial. The patients receiving Dragon's blood cream showed significant wound healing. The phenolic compounds present in Dragon's blood cream reportedly contribute to its effective wound healing property.

3.3. Clinical study on ozone therapy

3.3.1. Adjuvant ozone therapy

Shah *et al.* [87] presented a case study of a 59-year-old female patient with an extensively infected wound and exposed tibia to about $^4/_5$th of its extent. Topical ozone therapy twice a day and ozone hemotherapy once a day along with daily dressings and parenteral antibiotics showed significant improvement in 15 days in the patient. After a follow-up of 20 months, the patient was able to walk with minimal disability. Ozone disintegrates into reactive oxygen species which further lead to increased growth factors contributing to faster wound healing. The study stated that oxidative injury is a possible side effect of ozone therapy but at thera-peutic doses oxygen radicals are removed by the blood antioxidants and thus side effects are rare and only observed in overdose or compromised anti-oxidant system.

4. Conclusion

The folklore knowledge is abundant with mention of various herbs and medicines as wound healers across different civilizations and systems of medicines. Modern medicine is fast attempting to explore the ancestral data and test its effectiveness using current experimental methods. The focus is on analyzing the molecular basis of the effectiveness of the concerned plants. Proteomic and genomic-based evidences using robust markers blended with tradi-tional knowledge can provide relevant answers and solutions for healing of wounds which affect the largest organ of human body. Although more randomized clinical trials are the need of the day to validate the ancient claims.

Author details

Anuradha Majumdar* and Prajakta Sangole

*Address all correspondence to: anuradha.majumdar@bcp.edu.in

Department of Pharmacology, Bombay College of Pharmacy, Kalina, Mumbai, India

References

[1] Robson MC, Steed DL and Franz MG. Wound healing: biologic features and approaches to maximize healing trajectories. Curr Probl Surg 2001; 38: 72–140. doi:10.1067/j.cpsurg. 2008.10.004.

[2] Robson MC, Steed DL and Franz MG. The management of complex orthopaedic injuries. Surg Clin North Am 1996; 76: 879–903. doi:10.1016/S0039-6109(05)70486-2.

[3] Vanwijck R. Surgical biology of wound healing. Bull Mem Acad R Med Belg 2001; 115: 175–84. PMID: 11789398.

[4] Degreef H. How to heal a wound fast. Dermatol Clin 1998; 16 (2): 365-375. doi:10.1016/S0733-8635(05)70019-X.

[5] Attinger CE, Janis JE, Steinberg J, et al. Clinical approach to wounds: debridement and wound bed preparation including the use of dressings and wound-healing adjuvants. Plast Reconstr Surg 2006; 117(7 suppl): 72S–109S. doi:10.1097/01.prs. 0000225470.42514.8f.

[6] Broughton G 2nd, Janis JE, Attinger CE, et al. Wound healing: an overview. Plast Reconstr Surg 2006; 117(7 suppl):1e–S–32e–S. doi:10.1097/01.prs.0000222562.60260.f9.

[7] Hunt TK, Hopf H, Hussain Z, et al. Physiology of wound healing. Adv Ski Wound Care 2000; 13: 6–11. PMID: 11110286.

[8] General Guidelines for Methodologies on Research and Evaluation of Traditional Medicine. WHO/EDM/TRM/2000.1: 1–71.

[9] Santhosh Aruna M, Shravanthi V, Jhansi Sri U, et al. An Overview of herbs possessing wound healing activity. Eur J Pharm Med Res 2015; 2(7): 329–332.

[10] Haritha Yadav K, Ravi Kumar J, Ilias Basha S, et al Wound healing activity of topical application of aloe Vera Gel in experimental animal models. Int J Pharma Bio Sci 2012; 3: 63–73.

[11] Mondal S, Dash GK and Bal SK. Anthelmintic activity of Cleome rutidosperma DC. roots. Indian Drugs 2009; 46: 47–49.

[12] Gangopadhyay KS, Khan M, Pandit S, et al. Pharmacological evaluation and chemical standardization of an ayurvedic formulation for wound healing activity. Int J Low Extrem Wounds 2014; 13: 41–49. doi:10.1177/1534734614520705.

[13] Dudhamal T, Gupta S, Mahanta V, et al. Katupila Securinega leucopyrus as a potential option for diabetic wound management. J Ayurveda Integr Med 2014; 5: 60. doi: 10.4103/0975-9476.128872.

[14] Rawat S and Gupta A. Development and study of wound healing activity of an ayurvedic formulation. Asian J Res Pharm Sci 2011; 1 : 26–28. ISSN: 2231-5659.

[15] Gupta N and Jain UK. Investigation of Wound Healing Activity of Methanolic Extract of Stem Bark of Mimusops Elengi Linn. Afr J Tradit Complement Altern Med. 2011; 8(2): 98–103.

[16] Azarkan M, El Moussaoui A, Van Wuytswinkel D, *et al.* Fractionation and purification of the enzymes stored in the latex of *Carica papaya*. J Chromatogr B Anal Technol Biomed Life Sci 2003; 790: 229–238. doi:10.1016/S1570-0232(03)00084-9.

[17] Deshpande SS, Shah GB and Parmar NS. Antiulcer activity of *Tephrosia purpurea* in rats. Ind J Pharmacol 2000; 35: 168–172.

[18] Subhashini S and Arunachalam K. Investigations on the phytochemical activities and wound healing properties of *Adhatoda vasica* leave in Swiss albino mice. Afr J Plant Sci 2011;5: 133–145.

[19] Verma A, Kumar N and Ranade SA. Genetic diversity amongst landraces of a dioecious vegetatively propagated plant, betelvine (*Piper betle L.*). J Biosci 2004; 29: 319–328. doi: 10.1007/BF02702614.

[20] Rathi BS, Bodhankar SL and Baheti AM. Evaluation of aqueous leaves extract of *Moringa oleifera Linn* for wound healing in albino rats. Indian J Exp Biol 2006; 44: 898–901.

[21] Hukkeri VT, Kardi RV, Akki KS, *et al.* Wound healing property of *Eucalyptus globulus* leaf extract. Indian Drugs 2002; 39: 481–483.

[22] Singh D, Singh D, Choi SM, *et al.* Effect of extracts of *Terminalia chebula* on Proliferation of Keratinocytes and Fibroblasts Cells: an Alternative Approach for Wound Healing. Evid Based Complement Alternat Med 2014; 2014: 1–13. doi:http://dx.doi.org/ 10.1155/2014/701656.

[23] Jaswanth A, Loganathan V, Manimaran S, *et al.* Wound healing activity of *Aegle marmelos*. Ind J Pharm Sci 2001;63: 41–44.

[24] Jalalpure S, Agrawal N, Patil M, *et al.* Antimicrobial and wound healing activities of leaves of *Alternanthera sessilis Linn*. Int J Green Pharm 2008; 2: 141. doi: 10.4103/0973-8258.42729.

[25] Patil SA, Joshi VG, Sutar PS, *et al.* Screening of alcoholic extract of *Mussaenda frondosa* leaf for wound-healing and antibacterial activities in albino rats. Pharmacologyonline 2010; 2: 761–773.

[26] Jayasutha A and Nithila SMJ. Evaluation of wound healing activity of Ethanolic extract of *Aristolochia bracteata* and *Cassia tora* on wistar Albino rats. Int J Pharmtech Res 2011; 3: 1547–1550.

[27] Pawaskar SM and Kale KU. Antibacterial activity of successive extracts of *Mimosa pudica*. Ind Drugs 2006; 43: 476–480.

[28] Sanjay PU, Kumar GS, Jayaveera KN, *et al.* Antimicrobial, wound healing and antioxidant activities of *Anthocephalus cadamba*. African J Tradit Complement Alternat Med 2007; 4: 481–487. doi:10.1089/ast.2006.0095.

[29] Nayak BS, Raju SS and Ramsubhag A. Investigation of wound healing activity of *Lantana camara L.* in Sprague Dawley rats using a burn wound model. Int J Appl Res Nat Prod 2008; 1: 15–19.

[30] Nayak BS, Kanhai J, Milne DM, *et al.* Experimental evaluation of ethanolic extract of *Carapa guianensis L.* leaf for its wound healing activity using three wound models. Evid Based Complement Alternat Med 2011; 2011. Article ID 419612: 1–6. doi:10.1093/ecam/nep160.

[31] Mehra KS, Mikuni I, Gupta U, *et al. Curcuma longa (Linn)* drops in corneal wound healing. Tokai J Exp Clin Med 1984; 9: 27–31.

[32] Saini N, Singhal M and Srivastava B. Evaluation of wound healing activity of *Tecomaria capensis* leaves. Chin J Nat Med 2012; 10(1 suppl): 138–141. doi:10.3724/SP.J. 1009.2012.00138.

[33] Shenoy C, Patil MB, Kumar R., *et al.* Wound Healing Activity of *Hyptis suaveolens (L.) Poit* (Lamiaceae). Int J Pharm Tech Res 2009; 1: 737–744. ISSN: 0974-4304

[34] Kosger HH, Ozturk M, Sokmen A, *et al.* Wound healing effects of *Arnebia densiflora* root extracts on rat palatal mucosa. Eur J Dent 2009; 3: 96–99.

[35] Shenoy C, Patil MB, Kumar R, *et al.* Preliminary phytochemical investigation and wound healing activity of *Allium Cepa linn.* (Liliaceae). Int J Pharm Sci 2009; 2: 167–175.

[36] Jain S, Jain N, Tiwari A, *et al.* Simple evaluation of wound healing activity of polyherbal formulation of roots of *Ageratum conyzoides Linn.* Asian J Res Chem 2009; 2 (2): 135–138. ISSN: 0974–4169.

[37] Reddy JS, Rao PR and Reddy MS. Wound healing effects of *Heliotropium indicum, Plumbago zeylanicum* and *Acalypha indica* in rats. J Ethnopharmacol 2002; 79: 249–251. doi:10.1016/S0378-8741(01)00388-9.

[38] Udupa SL, Shetty S, Udupa AL, *et al.* Effect of *Ocimum sanctum Linn.* on normal and dexamathasone suppressed wound healing. Indian J Exp Biol 2006:49–54.

[39] Velmurugan C, Bhargava A, Vijaya Kumar S, *et al. Gossypium Herbaceum* hasten wound healing in dexamethasone delayed wound healing model in rats. Int J Phytopharm 2013; 4: 152–157.

[40] Murti K, Lambole V, Panchal M Effect of *Ficus hispida L.* on normal and dexamethasone suppressed wound healing. Brazilian J Pharm Sci 2011; 47: 855–860.

[41] Anitha KN, Reddy BS, Velmurugan C, *et al.* Pear fruit velocity of wound healing in dexamethasone delayed wound healing model in rats. Der Pharm Lett 2015; 7: 310–319.

[42] Tsala DE, Habtemariam S, Simplice FH, *et al.* Topically applied *Tetrapleura tetraptera* stem-bark extract promotes healing of excision and incision wounds in rats. J Intercult Ethnopharmacol 2014; 3: 63–67. doi:10.5455/jice.20140129034637.

[43] Tsala DE, Nga N, Joseph MN, *et al*. A dermal wound healing effect of water extract of the stem bark of *Alafia multiflora Stapf*. Phytopharmacology 2013; 4: 114–122.

[44] Barrett B. Medicinal properties of *Echinacea*: a critical review. Phytomedicine 2003; 10: 66–86.

[45] Wicke C, Halliday B, Allen D, *et al*. Effects of steroids and retinoids on wound healing. Arch Surg 2000; 135: 1265–1270. doi:10.1001/archsurg.135.11.1265.

[46] Maurer IIR. Bromelain: biochemistry, pharmacology and medical use. Cell Mol Life Sci 2001; 58: 1234–1245.

[47] Miller ER, Pastor-Barriuso R, Dalal D, *et al*. Meta-analysis: high-dosage vitamin E supplementation may increase all-cause mortality. Ann Intern Med 2005; 142 (1): 37–46.

[48] Bagchi D, Bagchi M, Stohs SJ, *et al*. Free radicals and grape seed proanthocyanidin extract: importance in human health and disease prevention. Toxicology 2000; 148: 187–197. doi:S0300483X00002109 [pii].

[49] Merish S, Tamizhamuthu M and Thomas W. Styptic and wound healing properties of siddha medicinal plants – a review. Int J Pharm Bio Sci 2014; 5: 43–49.

[50] Thomas W, Merish S, Tamizhamuthu M. Review of *Alternanthera sessilis* with reference to traditional siddha medicine. Int J Pharmacogn Phytochem Res 2014; 6: 249–254.

[51] Sabarianandh JV, Uma VK, Fernandes DL, *et al*. Wound healing effect of three traditional medicated oils (*Kayathirumeniennai*, *Punguthailam* and *Mathanthailam*) on experimentally induced burn wounds in Wistar rats . World J Pharm Pharm Sci 2014; 3: 1307–1313.

[52] Pugalendhi V, Panicker TMR, Korath MP, *et al*. Effect of heritage sanjeevi (a siddha combination drug) on wound healing in Wistar rats. JIMSA 2010; 23: 233–234.

[53] Devi M, Kumar B. Evaluation of wound healing activity of polyherbal Siddha formulation. J Pharm Biomed Sci 2011; 5: 6–8.

[54] Krishnamoorthy JR, Sumitira S, Ranjith MS, *et al*. An in vitro study of wound healing effect of a poly-herbal formulations as evidenced by enhanced cell proliferation and cell migration. Egypt Dermatology Online J 2012; 8: 1–7.

[55] Bhat V, Amuthan A, Rosli BBM, *et al*. Effect of *Kungiliya vennai* and *Kalchunna thailam* on excision wound healing in albino Wistar rats. Int J Pharmacol Clin Sci 2015; 4: 52–57. doi:10.5530/ijpcs.4.3.4.

[56] Murti K, Kumar U, Panchal M. Healing promoting potentials of roots of *Ficus benghalensis L*. in albino rats. Asian Pac J Trop Med 2011; 4: 921–924. doi:10.1016/S1995-7645(11)60219-8.

[57] Akilandeswari S, Senthamarai R, Valarmathi R, *et al*. Wound healing activity of *Sida acuta* in rats. Int J Pharm Tech Res 2010; 2: 585–587. ISSN: 0974-4304.

[58] Saroja M, Santhi R and Annapoorani S. Wound healing activity of Flavanoid fraction of *Cynodon dactylon* in Swiss albino Mice. Int Res J Pharm 2012; 3 (2). 230–231.

[59] Murti K and Kumar U. Enhancement of wound healing with roots of *Ficus racemosa L.* in albino rats. Asian Pacific J Trop Med J Trop Med 2012: 276–280. doi:10.1016/S2221-1691(12)60022-7.

[60] Shetty S, Udupa SL, Udupa AL, *et al*. Wound healing activities of Bark Extract of *Jatropha curcas Linn* in albino rats. Saudi Med J 2006; 27: 1473–1476.

[61] Umachigi SP, Jayaveera KN, Ashok Kumar CK, *et al*. Studies on wound healing properties of *Quercus infectoria*. Trop J Pharm Res 2008; 7: 913–919.

[62] Pirbalouti AG, Azizi S, Koohpayeh A, Hamedi B. Wound healing activity of *Malva sylvestris* and *Punica granatum* in alloxan-induced diabetic rats. Acta Pol Pharm 2010; 67: 511–516. PMID: 20210088.

[63] Udaya chandrika P, Girija K, Lakshman K, *et al*. Evalution of wound healing activity of bark of *Bombax malabaricum*. Int J Bio Pharm Res 2010; 1: 50–55.

[64] Sathish R, Ahmed MH, Natarajan K, *et al*. Evaluation of wound healing and antimicrobial activity of *Lannea coromandelica* (*Houtt*) *Merr*. J Pharm Res 2010; 3: 1225–1228.

[65] Goel RK and Sairam K. Anti-ulcer drugs from indigenous sources with emphasis on *Musa sapientum, tamrabhasma, Asparagus racemosus* and *Zingiber officinale*. Indian J Pharmacol 2002; 34: 100–110.

[66] Gupta M, Soni R, Singhal A, *et al*. Evaluation of wound healing potential of *Pterocarpus marsupium* heart wood extract in normal and diabetic rats. Chronicles Young Sci 2012; 3 (1): 42–47. doi:10.4103/2229-5186.94313.

[67] Pirbalouti AG, Azizi S, Koohpayeh A. Healing potential of Iranian traditional medicinal plants on burn wounds in alloxan-induced diabetic rats. Brazilian J Pharmacogn 2012; 22: 397–403. doi:10.1590/S0102-695X2011005000183.

[68] Mokhtar MA, Ahmad MA, Nizami Q, *et al*. Wound healing effect of a unani formulation *Marham-e-Ral*. Int J Adv Pharm Med Bioallied Sci 2014; 2 (1): 20–24.

[69] Oryan A, Naeini AT, Nikahval B, *et al*. Effect of aqueous extract of *Aloe vera* on experimental cutaneous wound healing in rat. Vet Arch 2010; 80: 509–522. ISSN: 0372-5480.

[70] Pirbalouti AG, Koohpayeh A and Karimi I. The wound healing activity of flower extracts of *Punica granatum* and *Achillea kellalensis* in Wistar rats. Acta Pol Pharm Ñ Drug Res 2010; 67: 107–110.

[71] Wani T, Chandrashekara H and Kumar D. Wound healing activity of ethanolic extract of *Shorea robusta Gaertn. f.* resin. Indian J Exp Biol 2012; 50: 277–281. PMID: 22611916

[72] Tam JCW, Lau KM, Liu CL, *et al.* The in vivo and in vitro diabetic wound healing effects of a 2-herb formula and its mechanisms of action. J Ethnopharmacol 2011; 134: 831–838. doi:10.1016/j.jep.2011.01.032.

[73] Hsiao CY, Hung CY, Tsai TH, *et al.* A study of the wound healing mechanism of a Traditional Chinese Medicine, *Angelica sinensis*, using a proteomic approach. Evid Based Complement Alternat Med 2012; 2012. doi:10.1155/2012/467531.

[74] Qian H, Wen-Jun H, Hao-Jie H, *et al.* The four-herb chinese medicine ANBP enhances wound healing and inhibits scar formation via bidirectional regulation of transformation growth factor pathway. PLoS One 2014; 9: 1–15. doi:10.1371/journal.pone.0112274.

[75] Zhang Z, Wang S, Diao Y, *et al.* Fatty acid extracts from *Lucilia sericata* larvae promote murine cutaneous wound healing by angiogenic activity. Lipids Health Dis 2010; 9. doi: 10.1186/1476-511X-9-24.

[76] Chak K-F, Hsiao C-Y and Chen T-Y. A study of the effect of shiunko, a traditional Chinese herbal medicine, on fibroblasts and its implication on wound healing processes. Adv Wound Care 2013; 2: 448–455. doi:10.1089/wound.2012.0368.

[77] Li K, Diao Y, Zhang H, *et al.* Tannin extracts from immature fruits of *Terminalia chebula Fructus Retz.* promote cutaneous wound healing in rats. BMC Complement Alternat Med 2011; 11: 86. doi:10.1186/1472-6882-11-86.

[78] Zhang J, Guan M, Xie C, *et al.* Increased growth factors play a role in wound healing promoted by noninvasive oxygen-ozone therapy in diabetic patients with foot ulcers. Oxid Med Cell Longev 2014; 2014, Article ID 273475: 1–8. doi:10.1155/2014/273475.

[79] Wainstain J, Feldbrin Z, Boaz M, *et al.* Efficacy of ozone-oxygen therapy for the treatment of diabetic foot ulcers. Diabetes Technol Ther 2011; 13: 1255–1260. doi: 10.1089/dia.2011.0018.

[80] Pai SA, Gagangras SA, Kulkarni SS, *et al.* Potential of ozonated sesame oil to augment wound healing in rats. Ind J Pharm Sci 2014; 76: 87–92. PMID: 24799744.

[81] Kim HS, Noh SU, Han YW, *et al.* Therapeutic effects of topical application of ozone on acute cutaneous wound healing. J Korean Med Sci 2009; 24:368–374. doi:10.3346/jkms. 2009.24.3.368.

[82] Travagli V, Zanardi I, Valacchi G, *et al.* Ozone and ozonated oils in skin diseases: a review. Mediators Inflamm 2010; 2010. doi:10.1155/2010/610418.

[83] Baria J, Gupta SK and Bhuyan C. Clinical study of *Manjishthadi Ghrita* in *vrana ropana*. Ayu 2011;32:95–9. doi:10.4103/0974-8520.85738.

[84] Vijaya KK and Nishteswar K. Wound healing activity of honey: a pilot study. Ayu 2012; 33: 374–347. doi:10.4103/0974-8520.108827.

[85] Dudhamal TS, Gupta SK and Bhuvan C. Role of honey (madhu) in management of wounds (*Dushta vrana*). Int J Ayur Res 2010; 1: 271–273. doi:10.4103/0974-7788.76793.

[86] Namjoyan F, Kiashi F, Beigom Moosavi Z, *et al.* Efficacy of Dragon's blood cream on wound healing: a randomized, double-blind, placebo-controlled clinical trial. J Tradit Chinese Med Sci 2014. doi:10.1016/j.jtcme.2014.11.029.

[87] Shah P, Shyam AK and Shah S. Adjuvant combined ozone therapy for extensive wound over tibia. Indian J Orthop 2011; 45: 376–379.

Antimicrobial Dressings for Improving Wound Healing

Omar Sarheed, Asif Ahmed, Douha Shouqair and
Joshua Boateng

Abstract

Wound healing occurs by a series of interrelated molecular events which work together to restore tissue integrity and cellular function. These physiological events occur smoothly in normal healthy individual and/or under normal conditions. However, in certain cases, these molecular events are retarded resulting in hard-to-heal or chronic wounds arising from several factors such as poor venous return, underlying physiological or metabolic conditions such as diabetes as well as external factors such as poor nutrition. In most cases, such wounds are infected and infection also presents as another complicating phenomenon which triggers inflammatory reactions, therefore delaying wound healing. There has therefore been recent interests and significant efforts in preventing and actively treating wound infections by directly targeting infection causative agents through direct application of antimicrobial agents either alone or loaded into dressings (medicated). These have the advantage of overcoming challenges such as poor circulation in diabetic and leg ulcers when administered systemically and also require lower amounts to be applied compared to that required via oral or iv administration. This chapter will review and evaluate various antimicrobial agents used to target infected wounds, the means of delivery, and current state of the art, including commercially available dressings. Data sources will include mainly peer-reviewed literature, clinical trials and reports, patents as well as government reports where available.

Keywords: antimicrobial, bioburden, dressings, infection, wounds, wound healing, bacterial resistance

1. Introduction

A wound may be defined as a disruption to the physiological arrangement of the skin cells and a disturbance to its function in connecting and protecting underlying tissues and organs. It may be primary caused by accidental cut, tear, scratch, pressure, extreme temperatures, chemicals, and electrical current, or secondary to surgical intervention or disease (i.e., diabetes, ulcers, or carcinomas) [1]. It ranges from superficial (affecting the epidermis) to partial-thickness (affecting both epidermis and parts of the dermis) and full-thickness (including subcutaneous fat and bones) wounds [2]. Wound healing is a physiological process, by which the living body repairs tissue damages, restores its anatomical integrity, and regains the functionality of the injured parts. A wound can be closed by primary intention or left to heal by secondary intention, and in both ways the healing process occurs through a series of overlapping events and is influenced by a number of intrinsic and extrinsic factors [3].

1.1. Acute wounds

Acute wounds can heal within a limited amount of time, usually show no complications, and are characterized by the loss of skin integrity (injury) that occurs suddenly. The injured tissue heals in a predictable manner where platelets, keratinocytes, immune surveillance cells, microvascular cells, and fibroblasts play major roles in the restoration of tissue integrity [4]. These wounds are either surgical or traumatic [5].

1.2. Chronic wounds

Chronic wounds are wounds that do not heal within normal period and are associated with predisposing factors that weaken the integrity of dermal and epidermal tissues. Those factors either disrupt the balance between wound bioburden and the patient's immune system or impair the wound healing cycle. In terms of duration, if the wound fails to heal or shows no sign of recovery within 12 weeks, it is considered a chronic wound. Predisposing factors may affect the tissue perfusion causing chronic wounds such as vascular ulcers, associated with metabolic disorders such as diabetes causing diabetic foot ulcers [6]. They can be identified by criteria such as delayed healing and friable granulation tissue, prolonged inflammatory phase, persistent infection, and presence of resistant microorganisms [7–10].

1.3. Wound healing

The repair (wound healing) process involves four overlapping biochemical, physiological, and molecular phases.

I. Hemostasis

> This stage is characterized by microvascular injury and release of blood components at the wound site. Platelets come into contact with and adhere to the wall of the injured blood vessels. This adherence activates the platelets to release cytokines, growth factors, and numerous pro-inflammatory mediators, resulting in platelet aggregation and triggering the intrinsic and extrinsic coagulation path-

ways to form a fibrin clot which limits further blood loss. Growth factors produced by the platelets initiate the healing cascade [11, 12].

II. Inflammatory phase

The inflammatory phase starts at the same time as hemostasis sometime between a few minutes after injury up to 24 h and lasts for about 3 days. Aggregated platelets store vasoactive amines such as prostaglandins and histamine while other amines from granules released by mast cells, in response to injury, result in increased microvascular permeability and vasodilation, leading to exudation of fluid into the extravascular space [13]. This allows the migration of monocytes and protein-rich exudate into the wound and surrounding tissue, resulting in edema. These are typical signs of the inflammation process, and patients start complaining about pain at the site of injury within 24 h.

III. Proliferative phase

This phase commences after the inflammatory phase wanes. The remaining inflammatory cells produce growth factors to initiate angiogenesis, which is important to keep adequate blood supply within the wound bed [14]. Newly formed blood vessels will contribute to granulation tissue (composed of collagen and extracellular matrix) formation and provide the required nutrients.

IV. Maturation phase

This commences when the wound is superficially sealed. It involves the re-epithelialization and remodeling of newly formed tissues in the proliferative phase and restoration of epidermal integrity [15]. It also involves transferring collagen III to collagen I.

1.4. Factors affecting wound healing

Multiple factors affect wound healing and lead to the impairment of healing classified into local and systemic factors [16].

1.4.1. Oxygenation

Oxygen is crucial to wound healing and for resistance to infection, and used for cellular energy production by adenosine triphosphate [17]. It acts on different levels of wound healing by inducing angiogenesis, keratinocytes differentiation, migration, re-epithelialization, fibroblast proliferation, and collagen synthesis, and promotes wound contraction [18]. When injury occurs, temporary hypoxia and oxygen are useful to trigger wound healing by inducing the production of cytokines and growth factors from macrophages, keratinocytes, and fibroblasts [16]. Chronic wounds are generally hypoxic with oxygen tissue tension of 5–20 mm Hg compared to normal levels of 30–50 mm Hg [19]. Factors predisposing chronic wounds such as advancing age and diabetes can induce poor oxygenation through impaired vascular flow. Interventional revascularization therapies have been used to reverse hypoxic conditions in diabetic foot ulcers [20]. However, it has also been reported that such procedures can cause adverse effects to diabetic patients [21]. Recently, some topical foam dressings containing dissolved oxygen were developed to increase oxygen perfusion into the chronic wound area [22]. Results showed that dissolved oxygen from topical foam dressing penetrates into skin layers compared to topical gaseous oxygen.

1.4.2. Wound bioburden and infection

1.4.2.1. Bioburden

The intact skin acts to control the microbial population on the skin surface itself [23]. Once the integrity is lost through injury, the subcutaneous tissue becomes exposed, providing an environment for colonization and growth of microbes. However, this does not necessarily lead to an infection as there is a balance between the wound bioburden and the immune system [24].

1.4.2.2. Wound infection

Skin microflora is present to about 10^5 colonies without any clinical problems [25]. However, if the balance is disrupted, microorganisms will proliferate and start a microbiological chain of events by invading tissues resulting in an inflammatory response which may lead to tissue damage and delayed healing [7]. Once it causes damage to the host tissue, infection will arise. One of the consequences of infection is the prolonged inflammation due to prolonged elevation of pro-inflammatory cytokines, which causes the wound to enter the chronic stage and fail to heal within the expected 8–12 weeks [26]. This prolonged inflammation is also associated with increased levels of matrix metalloproteases which are capable of degrading the extracellular matrix which is the key component of proliferative phase of wound healing [9]. This increase in protease levels happens at the expense of the naturally occurring protease inhibitor levels that are decreased. From a microbiological perspective, wound infection is described as the presence of replicating microorganisms at the wound site overwhelming the host's immune system. It delays wound healing due to the release of toxins and exhibits active signs and symptoms of infections.

1.4.2.3. Common bacterial species present in chronic wounds

Generally, most infected wounds are polymicrobial and are commonly contaminated by pathogens found in the immediate environment, the endogenous microbes living in the mucous membranes, and the microflora on adjacent skin. Bacteria are the main cause of wound infection among other microorganisms present in the skin, though other microorganisms such as fungi have been implicated in certain mixed infections. In the initial stages of chronic wound formation, Gram-positive organisms such as *Staphylococcus aureus* and *Escherichia coli* are predominant [9]. In the later stages, Gram-negative *Pseudomonas* species are common and tend to invade deeper layers in the wound causing significant tissue damage [27]. Other aerobes implicated include *Staphylococci* and *Streptococci* species as well as anaerobic bacteria and are estimated in 50% of chronic wounds [28, 29].

1.4.3. Chronic wounds and biofilm

Biofilm is defined as "a microbially derived sessile community characterized by cells that are irreversibly attached to a substratum or interface or to each other, are embedded in a secreted matrix of extracellular polymeric substances (EPSs), and exhibit an altered phenotype with respect to growth rate and gene transcription" [30]. Firstly, conditioning film forms and is composed of proteins and polysaccharide molecules adsorbed onto the solid surface. This makes the surface ready to receive the first cells of the insipient biofilm. Secondly, bacteria will start to approach and attach onto the surface by forces such as van der Waals forces and the negative electrostatic charges of bacterial surface [31]. The attached bacteria become encased in a polymeric matrix called extracellular polymeric substance (EPS). This bacterial attachment induces a phenomenon called quorum sensing, which is responsible for "the regulation of gene expression in response to fluctuations in cell population density" [32]. This causes the bacteria within biofilm to alter their phenotypes resulting in the production of more virulent factors in response to signals from other bacteria within biofilm. These factors with barrier made from EPS contribute to the increased resistance to antibiotics. It has been suggested that EPS can interact with antibiotics spontaneously thereby preventing them reaching the bacteria to exert their antimicrobial activity [33]. The biofilm also protects the bacteria from host defenses by the covering of glycocalyx while bacteria secrete products within the film which makes phagocytic penetration poor [34].

This understanding is of great importance for intervention modalities in chronic wounds especially the use of antimicrobial wound dressing. For example macrolides can have inhibitory effect on the film formation or induce phagocytic invasion into biofilms [35]. Furthermore, in clinical wound management, it is always essential to promptly clean the wound and remove necrotic tissue and foreign material (e.g. bacteria and biofilms) from areas around the wound to improve the chances of enhanced wound healing, and this is known as debridement [1]. This is important because the presence of necrotic tissue increases the risk of infection and sepsis, which prolongs the inflammatory phase. Several approaches are employed including surgical removal, wound irrigation (e.g. saline and antiseptics such as chlorhexidine), autolytic rehydration using hydrogel dressings, applying enzymes such as collagenases or streptokinase preparations as well as using maggots to selectively dissolve necrotic and infected tissue (including biofilms) without destroying healthy or newly formed tissue [1].

2. Wound dressings

Wound dressings can maintain a moist environment in the wound which helps in proliferation and migration of fibroblast and keratinocytes. Moisture in the wound serves as a transporter for enzymes, growth factors, and hormones, thus inducing cell growth. Moist wound dressings promote collagen synthesis and decrease scar formation [36] which help wounds to heal faster [37]. Modern moist wound dressings can be classified depending on their materials (synthetic and natural polymers) and physical forms (hydrogels, hydrocolloids, films, and wafers).

Hydrogels consist of hydrated polymers which make them hydrophilic in nature. Water content is higher than 95%, and as a result they cannot absorb much exudate and cause maceration. But, this dressing is very useful in dry wound which can maintain moisture within wounds [36]. A Cochrane Review [38] of hydrogel dressings for healing diabetic foot ulcers suggests that hydrogel dressings are more effective than basic wound contact dressing. Hydrogels have advantages of autolytic debridement of slough and necrotic tissue and do not support bacterial growth [39, 40]. Hydrocolloid dressings are occlusive and can absorb wound exudate into the matrix to help improve healing. It can work for a sustained period of time, thus reducing the frequency of dressing changes. It also assists autolysis of necrotic materials [40]. Due to its extra absorbent nature, it is widely used in the treatment of cavity wounds [41]. A Cochrane Review [42] reported that any type of hydrocolloid and other dressings have no difference in efficacy. Foam dressings are highly absorptive, protective, and comfortable to the body surface. They promote thermal insulation, angiogenesis, and autolysis [43]. Film dressings are adhesive, transparent, durable, comfortable, and cost effective. Due to their transparency, the wound bed can be monitored without removing the dressing. However, films are suitable for superficial pressure wounds. The disadvantage of film dressing is maceration of wound exudate [36]. Lyophilized wafers are one of the most recent moist dressings proposed for wound care. Due to their highly porous nature, they can absorb high amounts of exudate rapidly which improves wound healing. Wafers can carry both antibacterial and anti-inflammatory drugs at the same time which give dual effects of inhibiting bacteria and reducing inflammation [44]. Wafers have good adhesion and diffusion properties [45] while Labovitiadi et al. [46] reported that wafers are a compatible delivery system for both insoluble and soluble antimicrobial drugs that exhibit better antimicrobial activity.

3. Antimicrobial wound dressings

3.1. Need for antimicrobial wound dressing

The major need for antimicrobial dressing is drug resistance to bacteria. Zubair et al. [47] isolated bacteria from diabetic foot ulcer patients and their resistance to different classes of drugs with the penicillins showing highest susceptibility to resistance followed by cephalosporins (54%), quinolones and fluoroquinolones (52.8%), aminoglycosides (38.5%), beta lactams (32.2%), and carbapenems (18.4%). Further, most chronic wound sufferers such as older patients and diabetics with leg and foot ulcers suffer from complications of poor circulation at the lower extremities, which makes oral and IV antibiotics ineffective. In addition, topical dressings are able to avoid the adverse effects of systemic administration (oral and IV) of high antibiotic doses including nausea, vomiting, diarrhea, allergic reactions, leukocyturia, insomnia, headache, and vaginosis, when only small doses above the minimum inhibitory concentration are required at the infected wound site. Finally, production costs of most dressings are less than those of IV or oral products.

3.2. Advanced medicated antimicrobial wound dressings

Antimicrobial dressings can be broadly classified into two groups as antiseptic or antibiotic dressings. Antiseptic dressings have broad spectrum activity which can kill or inhibit bacteria, fungus, protozoa, viruses, and prions [48]; however, some antiseptic dressings often show dose-dependent cytotoxicity to the host cells including keratinocytes, fibroblasts, and leuko-cytes [49, 50]. The concentration of povidone iodine greater than 0.004 and 0.05% is completely toxic to keratinocytes and fibroblasts, respectively [51]. Cadexomer iodine is reported to be nontoxic to fibroblasts *in vitro* at concentrations of up to 0.45% [52]. Chlorhexidine also shows dose-dependent toxicity to fibroblasts at concentrations between 0.2 and 0.001% [53, 54]. Moreover, silver-impregnated dressings have been reported to be more cytotoxic to epidermal keratinocytes and dermal fibroblasts than honey-based dressings [55]. On the other hand,

Dressing type	Polymers	Drug	Reference
Pads	Bovine serum albumin	Ciprofloxacin	[58]
Nanofibers patch	PVA/sodium alginate	Ciprofloxacin	[59]
Hydrogel	Polyethylene glycol	Ciprofloxacin	[60]
Sponges	Alginate/chitosan	Ciprofloxacin	[61]
Films	Chitosan/gelatin	Ciprofloxacin	[62]
Nanofibers	PVA/regenerated silk fibroin	Ciprofloxacin	[63]
Nanofiber mats	Polyurethane/dextran	Ciprofloxacin	[64]
Nanofiber mats	PVA/poly(vinyl acetate)	Ciprofloxacin	[65]
Films	Poly (2-hydroxymethacrylate)	Ciprofloxacin	[66]
Films	PVA/aminophenylboronic acid	Ciprofloxacin	[67]
Collagen dressing	Collagen	Ciprofloxacin	[68]
Hydrogels	Keratin	Ciprofloxacin	[69]
Films	Sodium carboxymethyl cellulose/gelatin	Ciprofloxacin	[70]
Scaffolds	Chitosan/polyethylene glycol	Ciprofloxacin	[71]
Hydrogel films	Carboxymethyl chitin	Chlorhexidine gluconate	[72]
Gel	Chitosan	Ofloxacin	[73]
Wafers and films	Polyox/carrageenan	Streptomycin	[74–76]
Films	PVA/sodium alginate	Clindamycin and nitrofurazone	[77, 78]
Films	PVA/dextran	Gentamicin	[79]
Scaffolds	Collagen	Doxycycline	[80]
Microspheres	Gelatin	Doxycycline	[81]
Microspheres	Chitosan	Levofloxacin	[82]
Nanofibrous scaffolds	Chitosan/poly(e-caprolactone)	Levofloxacin	[82]
Hydrogels	Polyvinylalcohol	Nitric oxide	[83]
Hydrogels	poly(2-hydroxyethyl methacrylate)	Nitric oxide	[84]
Hydrogels	S-Nitrosothiol	Nitric acid	[85]

Table 1. Summary of antibiotic dressings reported in the literature.

antibiotic dressings (**Table 1**) are nontoxic and can work effectively on the target sites without damaging host tissues [49]. The ideal antimicrobial dressing should have broad spectrum activity against all major microorganisms, be nonallergic and nontoxic to host cells, have the ability to drain exudate and maintain a moist wound environment, should release drugs rapidly in a sustained manner, should reduce malodor, and be cost effective [56, 57].

3.3. Silver-based dressings

Silver is a natural broad spectrum antibiotic, and its dressings have not yet shown any bacterial resistance. Silver exists in different forms such as silver oxide, silver nitrate, silver sulfate, silver salt, silver zeolite, silver sulfadiazine (SSD), and silver nanoparticles (AgNPs). Before the eighteenth century, silver nitrate was used for leg ulcers, epilepsy, acne, and venereal infections [86]. Currently different forms of silver are widely used in acute wound (burns, partial-thickness burns, freshly grafted burns, second-degree burns, surgical/traumatic wounds, colorectal surgical wounds, pilonidal sinus, and donor site), and chronic wound (pressure ulcers, leg ulcers, and diabetic foot ulcers) healing [87].

3.3.1. Antimicrobial activity of silver dressings

Antimicrobial activity of silver dressings depends on the amount and rate of silver release and its toxicity to bacterial, fungal, and algal cells. Silver works by interacting with thiol groups present in bacterial cells thus stop their respiration process. In the case of *E. coli*, silver prevents phosphate uptake and catalysation of disulfide bonds with silver tending to change the nature of protein structure in *E. coli*. The degenerative changes in cytosolic protein cause cell death [86, 88]. Feng et al. [89] reported antibacterial mechanism of action of silver ions on *E. coli* and *S. aureus* and showed that silver ions penetrate into bacterial cells and condense DNA molecules which inhibit their replication capabilities leading to cell death. Matsumura et al. [90] introduced two bactericidal mechanism actions of silver zeolite on *E. coli*. Firstly, silver ions released from silver zeolite come into contact with cells and penetrate into cells, altering the cellular functions that cause cell death. Secondly, silver ions inhibit respiration process through the generation of reactive oxygen molecules. Silver zeolite has also been reported against oral microorganisms (*Streptococcus mutans, Lactobacillus casei, Candida albicans, and S. aureus*) [91].

Silver nanoparticles show the most efficient antimicrobial activity amongst all forms of silver. The bactericidal effects of AgNPs depend on the size, shape, surface characteristics, and their dose [88, 92–101]. It has been reported that 75 µg ml⁻¹ of AgNPs having 1–100 nm particle size inhibits all bacterial strains (specifically, *E. coli, Vibrio cholerae, Salmonella typhi, and Pseudomonas aeruginosa*). It has also been reported nanoparticles having particle size ~1–10 nm have higher affinity of attaching to the surface of the cell membrane as compared to larger nanoparticles. Because of this nature, AgNPs can attach to the larger surface area of bacterial cell membrane and cause native membrane porations which cause cell damage [92]. Ivask et al. [93] examined toxicity of silver nanoparticles to bacteria (*E. coli*), yeast (*Saccharomyces cerevisiae*), algae (*Pseudokirchneriella subcapitata*), crustacean (*Daphnia magna*), and mammalian cells (murine fibroblast) according to their particle sizes ranging from 10 to 80 nm. They confirmed that the smaller-sized nanoparticles showed highly toxic effect. The review of Rai et al. [88] and Rizzello et al. [92] explained that truncated triangular nanoparticles are the strongest biocidal active products compared to spherical- and rod-shaped nanoparticles. 1 µg of truncated triangular nanoparticles shows greater activity than 12.5 µg of spherical-shaped nanoparticles and 50–100 µg of rod-shaped nanoparticles due to the enhancement of electrostatic interaction with bacterial cells (**Table 2**).

Dressing type	Brand name	Silver form
Contact layer dressings	Restore contact layer	Silver sulfate
	Acticoat Flex 3; Acticoat Flex 7	Elemental silver
	KerraContact Ag	Silver salt
	SilverDerm 7	Ionic silver
	Silverlon Wound & Burn Contact Dressings	Ionic silver
	Therabond 3D with Silvertrak™ Technology	Silver
Foams	RTD	Silver zirconium phosphate
	Acticoat Moisture Control	Elemental silver
	Allevyn Ag	Silver sulfadiazine
	Aquacel Ag	Ionic silver
	Biatain Ag Adhesive	Silver
	HydraFoam/Ag	Silver
	MediPlus Comfort Border Foam Ag+	Silver
	Mepilex Ag	Silver
	Optifoam Ag Adhesive	Ionic silver
	PolyMem MAX Silver Non-Adhesive Dressing	Silver
	Silverlon Negative Pressure	Ionic silver
	UrgoCell Silver/Cellosorb Ag	Silver salts
	V.A.C GranuFoam Silver	Silver
	Silverlon Acute Burn Glove	Silver
	Silvercel	Elemental silver
Fibers/clothes/mats /pads/others	Tegaderm Ag Mesh Dressing	Silver sulfate
	Absorbent Dermanet Ag+ Border	Silver
	Acticoat	Elemental silver
	Allevyn Ag Non-Adhesive	Silver sulfadiazine
	Durafiber Ag	Ionic silver
	Exsalt SD7	Silver

Dressing type	Brand name	Silver form
	Gentell Calcium Alginate Ag	Silver
	Silverlon Calcium Alginate	Silver
	Simpurity Silver Alginate Pads	Silver particles
	Urgotul SSD	Silver sulfadiazine
	Vliwaktiv Ag	Silver
	Acticoat 7	Elemental silver
	Arglaes film	Silver
Films/meshes	Avance	Silver
	Acticoat Absorbent	Elemental silver
	Algicell Ag	Silver
Alginate based	Algidex Ag	Ionic silver
	Biatain Alginate Ag	Silver
	CalciCare	Silver zirconium
	DermaGinate/Ag	Silver
	Dermanet Ag+	Silver
	Maxorb ES Ag+	Silver
	Maxorb Extra Ag+	Silver zirconium phosphate
	McKesson Calcium Alginate with Antimicrobial Silver	Silver
	Opticell Ag+	Ionic silver
	Restore Calcium Alginate Dressing with Silver	Ionic silver
	Sofsorb Ag	Silver
	Sorbalgon Ag	Ionic silver
	Suprasorb A + Ag Calcium Alginate	Silver
	Askina Calgitrol Ag	Silver alginate
	Invacare Silver Alginate	Silver sodium hydrogen zirconium phosphate
	Melgisorb Ag	Silver
	SeaSorb Ag	Ionic silver
	Silvasorb	Ionic silver
	Sorbsan Silver	Silver Sorbsan
	Algidex Ag	Ionic silver
	Urgotul SSD/S.Ag	Silver sulfadiazine

Dressing type	Brand name	Silver form
Gauze	Aquacel Ag	Ionic silver
	Arglaes Powder	Silver
Hydrofiber	Cardinal Health Hydrogel +Ag	Silver
Powder	DermaSyn/Ag	Ionic silver
Hydrogel	Elta Silver Gel	Silver
	ExcelGinate Ag	Silver
	Gentell Hydrogel Ag	Silver sulfadiazine
	SilvaSorb Antimicrobial Silver Dressing	Ionic silver
	Silver-Sept Silver Antimicrobial Skin & Wound Gel	Silver
	SilverMed Amorphous Hydrogel	Silver
	Silverseal	Silver
	SilvrSTAT Gel	Silver nanoparticles
	Viniferamine Hydrogel Ag	Silver
	Silverseal	Silver oxide
	Silver-Sept Antimicrobial Gel	Silver salt
	DermaCol Ag Collagen Matrix	Silver
	Puracol Plus Ag+ MicroScaffold Collagen	Silver
Collagen based	SilvaKollagen Gel	Silver
	Silverlon Adhesive Strips	Silver
	Contreet Hydrocolloid	Silver
Adhesive strips	Silverseal Hydrocolloid	Silver
Hydrocolloid	SilverMed Antimicrobial Wound Cleanser	Silver microparticles

Table 2. List of selected commercially available antimicrobial silver-containing dressings [22, 102, 103].

3.3.2. Silver dressings in wound healing

AgNPs (~11 to ~12 nm) containing gelatin fiber mats were prepared by electrospinning process and inhibited major microorganisms present in wounds [104]. Lin et al. [105] compared silver-containing carbon-activated fibers with commercially available silver-containing dressings and showed the silver-containing carbon-activated fibers to exhibit antibacterial activity and biocompatibility and promoting granulation and collagen deposition. A novel chitosan–hyaluronic acid composite with nanosilver was reported as a potential antimicrobial wound healing dressing for diabetic foot ulcers possessing high porosity, swelling, water uptake abilities, and biodegradable and potential blood clotting ability. The authors proved the inhibitory effects on *S. aureus*, *E. coli*, MRSA, *P. aeruginosa*, and *Klebsiella pneumoniae* [106].

In a related study, chitosan incorporated with polyphosphate and AgNPs was studied. The polyphosphate acts as a procoagulant which boosts blood clotting, platelet adhesion, and thrombin generation [107]. A similar scaffold dressing was developed by incorporating silver nanoparticles with chitin and showed antibacterial and blood clotting activity [108]. In another study, AgNPs containing hydrogel without any cytotoxicity but with antibacterial activity were reported [109]. Various inorganic forms of silver including silver zeolite, silver zirconium phosphate silicate, and silver zirconium phosphate demonstrate antimicrobial activity against oral microorganisms [91]. Pant et al. [110] stated AgNPs containing nylon-6 nanofibers prepared by one-step electrospinning process could be an effective antimicrobial wound dressing to kill both Gram-negative *E. coli* and Gram-positive *S. aureus*. Archana et al. [111] evaluated chitosan-blended polyvinyl pyrrolidone (PVP)–nano silver oxide (CPS) as an effective wound dressing *in vitro* and *in vivo*.

Lansdown et al. [112] investigated two forms of silver-containing dressings (Contreet foam and Contreet hydrocolloid) and found these promoted healing in chronic venous leg ulcers and diabetic foot ulcers. Polyvinylpyrolidone and alginate-based hydrogel-containing nanosilver has been functionally evaluated for efficient fluid handling capacity and strong antimicrobial activity against all major microorganisms such as *Pseudomonas, Staphylococcus, Escherichia, and Candida* [113]. Jodar et al. [114] demonstrated silver sulfadiazine-impregnated hydrogel for antimicrobial topical application for wound healing. Silver sulfadiazine (SSD)-impregnated hydrogel was prepared by polyvinyl alcohol (PVA) and dextran blending. Boateng et al. [115] formulated an ideal lyophilized wafer dressing composed of alginate and gelatin containing silver sulfadiazine for wound healing and showed the controlled release of SSD over 7 h and expected to diminish microbial load in the wound area. A novel SSD-loaded bilayer chitosan membrane was prepared with sustained release of silver which inhibits the growth of *P. aeruginosa and S. aureus* [116]. Shanmugasundaram et al. [117] formulated SSD-impregnated collagen-based scaffold with strong antibacterial activity *in vitro*. Ammons et al. [118] formulated dressings by combining commercial silver dressings (Acticoat™ Absorbent, Aquacel® Ag, and Tegaderm™Ag) with lactoferrin and xylitol and demonstrated greater efficacy against MRSA and *P. aeruginosa*.

There are several clinical studies with silver-containing dressings in the treatment of infected wounds to enhance wound healing, and the reader is referred to these [119–125].

3.4. Iodine and other antiseptics

Iodine is an old agent used in the treatment of chronic wounds and was used by soldiers during wars. The antibacterial activity of iodine was first investigated by Davaine in 1880 [126]. Iodine penetrates into the cell wall of microorganisms and damages the cell membrane by blocking hydrogen bond. This phenomenon alters the structure and function of cell proteins and enzymes, leading to cell death [127]. Iodine is active against a broad spectrum of microorganisms including *S. aureus, E. coli, Pseudomonas, Streptococcus, Salmonella, Candida, Enterobacter, Klebsiella, Clostridium, Corynebacterium, and Mycobacterium* [126]. Iodine dressings can be found in two preparations as povidone iodine and cadexomer iodine, and the various commercial formulations are summarized in **Table 3**.

Polyhexamethylene biguanide (PHMB) is an another antiseptic and widely used as antimicrobial dressing in wound healing. PHMB is known to be effective against *E. coli. S. aureus* and *S. epidermidis*. PHMB also works like iodine as it attaches to the bacterial cells and disrupts cell membrane resulting in leakage of potassium ions and cytosolic components that lead to cell death [128]. A study by Eberlein et al. [129] confirmed that PHMB containing biocellulose wound dressings were more effective than silver-containing dressing in retarding microbial loads present in locally infected wounds. Loke et al. [130] developed a two-layer dressing with sustained release of chlorhexidine which showed activity against *S. aureus* and *P. aeruginosa in vitro*.

Dressing type	Product name	Antiseptic
Pad	Iodoflex 0.9% Cadexomer Iodine Pad	Cadexomer iodine
Foam	IodoFoam	Iodine
Fibers	**Inadine**	Povidone iodine
Colloidal ointment base	Braunovidon ointment/ointment gauze	Povidone
Hydrogel dressing	Iodozym	Iodine
Liposome hydrogel	Repithel	Povidone
Foam	Kerlix AMD	PHMB
Sponges	Telfa AMD	PHMB
Foam	Kendall AMD	PHMB
Gauzes sponges	Curity AMD Antimicrobial Gauze Sponges	PHMB

Table 3. List of other commercially available antiseptics [36, 127].

3.5. Honey dressings

Honey has been used as wound dressing over centuries [131]. Honey has been reported in several clinical studies for treating chronic diabetic foot ulcers [132–135] and has antimicrobial and anti-inflammatory activity [136–138]. It is reported that honey can inhibit around 60 species of bacteria including *Alcaligenes faecalis, Citrobacter freundii, E. coli, Enterobacter aerogenes, Klebsiella pneumoniae, Mycobacterium phlei, Salmonella california, Salmonella enteritidis, Salmonella typhimurium, Shigella sonnei, S. aureus,* and *Staphylococcus epidermidis* [139]. In addition, it is reported Manuka honey and Cameroonian honey have an effect on *Pseudomonas aeruginosa*, methicillin-resistant *S. aureus* (MRSA), and vancomycin-resistant *Enterococcus* species [137, 140]. The antimicrobial properties of honey are ascribed to its low pH, hygroscopic nature, and peroxide-containing compounds [141]. The rich contents of sugar in honey generate high osmotic pressure and present an unsuitable environment to bacterial growth and cell proliferation [139]. Van den Berg et al. [142] investigated the anti-inflammatory properties of different types of honey *in vitro* by testing reactive oxygen species (ROS) inhibition capability and found American buckwheat honey exhibits high ROS inhibition ability. Many clinical studies have been performed on the basis of the antimicrobial effect of honey [143–145]. Clinical studies and bioactivity demonstrate the efficiency of honey in wound healing, maintaining a moist environment, promoting drainage of wound exudate and autolytic debridement [144]. It has been reported in minimizing malodour and scar formation of the wound [145] as well as angiogenic activity [146].

Sasikala et al. [147] developed a chitosan-based film dressing loaded with Manuka honey. They identified chitosan–lactic acid with 6% honey showed ideal dressing properties in terms of water vapor transmission rate, water absorption, tensile strength, elongation, and antibacterial activity against *E. coli* and *S. aureus*. **Table 4** summarizes the commercially available honey-based dressings currently sold on the market.

Dressing type	Product Name	Honey type
Hydrocolloid	MediHoney	Leptospermum honey
Alginate-based	MediHoney	Leptospermum honey
Fibers	MANUKAhd	Manuka honey
Pure honey	Surgihoney	Bioengineered honey
Foam	Ligasano	Honeycomb
Pure honey	MGO Manuka Honey	Manuka honey
Sterile Manuka honey	ManukaFill	Manuka honey
Honey-impregnated gauze	Manuka IG	Manuka honey
Sheets, ribbon, gel	TheraHoney	Manuka honey
Knitted viscose mesh dressing, pure honey	Activon	Manuka honey
Alginate ribbon and dressing	Algivon	Manuka honey
Composite, foam/silicone dressings	Actilite	Manuka honey
Nonadherent gauze fibers	MelDra	Buckwheat honey

Table 4. List of selected commercially available honey dressings used in wound healing [22, 148, 149].

3.6. Polymer-based antimicrobial dressings

Natural and synthetic polymers are widely used in acute and chronic wound healing due to their biodegradability, biocompatibility, and wound exudate handling capacity. However, some polymers themselves have an antimicrobial activity [150]. The combination of polymers and antimicrobial drugs provides effective dressings to improve wound healing. Biazar et al.

[151] evaluated a synthetic polymer-based hydrogel dressing that exhibits biocompatible and antimicrobials activity. In another study, synthetic polyvinyl alcohol was blended with calcium alginate to produce nano fiber matrix by electrospinning technique. *In vitro* antibacterial test showed the rate of inhibition of *S. aureus* depends on the concentration of calcium alginate [152]. Chitosan is a cationic polymer whose positive charge interacts with a negative charge of the microbial cell membrane, resulting in disruption and agglutination [153]. Carboxymethyl chitosan has been reported as a broad spectrum antibiofilm agent which can prevent biofilm formation for *E. coli and S. aureus* by 81.6 and 74.6%, respectively [154].

4. Summary

In this chapter, wound healing processes and types of dressings incorporating antimicrobial agents have been briefly discussed. Antimicrobials loaded into dressings for direct application to infected wound sites are becoming more popular worldwide in terms of safety, efficacy, cost effective, and convenience. The key antimicrobial agents ranging from antiseptics such as iodine, metals such as silver, antibiotics such as cephalosporins and aminoglycosides as well as natural products such as honey have been covered. In addition, the driving forces behind the developing of advanced therapeutic dressings have been reviewed. Furthermore, this review has demonstrated different and wide range of antimicrobial-loaded dressings, and a few clinical studies and commercially available antimicrobial dressings have been highlighted. Given the wide range of scientific studies and commercial products publicly available, it is evident that more evidence-based clinical trials are required to select appropriate dressings for the patients. It is also important to note the interdisciplinary fields (including formulation technology, biopharmaceutics, microbiology, materials and polymer chemistry and molecular biology) required for developing an effective antimicrobial dressing able to treat infection and also contribute towards enhanced wound healing.

Author details

Omar Sarheed[1*], Asif Ahmed[2], Douha Shouqair[1] and Joshua Boateng[2*]

*Address all correspondence to: sarheed@rakmhsu.ac.ae and j.s.boateng@gre.ac.uk

1 RAK College of Pharmaceutical Sciences, RAK Medical and Health Sciences University, Ras Al Khaiamah, United Arab Emirates

2 Department of Pharmaceutical, Chemical and Environmental Sciences, Faculty of Engineering and Science, University of Greenwich, Kent, UK

References

[1] Boateng JS, Matthews KH, Stevens HN, Eccleston GM. Wound healing dressings and drug delivery systems: a review. J Pharm Sci. 2008;97(8):2892–2923.

[2] Flanagan M. Wound care. Assessment criteria. Nurs Times. 1994;90(35):76–88.

[3] Hutchinson J. The Wound Programme. Centre for Medical Education: Dundee; 1992.

[4] Singer AJ, Clark RA. 1999. Cutaneous wound healing. N Engl J Med. 1999;341:738–746.

[5] Gottrup F, Melling A, Hollander DA. An overview of surgical site infections: aetiology, incidence and risk factors. EWMA J. 2005;5(2):11–15.

[6] Alavi A, Sibbald RG, Phillips TJ, Miller OF, Margolis DJ, Marston W, Woo K, Romanelli M, Kirsner RS. What's new: management of venous leg ulcers: approach to venous leg ulcers. J Am Acad Dermatol. 2016;74(4):627–640.

[7] Moffatt C. Identifying criteria for wound infection. EWMA Position document: 1–5 [Internet]. 2005. http://ewma.org/fileadmin/user_upload/EWMA/pdf/Position_Documents/2005__Wound_Infection_/English_pos_doc_final.pdf. [Accessed 17 Mar 2016].

[8] Eming SA, Krieg T, Davidson JM. Inflammation in wound repair: molecular and cellular mechanisms. J Invest Dermatol. 2007;127(3):514–525.

[9] Edwards R, Harding KG. Bacteria and wound healing. Curr Opin Infect Dis. 2004;17:91–96.

[10] Wolcott RD, Rhoads DD, Dowd SE. Biofilms and chronic wound inflammation. J Wound Care. 2008;17(8):333–341.

[11] Weyrich AS, Zimmerman GA. Platelets: signaling cells in the immune continuum. Trends Immunol. 2004;25(9):489–495.

[12] Reinke JM, Sorg H. Wound repair and regeneration. Eur Surg Res. 2012;49(1):35–43.

[13] Singer AJ, Clark RA. Cutaneous wound healing. N Engl J Med. 1999;341:738–746.

[14] Li J, Zhang YP, Kirsner RS. Angiogenesis in wound repair: angiogenic growth factors and the extracellular matrix. Microsc Res Tech. 2003;60(1):107–114.

[15] Steed, DL. The role of growth factors in wound healing. Surg Clin North Am. 1997;77(3): 575–586.

[16] Guo S, Dipietro LA. Factors affecting wound healing. J Dent Res. 2010;89(3): 219–229.

[17] Gottrup F. Oxygen in wound healing and infection. World J Surg. 2004;28(3):312–315.

[18] Rodriguez PG, Felix FN, Woodley DT, Shim EK. The role of oxygen in wound healing: a review of the literature. Dermatol Surg. 2008;34(9):1159–1169.

[19] Tandara AA, Mustoe TA. Oxygen in wound healing—ore than a nutrient. World J Surg. 2004;28(3):294–300.

[20] Faries PL, Teodorescu VJ, Morrissey NJ, Hollier LH, Marin ML. The role of surgical revascularization in the management of diabetic foot wounds. Am J Surg. 2004;187(5):S34–S37.

[21] Smith SC, Faxon D, Cascio W, Schaff H, Gardner T, Jacobs A, et al. Prevention conference VI: diabetes and cardiovascular disease: writing group VI: revascularization in diabetic patients. In: Proceeding of the American Heart Association; 18–20 January 2001; Circulation. 2002;105(18). p. 165–169.

[22] Boateng JS, Catanzano O. Advanced therapeutic dressings for effective wound healing—a review. J Pharm Sci. 2015;104(11):3653–3680.

[23] Bowler PG, Duerden BI, Armstrong DG. Wound microbiology and associated approaches to wound management. Clin Microbiol Rev. 2011;14 (2):244–269.

[24] Sue E. Gardner, Rita A. Frantz. Wound bioburden and infection-related complications in diabetic foot ulcers. Biol Res Nurs. 2008;10(1): 44–53.

[25] Noble WC. Ecology and Host Resistance in Relation to Skin Disease. 5th ed. New York: McGraw-Hill; 1999. p. 184–191.

[26] Menke NB, Ward KR, Witten TM, Bonchev DG, Diegelmann RF. Impaired wound healing. Clin Dermatol. 2007;25(1):19–25.

[27] Dow G, Browne A, Sibbald RG. Infection in chronic wounds: controversies in diagnosis and treatment. Ostomy Wound Manage. 1999;45(8):23–7, 29–40; quiz 41–2.

[28] Sun Y, Smith E, Wolcott R, Dowd SE. Propagation of anaerobic bacteria within an aerobic multi-species chronic wound biofilm model. J Wound Care. 2009;18(10):426–431.

[29] Stephens P, Wall IB, Wilson MJ, Hill KE, Davies CE, Hill CM, Harding KG, Thomas DW. Anaerobic cocci populating the deep tissues of chronic wounds impair cellular wound healing responses in vitro. Br J Dermatol. 2003;148(3):456–66.

[30] Donlan RM1, Costerton JW. Biofilms: survival mechanisms of clinically relevant microorganisms. Clin Microbiol Rev. 2002;15(2):167–193.

[31] Garrett TR, Bhakoo M, Zhang Z. Bacterial adhesion and biofilms on surfaces. Prog Natl Sci. 2008;18(9):1049–1056.

[32] Miller MB, Bassler BL. Quorum sensing in bacteria. Annu Rev Microbiol. 2001;55:165–199.

[33] Song C, Sun XF, Xing SF, Xia PF, Shi YJ, Wang SG. Characterization of the interactions between tetracycline antibiotics and microbial extracellular polymeric

substances with spectroscopic approaches. Environ Sci Pollut Res Int. 2014;21(3): 1786–1795.

[34] Costerton JW, Stewart PS, Greenberg EP. Bacterial biofilms: a common cause of persistent infections. Science. 1999;284(5418):1318–1322.

[35] Yamasaki O, Akiyama H, Toi Y, Arata J. A combination of roxithromycin and imipenem as an antimicrobial strategy against biofilms formed by *Staphylococcus aureus*. J Antimicrob Chemother. 2001;48(4):573–577.

[36] Moura LI, Dias AM, Carvalho E, de Sousa HC. Recent advances on the development of wound dressings for diabetic foot ulcer treatment—a review. Acta Biomater. 2013;9(7):7093–7114.

[37] Harding KG, Jones V, Price P. Topical treatment: which dressing to choose. Diabetes Metab Res Rev. 2000;16: S47–S50.

[38] Dumville JC, O'Meara S, Deshpande S, Speak K. Hydrogel dressings for healing diabetic foot ulcers. Cochrane Database Syst Rev. 2011;9:CD009101.

[39] Fonder M., Lazarus G, Cowan D, Aronson-Cook B, Kohli A, Mamelak A. Treating the chronic wound: a practical approach to the care of nonhealing wounds and wound care dressings. J Am Acad Dermatol. 2008;58(2):185–206.

[40] Hilton JR, Williams DT, Beuker B, Miller DR, Harding KG. Wound dressings in diabetic foot disease. Clin Infect Dis. 2004;39(Suppl 2):S100–S103.

[41] Lloyd LL, Kennedy JF, Methacanon P, Paterson M, Knill CJ. Carbohydrate polymers as wound management aids. Carbohydr Polym. 1998;37(3):315–322.

[42] Dumville JC, Deshpande S, O'Meara S, Speak K. Hydrocolloid dressings for healing diabetic foot ulcers. Cochrane Database Syst Rev. 2013; 8:CD009099.

[43] Skórkowska-Telichowska K, Czemplik M, Kulma A, Szopa J. The local treatment and available dressings designed for chronic wounds. J Am Acad Dermatol. 2013;68(4):117–126.

[44] Pawar HV, Boateng JS, Ayensu I, Tetteh J. Multifunctional medicated lyophilised wafer dressing for effective chronic wound healing. J Pharm Sci. 2014;103(6):1720–1733.

[45] Boateng JS, Pawar HV, Tetteh J. Evaluation of in vitro wound adhesion characteristics of composite film and wafer based dressings using texture analysis and FTIR spectroscopy: a chemometrics factor analysis approach. RSC Adv. 2015;5(129): 107064–107075.

[46] Labovitiadi O, Lamb AJ, Matthews KH. In vitro efficacy of antimicrobial wafers against methicillin-resistant *Staphylococcus aureus*. Ther Deliv. 2012; 3(4):443–55.

[47] Zubair M, Malik A, Ahmad J. Clinico-microbiological study and antimicrobial drug resistance profile of diabetic foot infections in North India. Foot (Edinburgh, Scotland). 2011;21(1):6–14.

[48] Gethin G. Role of topical antimicrobials in wound management. J Wound Care. 2009;Nov:4–8.

[49] Lipsky BA, Hoey C. Topical antimicrobial therapy for treating chronic wounds. Clin Infect Dis. 2009;49(10):1541–1549.

[50] Drosou A, Falabella A, Kirsner RS. Antiseptics on wounds: an area of controversy. Wounds Compend Clin Res Pract. 2003;15(5):149–166.

[51] Burks RI. Povidone-iodine solution in wound treatment. Phys Ther. 1998;78(2):212–218.

[52] Zhou LH, Nahm WK, Badiavas E, Yufit T, Falanga V. Slow release iodine preparation and wound healing: in vitro effects consistent with lack of in vivo toxicity in human chronic wounds. Br J Dermatol. 2002;146(3):365–374.

[53] Mirhadi H, Azar MR, Abbaszadegan A, Geramizadeh B, Torabi S, Rahsaz M. Cytotoxicity of chlorhexidine-hydrogen peroxide combination in different concentrations on cultured human periodontal ligament fibroblasts. Dent Res J. 2014;11(6):645–648.

[54] Severyns AM, Lejeune A, Rocoux G, Lejeune G. Non-toxic antiseptic irrigation with chlorhexidine in experimental revascularization in the rat. J Hosp Infect. 1991;17(3):197–206.

[55] Du Toit, DF, Page BJ. An in vitro evaluation of the cell toxicity of honey and silver dressings. J Wound Care. 2009;18:383–389.

[56] Vowden K, Vowden K, Carville K. Antimicrobials made easy. Wounds Int. 2011;2(1):1–6.

[57] Cutting K. Wound dressings: 21st century performance requirements. J Wound Care. 2010;19(Suppl 1):4–9.

[58] Phoudee W, Wattanakaroon W. Development of protein-based hydrogel wound dressing impregnated with bioactive compounds. Nat Sci. 2015;49(1):92–102.

[59] Kataria K, Gupta A, Rath G, Mathur RB, Dhakate SR. In vivo wound healing performance of drug loaded electrospun composite nanofibers transdermal patch. J Pharm Sci. 2014;469(1):102–110.

[60] Shi Y, Truong V, Kulkarni K, Qu Y, Simon G, Boyd R. Light-triggered release of ciprofloxacin from an in situ forming click hydrogel for antibacterial wound dressings. J Mater Chem B. 2015;3(45):8771–8774.

[61] Öztürk E, Ağalar C, Keçeci K, Denkba E. Preparation and characterization of ciprofloxacin-loaded alginate/chitosan sponge as a wound dressing material. J Appl Polym
Sci. 2006;101(3):1602–1609.

[62] Hima Bindu, TVL, Vidyavathi M, Kavitha K, Sastry T P, Kumar RVS. Preparation and
evaluation of chitosan-gelatin composite films for wound healing activity. Trends
Biomater Artif Organs. 2010;24(3):122–130.

[63] El-Shanshory A, Chen W, Mei M. Preparation of antibacterial electrospun PVA/
regenerated silk fibroin nanofibrous composite containing ciprofloxacin hydrochloride
as a wound dressing. J Donghua Univ. 2014;31(5):566–571.

[64] Unnithan AR, Barakat NA, Pichiah PB, Gnanasekaran G, Nirmala R, Cha YS, Jung CH,
El-Newehy M, Kim HY. Wound-dressing materials with antibacterial activity from
electrospun polyurethane–dextran nanofiber mats containing ciprofloxacin HCl.
Carbohydr Polym. 2012;90(4):1786–1793.

[65] Jannesari M, Varshosaz J, Morshed M, Zamani M. Composite poly(vinyl alcohol)/
poly(vinyl acetate) electrospun nanofibrous mats as a novel wound dressing matrix for
controlled release of drugs. Int J Nanomed. 2011;6:993–1003.

[66] Tsou TL, Tang ST, Huang YC, Wu JR., Young JJ, Wang HJ. Poly(2-hydroxyethyl
methacrylate) wound dressing containing ciprofloxacin and its drug release studies. J
Mater Sci Mater Med. 2005;16(2):95–100.

[67] Manju S, Antony M, Sreenivasan K. Synthesis and evaluation of a hydrogel that binds
glucose and releases ciprofloxacin. J Mater Sci. 2010;45(15):4006–4012.

[68] Puoci F, Piangiolino C, Givigliano F, Parisi OI, Cassano R, Trombino S, Curcio M.
Ciprofloxacin–collagen conjugate in the wound healing treatment. J Funct Biomater.
2012;3(2):361–371.

[69] Roy DC, Tomblyn S, Burmeister DM, Wrice NL, Becerra SC, Burnett LR.,
Saul J. Ciprofloxacin-loaded keratin hydrogels prevent infection and support
healing in a porcine full-thickness excisional wound. Adv Wound Care.
2015;4(8):457–468.

[70] Okoye EI, Okolie TA. Development and in vitro characterization of ciprofloxacin
loaded polymeric films for wound dressing. Int J Health Allied Sci. 2015;4(4):
234–42.

[71] Sinha M, Banik RM, Haldar C, Maiti P. Development of ciprofloxacin hydrochloride
loaded poly(ethylene glycol)/chitosan scaffold as wound dressing. J Porous Mater.
2013;20:799–807.

[72] Loke WK, Lau SK, Yong LL, Khor E, Sum CK. Wound dressing with sustained antimicrobial capability. J Biomed Mater Res. 2000;53(1):8–17.

[73] Kota S, Jahangir M, Ahmed M, Kazmi I, Bhavani P, Muheem A, Saleem M. Development and evaluation of ofloxacin topical gel containing wound healing modifiers from natural sources. Sch Res Library. 2015;7(10):226–233.

[74] Boateng JS, Pawar HV, Tetteh J. Polyox and carrageenan based composite film dressing containing anti-microbial and anti-inflammatory drugs for effective wound healing. Int J Pharm. 2013;1–2(441):181–191.

[75] Pawar HV, Boateng JS, Ayensu I, Tetteh, J. Multifunctional medicated lyophilised wafer dressing for effective chronic wound healing. J Pharm Sci. 2014;103(6):1720–1733.

[76] Pawar HV, Tetteh J, Boateng JS. Preparation, optimisation and characterisation of novel wound healing film dressings loaded with streptomycin and diclofenac. Colloid Surf B: Biointerfaces. 2013;102:102–110.

[77] Kim JO, Choi JY, Park JK, Kim JH, Jin SG, Chang SW, Li DX. Development of clinda-mycin-loaded wound dressing with polyvinyl alcohol and sodium alginate. Biol Pharm Bull. 2008;December(31):2277–2282.

[78] Kim JO, Park JK, Kim JH, Jin SG, Yong CS, Li DX, Choi JY. Development of polyvinyl alcohol–sodium alginate gel-matrix-based wound dressing system containing nitro-furazone. Int J Pharm. 2008;1–2(359): 79–86.

[79] Hwang MR, Kim JO, Lee JH, Kim YI, Kim JH, Chang SW, Jin SG. Gentamicin-loaded wound dressing with polyvinyl alcohol/dextran hydrogel: gel characterization and in vivo healing evaluation. AAPS PharmSciTech. 2010;11(3):1092–103.

[80] Adhirajan N, Shanmugasundaram N, Shanmuganathan S, Babu M. Collagen-based wound dressing for doxycycline delivery: in-vivo evaluation in an infected excisional wound model in rats. J Pharm Pharmacol. 2009; 61(12):1617–23.

[81] Adhirajan N, Shanmugasundaram N, Shanmuganathan S, Babu M. Functionally modified gelatin microspheres impregnated collagen scaffold as novel wound dressing to attenuate the proteases and bacterial growth. Eur J Pharm Sci. 2009;36(2–3):235–245.

[82] Guan J, Dong LZ, Huang SJ, Jing ML. Characterization of wound dressing with microspheres containing levofloxacin. In: Proceedings of the International Conference on Information Technology and Scientific Management; 20 December 2010; Tianjin, China: 2010;1–2. p. 344–348.

[83] Bohl MKS, Leibovich SJ, Belem P, West JL, Poole WLA. Effects of nitric oxide releasing poly(vinyl alcohol) hydrogel dressings on dermal wound healing in diabetic mice. Wound Repair Regen. 2002;10(5):286–294.

[84] Halpenny GM, Steinhardt RC, Okialda KA, Mascharak, PK. Characterization of pHEMA-based hydrogels that exhibit light-induced bactericidal effect via release of NO. J Mater Sci Mater Med. 2009;20(11):2353–2360.

[85] Li Y, Lee PI. Controlled nitric oxide delivery platform based on S-nitrosothiol conjugated interpolymer complexes for diabetic wound healing. Mol Pharm. 2010;7(1):254–266.

[86] Lansdown AB. Silver. I: its antibacterial properties and mechanism of action. J Wound Care. 2002;11(4):125–130.

[87] Leaper D. Appropriate use of silver dressings in wounds: international consensus document. Int Wound J. 2012;9(5):461–464.

[88] Rai M, Yadav A, Gade A. Silver nanoparticles as a new generation of antimicrobials. Biotechnol Adv. 2009;27(1):76–83.

[89] Feng QL, Wu J, Chen GQ, Cui FZ, Kim TN, Kim JO. A mechanistic study of the antibacterial effect of silver ions on Escherichia coli and Staphylococcus aureus. J Biomed Mater. 2000;52(4):662–668.

[90] Matsumura Y, Yoshikata K, Kunisaki SI, Tsuchido T. Mode of bactericidal action of silver zeolite and its comparison with that of silver nitrate. Appl Environ Microbiol. 2003;69(7):4278–4281.

[91] Saengmee-anupharb S, Srikhirin T, Thaweboon B, Thaweboon S, Amornsakchai T, Dechkunakorn S, Suddhasthira T. Antimicrobial effects of silver zeolite, silver zirconium phosphate silicate and silver zirconium phosphate against oral microorganisms. Asian Pac J Trop Biomed. 2013;3(1):47–52.

[92] Rizzello L, Pompa PP. Nanosilver-based antibacterial drugs and devices: mechanisms, methodological drawbacks, and guidelines. Chem Soc Rev. 2014;43(5):1501–18.

[93] Ivask A, Kurvet I, Kasemets K, Blinova I, Aruoja V, Suppi S, Vija H. Size-dependent toxicity of silver nanoparticles to bacteria, yeast, algae, crustaceans and mammalian cells in vitro. PLoS One. 2014;9(7):e1–14.

[94] Sondi I, Salopek-Sondi B. Silver nanoparticles as antimicrobial agent: a case study on E. coli as a model for Gram-negative bacteria. J Colloid Interface Sci. 2004;275(1):177–182.

[95] Shrivastava S, Bera T, Roy A, Singh G, Ramachandrarao P, Dash D. Characterization of enhanced antibacterial effects of novel silver nanoparticles. Nanotechnology. 2010;18(22):1–9.

[96] Kazachenko A, Legler A, Per'yanova O, Vstavskaya Y. Synthesis and antimicrobial activity of silver complexes with histidine and tryptophan. Pharm Chem J. 2000;34(5):257–258.

[97] Baker C, Pradhan A, Pakstis L, Pochan DJ, Shah SI. Synthesis and antibacterial properties of silver nanoparticles. J Nanosci Nanotechnol. 2005;5(2):244–249.

[98] Morones JR, Elechiguerra JL, Camacho A, Holt K, Kouri JB, Ram JT, Yacaman MJ. The bactericidal effect of silver nanoparticles. Nanotechnology. 2005;16(10):2346–53.

[99] Panacek A, Kvítek L, Prucek R, Kolar M, Vecerova R., Pizúrova N, Sharma VK. Silver colloid nanoparticles: synthesis, characterization, and their antibacterial activity. J Phys Chem B. 2006;110(33):16248–16253.

[100] Kim JS, Kuk E, Yu KN, Kim JH, Park SJ, Lee HJ, Kim SH. Antimicrobial effects of silver nanoparticles. Nanomed Nanotechnol Biol Med. 2007;3(1):95–101.

[101] Gade AK, Bonde P, Ingle AP, Marcato PD, Durán N, Rai MK. Exploitation of *Aspergillus niger* for synthesis of silver nanoparticles. J Biobased Mater Bioenergy. 2008;2(3):1–5.

[102] Lindsay S. Silver white paper—everything you ever wanted to know about the use of silver in wound therapy [Internet]. 2011. http://www.systagenix.co.uk/cms/uploads/1458_Silver_WhitePaperA4_LP3_060.pdf. [Accessed 10 Mar 2016].

[103] Wound Source [Internet]. http://www.woundsource.com/product-category/dressings/antimicrobial-dressings. [Accessed 10 Mar 2016].

[104] Rujitanaroj PO, Pimpha N, Supaphol P. Wound-dressing materials with antibacterial activity from electrospun gelatin fiber mats containing silver nanoparticles. Polymer. 2008;49(21):4723–4732.

[105] Lin YH, Hsu WS, Chung WY, Ko TH, Lin JH. Evaluation of various silver-containing dressing on infected excision wound healing study. J Mater Sci Mater Med. 2014;25(5): 1375–1386.

[106] Anisha BS, Biswas R, Chennazhi KP, Jayakumar R. Chitosan–hyaluronic acid/nano silver composite sponges for drug resistant bacteria infected diabetic wounds. Int J Biol Macromol. 2013;62:310–320.

[107] Ong SY, Wu J, Moochhala SM, Tan MH, Lu J. Development of a chitosan-based wound dressing with improved hemostatic and antimicrobial properties. Biomaterials. 2008;29(32):4323–4332.

[108] Madhumathi K, Sudheesh Kumar PT, Abhilash S, Sreeja V, Tamura H, Manzoor K, Nair SV. Development of novel chitin/nanosilver composite scaffolds for wound dressing applications. J Mater Sci Mater Med. 2010;21(2):807–813.

[109] Boonkaew B, Suwanpreuksa P, Cuttle L, Barber PM, Supaphol P. Hydrogels containing silver nanoparticles for burn wounds show antimicrobial activity without cytotoxicity. J Appl Polym Sci. 2014;131(9):40215.

[110] Pant B, Pant HR, Pandeya DR, Panthi G, Nam KT, Hong ST, Kim CS. Characterization and antibacterial properties of Ag NPs loaded nylon-6 nanocomposite prepared by one-step electrospinning process. Colloid Surf A: Physicochem Eng Aspects. 2012;395:94–99.

[111] Archana D, Singh BK, Dutta J, Dutta PK. Chitosan-PVP-nano silver oxide wound dressing: in vitro and in vivo evaluation. Int J Biol Macromol. 2015;73(1):49–57.

[112] Lansdown BG, Jensen K, Jensen MQ. Contreet foam and contreet hydrocolloid: an insight into two new silver-containing dressings. J Wound Care. 2003;12(6):205–210.

[113] Singh R., Singh D. Radiation synthesis of PVP/alginate hydrogel containing nanosilver as wound dressing. J Mater Sci Mater Med. 2012;23(11):2649–2658.

[114] Jodar KSP, Balcão VM, Chaud MV, Tubino M, Yoshida VMH, Oliveira JM, Vila MMDC. Development and characterization of a hydrogel containing silver sulfadiazine for antimicrobial topical applications. J Pharm Sci. 2015;104(7):2241–2254.

[115] Boateng JS, Burgos AR, Okeke O, Pawar H. Composite alginate and gelatin based bio-polymeric wafers containing silver sulfadiazine for wound healing. Int J Biol Macromol. 2015;79:63–71.

[116] Mi FL, Wu YB, Shyu SS, Schoung JY, Huang YB, Tsai YH, Hao JY. Control of wound infections using a bilayer chitosan wound dressing with sustainable antibiotic delivery. J Biomed Mater Res. 2002;59(3):438–449.

[117] Shanmugasundaram N, Sundaraseelan J, Uma S, Selvaraj D, Babu M. Design and delivery of silver sulfadiazine from alginate microspheres-impregnated collagen scaffold. J Biomed Mater Res B: Appl Biomater. 2006;77(2):378–388.

[118] Ammons M, Ward L, James G. Anti-biofilm efficacy of a lactoferrin/xylitol wound hydrogel used in combination with silver wound dressings. Int Wound J. 2011;8(3):268–273.

[119] Rayman G, Rayman A, Baker NR, Jurgeviciene N, Dargis V, Sulcaite R., Pantelejeva O. Sustained silver-releasing dressing in the treatment of diabetic foot ulcers. Br J Nurs (Mark Allen Publishing). 2005;14(2):109–114.

[120] Jude EB, Apelqvist J, Spraul M, Martini J, Jones G, Harding K, Benbow S. Prospective randomized controlled study of Hydrofiber® dressing containing ionic silver or calcium alginate dressings in non-ischaemic diabetic foot ulcers. Diabet Med. 2007;24(3):280–288.

[121] Gago M, Garcia F, Gaztelu V, Verdu J, Lopez P, Nolasco A. A comparison of three silver-containing dressings in the treatment of infected, chronic wounds. Wound Res. 2008;20(10):273–278.

[122] Hiro ME, Pierpont YN, Ko F, Wright TE, Robson MC, Payne WG. Comparative evaluation of silver-containing antimicrobial dressings on in vitro and in vivo processes of wound healing. Eplasty. 2012;12:48.

[123] Thomas S, McCubbin P. A comparison of the antimicrobial effects of four silver-containing dressings on three organisms. J Wound Care. 2003;12(3):101–107.

[124] Thomas S, McCubbin P. An in vitro analysis of the antimicrobial properties of 10 silver-containing dressings. J Wound Care. 2003;12(8):305–308.

[125] Gaisford S, Beezer AE, Bishop AH, Walker M, Parsons D. An in vitro method for the quantitative determination of the antimicrobial efficacy of silver-containing wound dressings. Int J Pharm. 2009;1–2(366):111–116.

[126] Sunil KP, Raja BP, Jagadish RG, Uttam A. Povidone iodine—revisited. Indian J Dent Adv. 2011;3(3):617–620.

[127] Sibbald R, Leaper D, Queen D. Iodine made easy. Wounds Int. 2011;2(2):1–6.

[128] Gilliver S. PHMB: a well-tolerated antiseptic with no reported toxic effects. J Wound Care. 2009; Active Health Care Suppl:9–14.

[129] Eberlein T, Haemmerle G, Signer M, Gruber MU, Traber J, Mittlboeck M, Abel M. Comparison of PHMB-containing dressing and silver dressings in patients with critically colonised or locally infected wounds. J Wound Care. 2012;21(1):13–19.

[130] Loke WK, Lau SK, Yong LL, Khor E, Sum CK. Wound dressing with sustained anti-microbial capability. J Biomed Mater Res. 2000;53(1):8–17.

[131] Forrest RD. Early history of wound treatment. J R Soc Med. 1982;75(3):198–205.

[132] Hammouri S. The role of honey in the management of diabetic foot ulcers. JRMS. 2004;11(2):20–22.

[133] Schumacher HH. Use of medical honey in patients with chronic venous leg ulcers after split-skin grafting. J Wound Care. 2004;13(10):451–452.

[134] Molan P, Betts J. Using honey to heal diabetic foot ulcers. Adv Skin Wound Care. 2008;21(7):313–316.

[135] Mclennan ASV, Henshaw FR, Twigg SM. What's the buzz: bee products and their potential value in diabetic wound healing. J Diabet Foot Complic. 2014;6(2):24–39.

[136] Boateng JS, Diunase K. Comparing the antibacterial and functional properties of Cameroonian and Manuka honeys for potential wound healing—have we come full cycle in dealing with antibiotic resistance? Molecules. 2015;20(9):16068–16084.

[137] Subrahmanyam M. A prospective randomised clinical and histological study of superficial burn wound healing with honey and silver sulfadiazine. Burns J Int Soc Burn Inj. 1998;24(2):157–161.

[138] Cooper RA, Halas E, Molan, PC. The efficacy of honey in inhibiting strains of Pseudomonas aeruginosa from infected burns. J Burn Care Rehabil. 2002;23(6):366–370.

[139] Aggad H, Guemour D. Honey antibacterial activity. Med Aromat Plants. 2014;2(3):1–2.

[140] Song JJ, Salcido R. Use of honey in wound care: an update. Adv Skin Wound Care. 2011;24(1):40–4; quiz 45–6.

[141] Karayil S, Deshpande SD, Koppikar GV. Effect of honey on multidrug resistant organisms and its synergistic action with three common antibiotics. J Postgrad Med. 1998;44(4):93–96.

[142] Van den Berg AJ, Van den Worm E, Van Ufford HC, Halkes SB, Hoekstra MJ, Beukelman CJ. An in vitro examination of the antioxidant and anti–inflammatory properties of buckwheat honey. J Wound Care. 2008;17(4):172–174, 176–178.

[143] Gethin G, Cowman S. Bacteriological changes in sloughy venous leg ulcers treated with Manuka honey or hydrogel: an RCT. J Wound Care. 2008;17(6):241–244, 246–247.

[144] Molan P, Betts J. Clinical usage of honey as a wound dressing: an update. J Wound Care. 2004; 13(9):353–356.

[145] Alam F, Islam M, Gan S, Khalil M. Honey: a potential therapeutic agent for managing diabetic wounds. Evidence Based Complement Altern Med. 2014; 2014:Article ID 169130

[146] Rossiter K, Cooper AJ, Voegeli D, Lwaleed BA. Honey promotes angiogeneic activity in the rat aortic ring assay. J Wound Care. 2010;19(10):440, 442–446.

[147] Sasikala L, Durai B, Rathinamoorthy R. Manuka honey loaded chitosan hydrogel films for wound dressing applications. Int J PharmTech Res. 2013;5(4):1774–1785.

[148] Halstead F, Webber M, Rauf M, Burt R, Dryden M, Oppenheim B. In vitro activity of an engineered honey, medical-grade honeys, and antimicrobial wound dressings against biofilm-producing clinical bacterial isolates. J Wound Care. 2016;25(2):93–102.

[149] Molan PC. The evidence and the rationale for the use of honey as a wound dressing. Wound Practice Res. 2011;19(4):204–220.

[150] Mogosanu GD, Grumezescu AM. Natural and synthetic polymers for wounds and burns dressing. Int J Pharm. 2014;463(2):127–136.

[151] Biazar E, Roveimiab Z, Shahhosseini G, Khataminezhad M, Zafari M, Majdi A. Biocompatibility evaluation of a new hydrogel dressing based on polyvinylpyrroli-done/polyethylene glycol. J Biomed Biotechnol. 2012; 2012:Article ID 343989.

[152] Tarun K, Gobi N. Calcium alginate/PVA blended nano fibre matrix for wound dressing. Indian J Fibre Textile Res. 2012;37(2):127–132.

[153] Dai T, Tanaka M, Huang YY, Hamblin MR. Chitosan preparations for wounds and burns: antimicrobial and wound-healing effects. Exp Rev Anti-infect Ther. 2011;9(7): 857–879.

[154] Tan Y, Han F, Ma S, Yu W. Carboxymethyl chitosan prevents formation of broad-spectrum biofilm. Carbohydr Polym. 2011;84(4):1365–1370.

Topical Wound Oxygen Versus Conventional Compression Dressings in the Management of Refractory Venous Ulcers

Sherif Sultan, Wael Tawfick, Edel P Kavanagh and Niamh Hynes

Abstract

Topical wound oxygen (TWO$_2$) proposes an innovative therapy option in the management of refractory non-healing venous ulcers (RVU) that aims to accelerate wound healing. TWO$_2$ accelerates epithelialisation. This leads to the development of a higher tensile strength collagen, which lessens scarring and the risk of recurrence. Sixty-seven limbs with 67 ulcers were managed using TWO$_2$ therapy, and 65 limbs with 65 ulcers were managed using conventional compression dressings (CCD). The proportion of ulcers completely healed by 12 weeks was 76% in patients managed with TWO$_2$, compared to 46% in patients managed with CCD ($p < 0.0001$). The mean reduction in ulcer surface area at 12 weeks was 96% in the TWO$_2$ therapy group, compared to 61% in patients managed with CCD. The median time to full ulcer healing was 57 days in the TWO$_2$ group, in contrast to 107 days in patients managed with CCD ($p < 0.0001$). TWO$_2$ patients had a significantly improved Quality-Adjusted Time Spent Without Symptoms of disease and Toxicity of treatment (Q-TWiST) compared to CCD patients, denoting an improved outcome ($p < 0.0001$). TWO$_2$ reduces the time needed for RVU healing and is successful in pain alleviation and MRSA elimination. TWO$_2$ therapy radically degrades recurrence rates. Utilising diffused oxygen raises the capillary partial pressure of oxygen (Po$_2$) levels at the wound site, stimulating epithelialisation, and granulation of new healthy tissue. Taking the social and individual aspects of chronic venous ulceration into account, the use of TWO$_2$ can provide an overwhelmingly improved quality of life for long-time sufferers of this debilitating disease.

Keywords: topical wound oxygen, conventional compression dressings, refractory venous ulcers, MRSA, epithelialisation

1. Introduction

Chronic venous ulceration is a common disease. Its prevalence is 1% of the total population, with 20% of venous ulcers presented in octogenarians [1–5]. Refractory venous leg ulceration is a common basis of morbidity [6, 7] and leads to a reduced quality of life [8], especially in the elderly population [4, 5]. It causes a considerable amount of work incapacity, social exclusion and lack of self-esteem [4]. There is a probable underestimation of the true extent of venous leg ulceration in the general population due to its underreporting [7]. Venous ulcers are characterised by a recurring pattern of healing and subsequent 70% recurrence rate at one year [9–14]. Venous ulceration places a huge monetary burden on the healthcare system [15]. The cost of managing venous ulcers accrues to £400 million sterling per year in the UK [16].

Ambulatory venous hypertension is one of the leading causes of chronic reperfusion injury. This in turn provokes venous ulceration with its habitual history of chronicity and recurrence [1]. Over the past 40 years, compression bandaging has been the gold standard form of therapy for treatment of venous ulceration. We have learned that compression will both improve perfusion and enhance healing [2, 17, 18]. Nevertheless, active healthy tissue granulation can take upwards to 3 weeks to cultivate [19]. Therefore, the following question is posed: How can we speed up epithelial coverage in a granulating wound?

1.1. Topical wound oxygen

Topical wound oxygen (TWO_2) proposes an innovative therapy option in the management of refractory non-healing venous ulcers (RVU) that aims to accelerate wound healing. The application of positive pressure oxygen to manage open wounds has been studied extensively and has demonstrated promising clinical results [20–28]. The systemic complications associated with the use of a full-body hyperbaric chamber have been overcome by the application of topical wound pure oxygen at an appropriate cycled pressure to only the specific wound site. This maximizes the beneficial wound healing effects and minimizes the negative systemic side effects [29].

Delivered through a targeted delivery system, a Hyper-Box, TWO_2 accelerates epithelialisation and eliminates MRSA within 72 h. This leads to the development of a higher tensile strength collagen, which lessens scarring and the risk of recurrence [29–32]. Hyperbaric oxygen promotes angiogenesis and increases the expression of angiogenesis-related growth factors [33, 34]. It promotes leukocyte function with enhanced bactericidal activity [35–40]. The intermittent cycled pressure, under which TWO_2 is delivered, stimulates circulation, reduces oedema and provides a sealed humidified environment essential for healing [41].

2. Materials and methods

The aim of this study is to scrutinise the use of TWO_2 when compared to conventional compression dressings (CCD) for managing RVU, with reference to technical and clinical outcomes from our tertiary referral leg ulcer clinic.

A 5-year study of TWO_2 versus CCD for chronic RVU was carried out at our tertiary referral leg ulcer clinic [42, 43]. This parallel group observational comparative study aimed at examining the safety and efficacy of TWO_2 in managing RVU in the short-term (12 weeks), and the mid-term (36 months).

Ethical approval was obtained from the local research ethics committee. Patients with chronic RVU, with an ulcer of more than two years duration, were recruited from the vascular unit. All patients must show no sign of improvement of the ulcer over the past 12 months, despite acceptable compliance with a suitable treatment, provided by community-based leg ulcer clinics. All patients were managed on an intention to treat basis and were given the choice of receiving CCD or TWO_2 therapy. Patients were informed on both CCD and TWO_2 therapies, and the treatment choice was discussed with their primary care physician and local tissue viability nurse. Treatment allocation was based on each patient's choice. All patients signed an informed consent form prior to beginning therapy.

2.1. Technical and clinical endpoints

The end points of this study were the proportion of ulcers healed at 12 weeks and recurrence rates at 36 months. Secondary end-points were time taken for full healing, percentage of reduction in the ulcer size at 12 weeks, methicillin-resistant *Staphylococcus aureus* (MRSA) elimination, pain reduction, recurrence rates and Quality-Adjusted Time Spent Without Symptoms of disease and Toxicity of treatment (Q-TWiST).

2.2. Inclusion criteria

Informed written consent was required from patient's aged ≥ 18 years.

The patients must be treated at a dedicated veins unit with $C_{6,s}$ in the Clinical, Etiological, Anatomical, and Pathophysiological (CEAP) classification [44, 45]. The venous ulcer must have been present for more than 2 years, with no improvement over the past 12 months despite adequate treatment at the veins unit. The patients must also have a normal ankle-brachial index (ABI) with a normal digital pressure.

2.3. Exclusion criteria

Patients who are bedridden, have ischemic or malignant ulcers, or osteomyelitis in the treated limb were primarily excluded. Patients with ischemic diabetic ulcers were excluded; however, it should be noted that diabetes in isolation was not considered an exclusion criterion. A prior study has shown that the AOTI Hyper-Box (AOTI Ltd., Galway, Ireland) is not sufficient in ischemic diabetic ulcers. It may induce iatrogenic deterioration of the affected diabetic limb due to the cyclic pressure of the Hyper-Box [46, 47].

2.4. Statistical analysis

Data was collected and analysed using SPSS 18 software (SPSS Inc., Chicago, IL). An independent sample *t*-test was used for continuous variables, while the Mann-Whitney *U* test was used to compare unpaired, non-parametric data. Categorical proportions were examined using the chi-squared test. Time for healing was examined using Kaplan-Meier with log-rank comparison.

2.5. Quality-Adjusted Time Spent Without Symptoms of disease and Toxicity of treatment (Q-TWiST)

The survival time for patients was divided into three separate phases: the time spent with toxicity of the disease or severe adverse events prior to disease progression known as Toxicity (TOX); the time spent without any symptoms of disease progression or toxicity of treatment known as TWiST; and finally the time spent with progression of the disease known as Progression (PROG). Ulcer recurrence in fully healed ulcers or an increase of size in ulcers that had not fully healed was defined as progression of disease. The Kaplan Meier method was used to determine the mean time spent in each of the TOX, TWiST and PROG periods for each treatment group. Mean Q-TWiST was calculated for each treatment.

2.6. Techniques

The anatomical location and duration of the ulcer, signs of infection, slough, and cellulitis, as well as any other vascular risk factors were observed in each patient. The leg ulcers were swabbed for culture as well as for level of sensitivity. Prior to therapy, a numerical rating scale in regards to pain was used. This was then repeated every three days. To record surface area, maximum length and maximum width of the ulcer, the ulcers were cleaned, debrided and digitally photographed using a Visitrak system (Smith & Nephew Ltd., Hull, United Kingdom). For all patients, ABI with big toe digital pressure measurement and punch biopsy were performed, as well as venous duplex ultrasound scan for full CEAP assessment [44, 45]. Venous Clinical Severity Score was recorded for each patient [48, 49].

2.6.1. TWO$_2$ therapy

Sixty-seven ulcers were treated with TWO$_2$ therapy. The limb was placed in the Hyper-Box for twice daily for a duration of 180 min and under pressure of 50 mbar. Oxygen supplied at 10 L/min with continuous humidification. Between each session, wounds were washed and left exposed with no dressings or compression. Wounds were cleaned, debrided and re-measured twice weekly [42, 46, 47].

2.6.2. Compression therapy

Sixty-five ulcers were treated with compression therapy. Full compression was performed using Profore ◊ multilayer compression bandage system with underlying non-adherent Profore◊ wound contact layer dressings (Profore◊, Smith & Nephew plc., London, United Kingdom). Dressings were applied by a wound care specialist nurse and changed as required, one to three times per week, depending on the amount of exudates.

Treatment was continued for 12 weeks or until complete healing of the ulcer or whichever can be first. As soon as the ulcer is healed, the leg was fitted with a class 3, closed toe, below knee elastic stocking during the day [50]. Patients were advised to revitalise the skin by soaking the leg with tap water, baby oil or olive oil to prevent itching and dry cracked skin. Patients were followed up at 3 monthly intervals following the end of the therapy. Patients without full healing of their ulcer by 12 weeks were considered failures of treatment. They were managed with CCD and continued to be seen on a weekly basis.

3. Results

Over the course of 5 years at our tertiary referral leg ulcer clinic, 1460 patients were diagnosed of chronic venous ulcers (**Figure 1**). Following application of the inclusion and exclusion criteria, 431 patients were enrolled in this study, but only 148 patients were eligible. One hundred and thirty-two patients consented to join the study, of which 67 limbs with 67 ulcers were treated using TWO_2 therapy, and 65 limbs with 65 ulcers were treated with CCD. Fifty-seven percent of the patients treated with TWO_2 were males ($n = 38$), and 54% of the patients treated with CCD were males ($n = 35$). Risk factors, such as age, gender, the presence of diabetes mellitus, smoking, hypertension and MRSA, were similar, with no statistical significance between each group. There was no significant difference between both the groups in the anatomical distribution of ulcers, size of the ulcers or the duration of the ulcer.

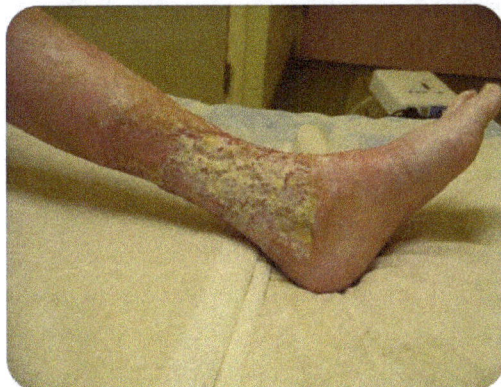

Figure 1. Patient with a chronic venous leg ulcer prior to therapy.

Twenty-four patients (36%) in the TWO_2 group and 19 patients (28%) in the CCD group were MRSA positive. Following treatment, MRSA was eliminated in 11 patients (46%), while zero cases of MRSA were eliminated in the CCD group.

The proportion of ulcers completely healed by 12 weeks was 76% ($n = 51/67$) in patients managed with TWO_2 compared to 46% ($n = 30/65$) in patients managed with CCD ($P < 0.0001$). The mean reduction in ulcer surface area at 12 weeks was 96% in the TWO_2 therapy group (**Figure 2**) compared to 61% in patients managed with CCD. The median time to full ulcer healing was 57 days in the TWO_2 group in contrast to 107 days in patients managed with CCD ($P < 0.0001$). Healing time for patients managed with TWO_2 was not affected by the extent of time of the ulcer and its size. In fact, ulcers managed with TWO_2 had a considerably shorter healing time, when compared to CCD ulcers, regardless of duration ($P < 0.0001$) or ulcer size ($P < 0.0001$). TWO_2 patients had a significantly improved Q-TWiST compared to CCD patients, denoting an improved outcome ($p < 0.0001$).

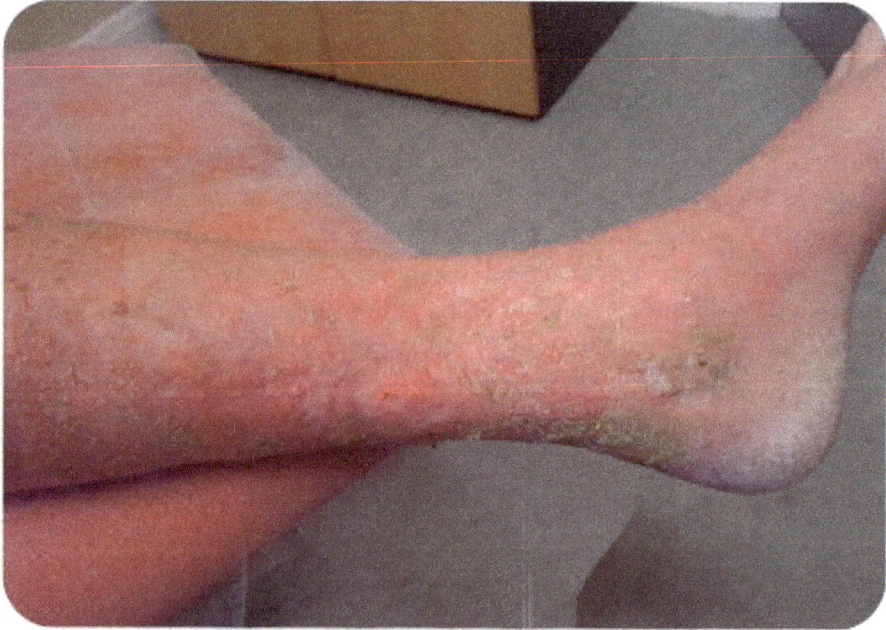

Figure 2. Significant healing and decrease in ulcer surface area post 9 weeks of TWO_2 therapy.

In all, three of the patients managed with TWO_2 were referred to our facility for primary amputation following the failure of other treatment modalities, including skin grafting. These three ulcers fully healed with no need for amputation in any case. After 36 months of follow-up, 14 of the 30 healed CCD ulcers showed recurrence compared to three of the 51 TWO_2-healed ulcers. Two CCD-managed ulcers that had not completely healed showed signs of deterioration and increase in surface area ($P < 0.0001$). All the cases that healed with TWO_2 showed reversed gradient healing phenomena where the ulcer healed from the centre to the periphery. This might be the reason for the absence of scarring and recurrence.

4. Discussion

The socio-economic consequences of management of RVU, merged with high recurrence rates, have encouraged the development of a disruptive technology innovative therapy, such as TWO_2 therapy. Compression therapy within the setup of a leg ulcer clinic is widely recognised as the main modality for managing venous leg ulcers [17, 18, 51, 52]. A previous study mentioned that contemporary dressing materials do not stimulate healing, and expenses are not clinically justified as they have no proven efficacy [19]. After 30 years of research, there is no data to defend using anything other than a simple, inexpensive, low-adherence dressing under multilayer compression [19].

The first publication on the use of TWO_2 was by Fischer in 1969 [20]. Fischer noted that lesions became aseptic and enhanced granulation was witnessed two days after TWO_2. In a prospective randomised study by Heng et al. red granulation tissue was present one week after TWO_2 [27]. Heng noted an absence of clinical scarring and most ulcers healed within 2–16 weeks. Gordillo et al. conducted a study on full-body hyperbaric oxygen (HBO) therapy versus TWO_2. Topical oxygen treatment showed a significant reduction in wound size and was associated with higher vascular endothelial growth factor (VEGF)165 expression in healing wounds [53].

Blackman et al. explored the efficacy of topical oxygen therapy as an adjunctive modality in repairing diabetic ulcers that failed to heal by best practice standard wound care. The healing rate after 12 weeks of topical wound oxygen therapy was 82.4%, and the mean time to complete healing was reduced. Patients also showed very low recurrence rates after 18 months [54].

Results from the Venous ULcer Cost-effectiveness of Antimicrobial dressings (VULCAN) trial showed that it took 101 days to heal 3-cm ulcers, while there was a 1-year recurrence rate of 14% in 86% of small ulcers [55], using silver dressings. These types of dressings are now rarely seen in a standard tertiary vein unit. In our unit, we have abandoned the use of silver dressing in any form as it showed a higher incidence of contacting eczema and an increase in the chronicity of the wounds.

Oxygen plays a major role in the promotion of vascular endothelial cell proliferation, collagen synthesis [56, 57] and infection control [58] by providing a direct microbial growth inhibitory effect [59] and also by activating neutrophils [60]. TWO_2 therapy evades the consequences of a full-body hyperbaric chamber [61], such as grand mal seizures and pulmonary oxygen toxicity [61, 62]. There is also the high associated cost of acquiring and maintaining a chamber to consider.

Utilising diffused oxygen raises the capillary partial pressure of oxygen (Po_2) levels at the wound site, stimulating epithelialisation and granulation of new healthy tissue [29, 32]. Oxygen generates reactive oxygen species at the wound site, acting as signalling substances, which increase the production of VEGF [63, 64]. Repeated treatment therefore accelerates wound closure.

TWO_2 therapy enhances both polymorph nuclear function and bacterial clearance and is fatal to anaerobic bacteria [35–37]. It reduces neutrophil adherence based on hindering the β-2 integrin function [38]. Eleven patients (46%) with MRSA were negative at the end of treatment with TWO_2. This informs us of its effectiveness against MRSA infection in comparison to CCD. TWO_2 therapy supports and strengthens antibiotic distribution for aminoglycosides, cephalosporins, quinilones and amphotericin [39, 40].

While TWO_2 therapy has been available for many years, there is paucity in clinical evidence for its safety and efficacy. Experience from our clinic shows that TWO_2 therapy is effective and valuable in managing RVU. Our course of therapy accomplished enhanced wound healing time, without complications, in a relatively large number of patients. TWO_2 therapy drastically reduced the time required for RVU healing and recurrence rates when compared to CCD. Quality of time spent without symptoms or toxicity of the disease was significantly improved in TWO_2 managed patients compared to CCD patients ($p < 0.0001$).

5. Conclusion

TWO_2 therapy is practical, effective and valuable in managing RVU without the risks associated with full-body hyperbaric chambers. TWO_2 therapy requires no further specialist skills by the primary care physician or local tissue viability nurse. It is therefore readily available for application under most circumstances, even for domiciliary use. The treatment has an extremely low risk of systemic complications when compared to HBO, and single-use devices greatly reduce the possibility of secondary infections.

TWO_2 slashes the time needed for RVU healing and is successful in pain alleviation, MRSA elimination and management. Utilising diffused oxygen raises the capillary partial Po_2 levels at the wound site, stimulating epithelialisation and granulation of new healthy tissue. TWO_2 therapy radically degrades recurrence rates. Taking the social and individual aspects of chronic venous ulceration into account, the use of TWO_2 can provide an overwhelmingly improved quality of life for long-time sufferers of this debilitating disease.

Author details

Sherif Sultan[1,2*], Wael Tawfick[1], Edel P Kavanagh[2] and Niamh Hynes[2]

*Address all correspondence to: sherif.sultan@hse.ie

1 Department of Vascular and Endovascular Surgery, Western Vascular Institute, University College Hospital Galway, Galway, Ireland

2 Department of Vascular and Endovascular Surgery, Galway Clinic, Doughiska, Galway, Ireland

References

[1] Trent JT, Falabella A, Eaglstein WH, Kirsner RS. Venous ulcers: pathophysiology and treatment options. Ostomy/Wound Management. 2005 May;51(5):38–54.

[2] O'Meara S, Cullum NA, Nelson EA. Compression for venous leg ulcers. Cochrane Database Systematic Review. 2009 Jan 21;1:CD000265.

[3] Moffatt CJ, Franks PJ, Doherty DC, Martin R, Blewett R, Ross F. Prevalence of leg ulceration in a London population. QJM. 2004 Jul 1;97(7):431–7.

[4] Graham ID, Harrison MB, Nelson EA, Lorimer K, Fisher A. Prevalence of lower-limb ulceration: a systematic review of prevalence studies. Advances in Skin & Wound Care. 2003 Nov 1;16(6):305–16.

[5] Margolisa DJ, Bilkerb W, Santannab J. Venous leg ulcer: incidence and prevalence in the elderly. Journal of the American Academy of Dermatology. 2002 Mar 31;46(3):381–6.

[6] Anand SC, Dean C, Nettleton R, Praburaj DV. Health-related quality of life tools for venous-ulcerated patients. British Journal of Nursing. 2003 Jan 9;12(1):48–59.

[7] Phillips TJ. Chronic cutaneous ulcers: etiology and epidemiology. Journal of Investigative Dermatology. 1994 Jun 1;102(6):38S–41S.

[8] Persoon A, Heinen MM, Van Der Vleuten CJ, De Rooij MJ, Van De Kerkhof P, Van Achterberg T. Leg ulcers: a review of their impact on daily life. Journal of Clinical Nursing. 2004 Mar 1;13(3):341–54.

[9] Armstrong SA. Compression hosiery. Professional Nurse (London, England). 1997 Apr; 12(7 Suppl):S10–1.

[10] Moffatt CJ, Dorman MC. Recurrence of leg ulcers within a community ulcer service. Journal of Wound Care. 1995 Feb;4(2):57–61.

[11] Monk BE, Sarkany I. Outcome of treatment of venous stasis ulcers. Clinical and Experimental Dermatology. 1982 Jul 1;7(4):397–400.

[12] Lees TA, Lambert D. Prevalence of lower limb ulceration in an urban health district. British Journal of Surgery. 1992 Oct 1;79(10):1032–4.

[13] Callam MJ, Ruckley CV, Harper DR, Dale JJ. Chronic ulceration of the leg: extent of the problem and provision of care. British Medical Journal (Clinical Research ed). 1985 Jun 22;290(6485):1855–6.

[14] Nelzen O, Bergqvist D, Lindhagen A. Venous and non-venous leg ulcers: Clinical history and appearance in a population study. British Journal of Surgery. 1994 Feb 1;81(2):182–7.

[15] Ragnarson Tennvall G, Hjelmgren J. Original research articles—clinical science: annual costs of treatment for venous leg ulcers in Sweden and the United Kingdom. Wound Repair and Regeneration. 2005 Jan 1;13(1):13–8.

[16] Ruckley CV. Socioeconomic impact of chronic venous insufficiency and leg ulcers. Angiology. 1997 Jan 1;48(1):67–9.

[17] Palfreyman SJ, Lochiel R, Michaels JA. A systematic review of compression therapy for venous leg ulcers. Vascular Medicine. 1998 Nov 1;3(4):301–13.

[18] Cullum N, Nelson EA, Fletcher AW, Sheldon TA. Compression for venous leg ulcers. Cochrane Database Syst Rev. 2001;(2):CD000265.

[19] Sultan MJ, McCollum C. Don't waste money when dressing leg ulcers. British Journal of Surgery. 2009 Oct 1;96(10):1099–100.

[20] Fischer B. Topical hyperbaric oxygen treatment of pressure sores and skin ulcers. The Lancet. 1969 Aug 23;294(7617):405–9.

[21] Olejniczak S. Employment of low hyperbaric therapy in management of leg ulcers. Michigan Medicine. 1966 Dec;65(12):1067–8.

[22] Gruber RP, Heitkamp DH, Billy LJ, Amato JJ. Skin permeability to oxygen and hyperbaric oxygen. Archives of Surgery. 1970 Jul 1;101(1):69–70.

[23] Fischer BH. Treatment of ulcers on the legs with hyperbaric oxygen. The Journal of Dermatologic Surgery and Oncology. 1975 Oct 1;1(3):55–8.

[24] Kalliainen LK, Gordillo GM, Schlanger R, Sen CK. Topical oxygen as an adjunct to wound healing: a clinical case series. Pathophysiology. 2003 Jan 31;9(2):81–7.

[25] Edsberg LE, Brogan MS, Jaynes CD, Fries K. Topical hyperbaric oxygen and electrical stimulation: exploring potential synergy. Ostomy/Wound Management. 2002 Nov; 48(11):42–50.

[26] Edsberg LE, Brogan MS, Jaynes CD, Fries K. Reducing epibole using topical hyperbaric oxygen and electrical stimulation. Ostomy/Wound Management. 2002 Apr;48(4):26.

[27] Heng MC, Harker J, Csathy G, Marshall C, Brazier J, Sumampong S, Paterno GE. Angiogenesis in necrotic ulcers treated with hyperbaric oxygen. Ostomy/Wound Management. 2000 Sep;46(9):18–28.

[28] Leslie CA, Sapico FL, Ginunas VJ, Adkins RH. Randomized controlled trial of topical hyperbaric oxygen for treatment of diabetic foot ulcers. Diabetes Care. 1988 Feb 1;11(2): 111–5.

[29] Heng MC. Topical hyperbaric therapy for problem skin wounds. The Journal of Dermatologic Surgery and Oncology. 1993 Aug 1;19(8):784–93.

[30] Prost-Squarcioni C, Fraitag S, Heller M, Boehm N. Functional histology of dermis. Annales de Dermatologie et de Venereologie 2008 Jan; 135(1 Pt 2):1S5–20.

[31] Wirthner R, Balamurugan K, Stiehl DP, Barth S, Spielmann P, Oehme F, Flamme I, Katschinski DM, Wenger RH, Camenisch G. Determination and modulation of prolyl-4-hydroxylase domain oxygen sensor activity. Methods in Enzymology. 2007 Dec 31;435:43–60.

[32] Upson AV. Topical hyperbaric oxygenation in the treatment of recalcitrant open wounds. A clinical report. Physical Therapy. 1986 Sep 1;66(9):1408–12.

[33] Knighton DR, Silver IA, Hunt TK. Regulation of wound-healing angiogenesis-effect of oxygen gradients and inspired oxygen concentration. Surgery. 1981 Aug;90(2):262–70.

[34] Scott G. Topical oxygen alters angiogenesis-related growth factor expression in chronic diabetic foot ulcers. Irish Journal of Medical Science. 2007;176:S2.

[35] Kaufman T, Alexander JW, Nathan P, Brackett KA, MacMillan BG. The microclimate chamber: the effect of continuous topical administration of 96% oxygen and 75% relative humidity on the healing rate of experimental deep burns. Journal of Trauma and Acute Care Surgery. 1983 Sep 1;23(9):806–15.

[36] Park MK, Myers RA, Marzella L. Oxygen tensions and infections: modulation of microbial growth, activity of antimicrobial agents, and immunologic responses. Clinical Infectious Diseases. 1992 Mar 1;14(3):720–40.

[37] Mandell GL. Bactericidal activity of aerobic and anaerobic polymorphonuclear neutrophils. Infection and Immunity. 1974 Feb 1;9(2):337–41.

[38] Thom SR. Effects of hyperoxia on neutrophil adhesion. Undersea & Hyperbaric Medicine. 2004 Apr 1;31(1):123.

[39] Mirhij NJ, Roberts RJ, Myers MG. Effects of hypoxemia upon aminoglycoside serum pharmacokinetics in animals. Antimicrobial Agents and Chemotherapy. 1978 Sep 1;14(3):344–7.

[40] Keck PE, Gottlieb SF, Conley J. Interaction of increased pressures of oxygen and sulfonamides on the in vitro and in vivo growth of pathogenic bacteria. Undersea Biomedical Research. 1980 Jun;7(2):95–106.

[41] Olejniczak S, Zielinski A. Topical oxygen promotes healing of leg ulcers. Medical Times. 1976 Dec;104(12):114–21.

[42] Tawfick W, Sultan S. Does topical wound oxygen (TWO 2) offer an improved outcome over conventional compression dressings (CCD) in the management of refractory venous ulcers (RVU)? A parallel observational comparative study. European Journal of Vascular and Endovascular Surgery. 2009 Jul 31;38(1):125–32.

[43] Tawfick WA, Sultan S. Technical and clinical outcome of topical wound oxygen in comparison to conventional compression dressings in the management of refractory nonhealing venous ulcers. Vascular and Endovascular Surgery. 2012 Dec 5:1538574412467684.

[44] Eklöf B, Rutherford RB, Bergan JJ, Carpentier PH, Gloviczki P, Kistner RL, Meissner MH, Moneta GL, Myers K, Padberg FT, Perrin M. American Venous Forum International Ad Hoc Committee for Revision of the CEAP Classification. Revision of the CEAP classification for chronic venous disorders: consensus statement. Journal of Vascular Surgery. 2004 Dec;40(6):1248–52.

[45] Meissner MH, Gloviczki P, Bergan J, Kistner RL, Morrison N, Pannier F, Pappas PJ, Rabe E, Raju S, Villavicencio JL. Primary chronic venous disorders. Journal of Vascular Surgery. 2007 Dec 31;46(6):S54–67.

[46] Tawfick W, Sultan S. Early results of topical wound oxygen (TWO2) therapy in the management of refractory nonhealing venous ulcers: superior role over conventional compression dressings. Vascular. 2008;16(Suppl 2):S156e7.

[47] Tawfick W, Sultan S. Topical wound oxygen versus conventional compression dressings in the management of refractory venous ulcers: a parallel observational pivotal study. Irish Journal of Medical Science. 2007;176(1):S2.

[48] Meissner MH, Moneta G, Burnand K, Gloviczki P, Lohr JM, Lurie F, Mattos MA, McLafferty RB, Mozes G, Rutherford RB, Padberg F. The hemodynamics and diagnosis of venous disease. Journal of Vascular Surgery. 2007 Dec 31;46(6):S4–24.

[49] Ricci MA, Emmerich J, Callas PW, Rosendaal FR, Stanley AC, Naud S, Vossen C, Bovill EG. Evaluating chronic venous disease with a new venous severity scoring system. Journal of Vascular Surgery. 2003 Nov 30;38(5):909–15.

[50] Nelson EA, Harper DR, Prescott RJ, Gibson B, Brown D, Ruckley CV. Prevention of recurrence of venous ulceration: randomized controlled trial of class 2 and class 3 elastic compression. Journal of Vascular Surgery. 2006 Oct 31;44(4):803–8.

[51] Ghauri AS, Taylor MC, Deacon JE, Whyman MR, Earnshaw JJ, Heather BP, Poskitt KR. Influence of a specialized leg ulcer service on management and outcome. British Journal of Surgery. 2000 Aug 1;87(8):1048–56.

[52] Fletcher A, Cullum N, Sheldon TA. A systematic review of compression treatment for venous leg ulcers. British Medical Journal. 1997 Sep 6;315(7108):576–80.

[53] Gordillo GM, Roy S, Khanna S, Schlanger R, Khandelwal S, Phillips G, Sen CK. Topical oxygen therapy induces vascular endothelial growth factor expression and improves closure of clinically presented chronic wounds. Clinical and Experimental Pharmacology and Physiology. 2008 Aug 1;35(8):957–64.

[54] Blackman E, Moore C, Hyatt J, Railton R, Frye C. Topical wound oxygen therapy in the treatment of severe diabetic foot ulcers: a prospective controlled study. Ostomy/Wound Management. 2010 Jun 1;56(6):24.

[55] Michaels JA, Campbell B, King B, Palfreyman SJ, Shackley P, Stevenson M. Randomized controlled trial and cost-effectiveness analysis of silver-donating antimicrobial dress-

ings for venous leg ulcers (VULCAN trial). British Journal of Surgery. 2009 Oct 1;96(10): 1147–56.

[56] Rodriguez PG, Felix FN, Woodley DT, Shim EK. The role of oxygen in wound healing: a review of the literature. Dermatologic Surgery. 2008 Sep 1;34(9):1159–69.

[57] Schreml S, Szeimies RM, Prantl L, Karrer S, Landthaler M, Babilas P. Oxygen in acute and chronic wound healing. British Journal of Dermatology. 2010 Aug 1;163(2):257–68.

[58] Asano S. Leukocyte. In: Uchiyama T, eds. Miwa Hematology 3rd edn, 292–5, Hakuhodo, Tokyo, 2006.

[59] McAllister TA, Stark JM, Norman JN, Ross RM. Inhibitory effects of hyperbaric oxygen on bacteria and fungi. The Lancet. 1963 Nov 16;282(7316):1040–2.

[60] Hohn DC. Host resistance of infection. In: Hunt TK, ed. Wound healing and wound infection. 264–80, Appleton-Century Crofts, New York, 1980.

[61] Leach RM, Rees PJ, Wilmshurst P. Hyperbaric oxygen therapy. British Medical Journal. 1998 Oct 24;317(7166):1140–3.

[62] Kindwall EP. A history of hyperbaric medicine. Hyperbaric medicine practice. Best Publishing Company, Arizona. 1994:2–16.

[63] Sheikh AY, Gibson JJ, Rollins MD, Hopf HW, Hussain Z, Hunt TK. Effect of hyperoxia on vascular endothelial growth factor levels in a wound model. Archives of Surgery. 2000 Nov 1;135(11):1293–7.

[64] Roy S, Khanna S, Nallu K, Hunt TK, Sen CK. Dermal wound healing is subject to redox control. Molecular Therapy. 2006 Jan 1;13(1):211–20.

4

Medicinal Plants and Natural Products with Demonstrated Wound Healing Properties

Christian Agyare, Emelia Oppong Bekoe,
Yaw Duah Boakye, Susanna Oteng Dapaah,
Theresa Appiah and Samuel Oppong Bekoe

Abstract

This section reviews the current literature on medicinal plants including extracts, fractions, isolated compounds and natural products that have been demonstrated to have wound healing properties. Various electronic databases such as PubMed, Science Direct, SciFinder and Google Scholar were employed to search for plants, natural plant constituents and natural products that have been scientifically demonstrated to have wound healing activity using *in vivo* and *in vitro* wound models. Parameters used in the evaluation of an agent with wound healing properties include rate of wound contraction, tensile strength, antioxidant and antimicrobial activities, hydroxyproline content assay and histological investigations including re-epithelization, collagen synthesis, granulation, proliferation and differentiation of fibroblasts and keratinocytes in excision and incision wound model studies. Eighty-five medicinal plants belonging to 45 families, phytoconstituents including phenolics, oils and other substances including honey were identified as potential wound healing agents or possess wound healing properties using various wound healing models.

Keywords: wounds, wound healing, medicinal plants, natural products, incision, excision

1. Introduction

Wounds are physical injuries that result in an opening or break of the skin that causes disturbance in the normal skin anatomy and function. They result in the loss of continuity of epithelium with or without the loss of underlying connective tissue [1, 2]. Wounds that are most difficult to heal include delayed acute wounds and chronic wounds. Current estimates indicate that nearly 6 million people suffer from chronic wounds worldwide [3, 4]. Foot and leg ulcer is a common disorder, and approximately 1% of the European population suffers from such chronic and recurrent ulceration [3, 5]. Non-healing or chronic wounds result in enormous health care expenditures, with the total cost estimated at more than $3 billion *per* year [3, 4]. Wounds such as injuries, cuts, pressure, diabetic, burns, gastric and duodenal ulcers continue to have severe impact on the cost of health care to patients as well as their families, dependents and health care institutions globally with increasing aging population.

Over the last decades, the search for newer and potent agents from nature (plants, marine environment, fungi and other microorganisms) to manage chronic wounds especially, in patients with underlying metabolic disorders has increased immensely. This is mainly due to the high risk of loss of function, loss of mobility, amputations and huge financial cost as well as death in some cases associated with chronic wounds [6, 7]. The situation is also compounded by the increase in the number of non-communicable diseases such as diabetes and ulcers and longer life expectancy in most developed countries where the prevalence and impact of chronic wounds are on the increase [8].

Most chronic wounds are ulcers that are associated with ischemia, diabetes mellitus, venous stasis disease, or pressure. Between 70% and 80% of people living in the developing countries especially in Africa and Asia depend on herbal medicine for their health needs including wounds, infectious and metabolic diseases [5]. For some time now, there have been increased use of herbal and natural products for the management and treatment of various disease conditions among people in the developed countries including the United States, Europe and Japan.

With respect to the use of medicinal plants and natural products for the treatment of various diseases including metabolic and infectious diseases, specific diagnoses using various modern tools and equipment are not normally made but the treatment is based on the signs and symptoms of the diseases with which these products have been used for over a long period of time with successful treatment outcomes.

This section highlights the importance of medicinal plants and natural products as a major source of wound healing agents with the potential to be developed into phytotherapeutic agents to treat and/or manage wounds and their associated complications. This will also provide a starting point for future studies aimed at isolation, purification, and characterization of bioactive compounds present in these plants as well as exploring the underlying pharmacological mechanisms of action and potential niche market of these medicinal plants and natural products.

2. Properties of a good wound healing agent from herbal or natural product

Wound healing agents are agents that can stimulate fibroblast proliferation, induce keratino-cytes proliferation and differentiation, increase collagen formation, exhibit antimicrobial, antioxidant and anti-inflammatory properties. In most cases, for an agent from medicinal plants or natural product to be classified as a good wound healing agent, it should possess two or more of the above properties [9, 10].

3. *In vivo* models for assessing wound healing activity

In vivo models include both artificial and tissue models. Artificial models include subcutaneous chamber/sponges and subcutaneous tubes. Tissue models such as excision wounds, incision wounds, superficial wounds, dead space and burn wounds are usually used to determine the degree of re-epithelialization, collagenation, neovascularization and tensile or breaking strength of wounds [11–13]. Models such as rabbit ear chamber, the hamster cheek pouch, the rabbit corneal pocket and the chick chorioallantoic membrane can also be employed to investigate the extent of re-epithelialization, neovascularization and dermal reconstitution [14].

4. *In vitro* models for assessing wound healing activity

In vitro models are generally simple, rapid and involve minimal ethical consideration compared to whole animal work and allow insight into the biochemical and physiological processes induced by the test agent. Many pharmacological agents at different concentrations can be evaluated concurrently without intrinsic heterogenecity associated with *in vivo* models [14]. As regenerative skin is characterized by connective as well as epithelial tissues, both cell types, dermal fibroblasts as well as human fibroblasts (either primary cells or cell lines), should be used for complete assessment of wound healing activity. *In vitro* models are relevant in study of cell-cell and cell-matrix interaction to mimic cell migration during wound healing. *In vitro* models can employ single cell systems, three dimensional systems, multicellular systems or organ cultures in assessing the wound healing properties of wound healing agents or compounds [14, 15].

5. Methods used for pinpointing herbal materials and natural products with wound healing property

Electronic databases such as PubMed, Scifinder® and Google Scholar were used to search medicinal plants that have been evaluated for wound healing. All filtered articles were appraised to determine whether they contain any validated *in vitro* or *in vivo* wound model. Primary search results were independently screened by two investigators. Included articles were reviewed concerning plant botanical names, part of plants used in the respective study and type of plant extracts, active constituents or compounds and wound models used (*in vivo* or *in vitro*) or standardized clinical trials with clearly demonstrated wound healing activity in the models used. Consideration was given to the significant differences between test group and control group with respect to wound contraction, wound tensile strength, period of epithelialization, neovascularization, collagenation, keratinization and fibrosis. In case of clinical studies, the respective design, number of patients, interventions, duration of treatment, and data related to the efficacy and tolerability of the patients to treatment were also monitored.

6. Medicinal plants used in wound care

6.1. Acanthaceae

Justicia flava (Forssk.) Vahl has widespread uses in tropical Africa. It is used in traditional medicine for the treatment of cough, paralysis, fever, epilepsy, convulsion and spasm, and skin infections and disorders. The roots are also used for diarrhea and dysentery [16, 17]. The methanol leaf extract of *J. flava* (7.5% w/w) has been found to reduce wound size significantly ($p < 0.01$) as compared to the untreated wounds in rats excision wound model. The extract also significantly ($p < 0.01$) increased the tensile strength of wounds compared to the untreated wounds. Wound tissues form animals treated with the test extract showed improved angiogenesis, collagenation, and re-epithelialization compared to the untreated wound tissue [16].

Adhatoda vasica L., commonly known as Chue Mue, grows in India. Leaves and stems of the plant have been reported to contain an alkaloid mimosine. Leaves also contain mucilage and root contains tannins. The methanol, chloroform and diethyl ether extract ointment (10% w/w) of *A. vasica* showed significant effect when compared to standard drug in excision wound model [18].

6.2. Amaranthaceae

Achyranthes aspera L., locally known as "Telenge or ambulale," is one of the traditionally used plants in the indigenous health care delivery system for the treatment of various kinds of wounds especially in Ethiopia and India. The leaves of *A. aspera* (2.5%, 5% and 10% w/w) simple ointment when applied topically have been shown to significantly ($p < 0.05$) enhance the rate of wound contraction, breaking strength and epithelization in excision wound model compared to the control. Histological evaluation of *A. aspera*-treated wound tissues revealed well organized epidermal layer, increased number of fibrocytes, improved neovascularization and epithelialization compared to the control group [19]. Barua et al. [20] further reported that 5% ointment of methanol leaf extract of *A. aspera* significantly ($p < 0.05$) increased the wound contraction rate, hydroproline and protein production, vitamin C content as well as elevates antioxidant enzymes such as superoxide dismutase and catalase levels in burn wound bed compared to control. The study via gelatin zymography also revealed an increased expression of matrix metalloproteinases (MMP-2 and 9) and improved granulation tissues, collagen and fibroblast deposition in wound bed of *A. aspera*-treated animals compared to control group in subsequent histological examinations.

Alternanthera sessilis (L.) R. Br. ex DC is a tropical plant which is traditionally used for the treatment of ulcers and cuts and wounds, fevers, ophthalmia, gonorrhea, pruritis, burning sensations, diarrhea, skin diseases, dyspepsia, hemorrhoids, liver and spleen diseases [21]. The oral application of chloroform extract from the leaves of *A. sessilis* at a dose of 200 mg/kg body weight significantly reduced wound area ($p < 0.005$) and increased re-epithelialization ($p < 0.0001$) compared to the untreated wound tissues. Furthermore, in excision wound model, scar area after complete epithelialization ($p < 0.0008$) with increased wound breaking strength ($p < 0.0001$) compared with the untreated wounds in incision wound model [22]. Antibacterial property of the leaves and aerial parts of *A. sessilis* has been reported by [23] and antibacterial activity is an ideal property of good wound healing agent [9].

Pupalia lappacea (L.) Juss is an annual or perennial herb found widespread in the tropics and subtropical regions in Africa and it is used in folklore medicine for treatment of boils, chronic wounds and skin infections [10, 24]. Histological studies of wound tissues treated with extracts revealed appreciable collagenation, re-epithelialization, granular tissue formation and angiogenesis for wounds treated with 2% and 10% (v/w) of ethanol leaf extract creams as well as 1% chloroform extract creams to untreated control wound tissues. The ethanol and chloroform extracts also exhibited high rate of wound closure [25]. However, Udegbunam et al. [26] also reported that higher concentrations (10% and 20% (w/v) ointment of methanol leaf extract of *P. lappacea*) significantly ($p < 0.05$) accelerated wound healing, thereby the 20% ointment having the highest percentage wound contraction and rate of epithelialization. The extract also exhibited antimicrobial activity with MIC of 3.0–9.0 mg/mL and MBC of 7–10 mg/mL against *Pseudomonas aeruginosa*, *Staphylococcus aureus* and *Bacillus subtilis*.

6.3. Anacardiaceae

Buchanania lanzan Spreng, commonly known as char, achar and chironji, is an evergreen tree commonly found in the dry deciduous tropical forests of India and it is used to treat cough, constipation, skin disorders and stomach disorders [27]. Topical application of methanol root extract of *B. lanzan* (10% (w/w) ointment) significantly ($p < 0.05$) increased the tensile strength in the incision wound model. *B. lanzan* also showed significant wound healing activity in excision wound model [28]. However, a study conducted by Chitra et al. [29] showed that the methanol fruit extract of *B. lanzan* did not significantly ($p > 0.05$) promote wound healing when compared to the control in excision, incision and dead space wound models.

Lannea welwitschii (Hiern.) Engl. is found growing in deciduous and secondary forests of Africa from Cote d'Ivoire to Cameroon and extending to Uganda and Angola. Decoction of the leaves is used traditionally for the treatment of diarrhea, dysentery, swellings, gout, gingivitis, topical infections, and wounds [10]. Methanol leaf extract of *L. welwitschii* (7.5%, w/w) significantly ($p < 0.05$) reduced wound size as compared to the untreated in excision wound model in rats. The extract also significantly ($p < 0.01$) increased the tensile strength, improved angiogenesis, collagenation, and re-epithelialization of wounds compared to the untreated wounds [16].

6.4. Apiaceae

Centella asiatica (L.) Urban is a tropical plant native to Southeast Asian countries such as India, Sri Lanka, China, Indonesia, and Malaysia as well as South Africa and Madagascar [30]. It is used for treatment of burns and postoperative hypertrophic scars [31, 32]. Asiaticoside, isolated from *C. asiatica*, has been studied in normal as well as delayed-type wound healing in guinea pigs. Topical applications of 0.2% (v/w) asiaticoside on wounds induced a 56% increase in hydroxyproline, 57% increment in tensile strength, increased collagen formation and improved re-epithelialization. Also in streptozotocin-diabetic rats, where wound healing is typically delayed, topical application of 0.4% (v/w) asiaticoside over punch wounds increased hydroxyproline content, tensile strength, collagen content and epithelialization thereby facilitating the healing. Asiaticoside was also found to be active by the oral route at a dose of 1 mg/kg in the guinea pig punch wound model. It promoted angiogenesis in the chick chorioallantoic membrane model at 40 µg/disk concentration [33]. Triterpene compounds such as asiatic acid, madecassic acid and madecassoside are the principal components of *C. asiatica*, responsible for wound healing. The action has been demonstrated both for the extracts as well as for the triterpene *in vitro* and *in vivo* studies [31, 32].

Cuminum cyminum L. is one of the oldest cultivated medicinal food herbs in Africa, Asia and Europe and seeds have been commonly used for culinary and flavoring purposes and folklore therapy since antiquity in various countries [34–36]. Alcoholic extract of the seeds and its petroleum ether fraction showed better re-epithelialization ($p < 0.001$), therefore promoted wound healing compared to the untreated wounds [37].

6.5. Apocyanaceae

Catharanthus roseus L. is native to the Caribbean Basin, Madagascar and has been found growing in tropical Africa. The fresh juice from the flowers of *C. roseus* made into a tea has been used by Ayurvedic physicians in India to treat skin infections, dermatitis, eczema and acne. Ethanol flower extract of *C. roseus* significantly ($p < 0.001$) increased the wound breaking strength in the incision wound model compared to controls. The extract-treated wounds were found to epithelialize faster, and wound contraction was significantly ($p < 0.001$) increased in comparison to control wounds and hydroxyproline content in a dead space wound model increased significantly ($p < 0.05$) [38].

Strophanthus hispidus DC. is found all over Africa including savannah forests in Ghana, Senegal, Sudan, Congo DR, Uganda, and Tanzania. It is used for the treatment of syphilis ulcers, bony syphilis, and guinea worm sores and wounds [39]. The influence of the leaf and root extracts of *S. hispidus* on rate of wound closure was investigated using the excision wound model. The extract (7.5%, w/w) showed significantly ($p < 0.05$) improved wound contraction compared to the untreated wounds. Extract-treated wound tissues with showed improved collagenation, re-epithelialization and rapid granulation formation compared with untreated wound tissues [40].

Wrightia tinctoria R. Br., commonly known as Indrajauis, is a small deciduous tree distributed in Asia and some tropical countries in Africa such as Ghana, Nigeria and Cameroun. It is used traditionally to treat various skin diseases and wounds [41–43]. *In vivo* investigations revealed that ethanol stem bark extract of *W. tinctoria* exhibited significant wound healing activity. The extract improved breaking strength ($p < 0.01$) increased the percentage wound closure and decreased epithelialization time ($p < 0.001$) compared to the control. It also significantly increased ($p < 0.001$) hydroxyproline content of ten-day-old granuloma of extract-treated animals compared to control animals in dead space wound model. The pro-healing action seems to be due to the increased synthesis of collagen and its cross-linking as well as better alignment and maturation [44].

Saba florida (Benth.) is widely distributed in tropical Africa in countries such as Senegal, Nigeria, Cameroon, Sudan and Tanzania. It is used to treat rheumatism, diarrhea, gonorrhea and as antidote against food poisoning as well as snake bites [45]. Alcohol extract of *S. florida* when administered topically (10%, w/w) and orally (100–400 mg/kg body weight) significantly stimulate wound healing in excision and incision wound models [46].

6.6. Asclepiadaceae

Calotropis gigantea R. Br. is a perennial under-shrub found chiefly in wastelands throughout India, and in some African countries such as Angola, Gabon, DR Congo, Kenya, Sudan, Tanzania and Mozambique. The whole plant is used for treatment of skin diseases, boils and sores. *C. gigantea* is also used in some parts of India for wound healing in combination with other plants [47–49]. The whole plant extract increased the percentage of wound contraction, scar area and decreased re-epithelialization time. Breaking strength of extract-treated wounds and hydroxyproline content increased compared to untreated [50].

Calotropis procera W. T. Aiton is a well-known plant in the Ayurvedic system of medicine. *C. procera* originated from the Afro-Asian monsoonal regions. It spreads on an arc expanding from north western Africa including Mauritania, Senegal, through the Arabian Peninsula and Middle-East to the Indian subcontinent. It was introduced to subtropical America, the Mascarene Islands, drier parts of Australia and probably Southeast Asia [51]. The latex of *C. procera* (1%, w/v) significantly facilitated the wound healing process by increasing collagen, DNA and protein synthesis and epithelialization leading to a marked reduction in wound area compared to the control [52].

6.7. Asteraceae

Achillea biebersteinii Afan is a perennial herb which is used in folkloric medicine in Turkey to treat abdominal pain, wounds and stomachache. N-hexane aerial parts extract of *A. biebersteinii* showed marked increase in wound contraction rate and tensile strength in excision and incision wound models, respectively. However ointment incorporated with 1% chloroform, ethyl acetate and methanol extract showed no significant influence on the wound healing process in both excision and incision wound models [53].

Ageratum conyzoides L. has long been known in herbal medicine as a remedy for various ailments in Africa [54], Asia, and South America [55, 56]. It is used by the Fipa in South Africa and central Africa for the treatment of fresh wounds and burns [57]. The wound healing activities of petroleum ether, chloroform, methanol and aqueous extracts of *A. conyzoides* were evaluated using the excision, incision and dead space wound models. Methanol and aqueous leaf extracts of *A. conyzoides* showed faster rate of wound healing compared to other extracts [58].

Chromolaena odorata L. is a perennial shrub that is native in Africa [59, 60]. Extracts from the leaves of *C. odorata* have been shown to be beneficial for treatment of wounds. The crude ethanol extract of the plant had been demonstrated to be a powerful antioxidant in protecting fibroblasts and keratinocytes *in vitro*. Phenolic acids including protocatechuic, p-hydroxybenzoic, p-coumaric, ferulic and vanillic acids and complex mixtures of lipophilic flavonoid aglycones (flavanones, flavonols, flavones and chalcones) were antioxidants found to protect cultured skin cells against oxidative damage in colorimetric and lactate dehydrogenase release assay [61].

Centaurea iberica Trev. ex Spreng also called Iberian star thistle is native to the Mediterranean region, southern Europe and northern Africa. Several *Centaurea* species are used in Turkish folk medicine to alleviate pain and inflammatory symptoms in rheumatoid arthritis, high fever, headache and wounds. Particularly, the aerial parts have found to improve wound healing. Histopathological evaluation of both ointment of aqueous and methanol extracts treated and untreated wound tissues from rats supported the healing process with remarkable increase in the proliferation of fibroblasts, differentiation of keratinocytes, re-epithilization and remodeling [62].

Sphaeranthus indicus L. is distributed throughout Africa, India, Sri Lanka and Australia. It is an important medicinal plant used for the treatment of styptic gastric disorders, skin diseases, anthelmintic, glandular swelling, and nervous depression. The decoction and powdered material of the plant are used for the treatment of bronchitis, asthma, leucoderma, jaundice, piles and scabies [63–65]. Extract of the aerial parts of *S. indicus* significantly enhanced the rate of wound contraction and the period of epithelialization comparable to neomycin in pigs [66].

Tridax procumbens L. is commonly known as 'coat buttons' among English folks. The plant is native to tropical America and naturalized in tropical Africa, Asia, Australia and India. The influence of whole plant extract and aqueous extract of *T. procumbens* on lysyl oxidase activity, protein and nucleic acid contents as well as the tensile strength which are relevant to wound healing resulted in significant ($p < 0.01$) increment in the above parameters in albino rat treated with whole plant aqueous extract and aqueous extract fractions compared to the untreated in dead space wound healing model. Butanol and petroleum ether fractions treated wound tissues showed a decrease in all these parameters except tensile strength. In these two groups, the hexosamine levels were increased ($p < 0.001$). Whole plant extract were more active as compared to the other extracts in dead space wound model [67]. Yaduvanshi et al. [68] reported that, excision wounds treated with extract of the juice of *T. procumbens* (1 mg/g) and VEGF (1 μg/mL) exhibited a significant ($p < 0.05$) increase of 38.81% and 47%, respectively in collagen biosynthesis compared to the vehicle-treated wounds. Histological investigations also showed increased infiltration of inflammatory cells, fibroblast proliferation and re-epithelialization with moderate vascularity in dermal wound tissues treated with extract of the juice of *T. procumbens*. However, dermal wounds treated with extract of the juice of *T. procumbens* at a dose of 4 mg/g induced inflammation, edematous tissue and decreased vascularity. Ethanolic and aqueous leaf extract *T. procumbens* significantly ($p < 0.05$) increase in wound tensile strength. In the excision model, biochemical markers such as hydroxyproline, collagen and hexosamine increased significantly ($p < 0.05$) compared to the untreated control group [69].

Calendula officinalis L., also known as pot marigold or garden marigold, is a common garden plant which is native to Southern Europe and Egypt. Traditionally it is used to treat various skin disorders such as burns and wounds, eczema, psoriasis and variety of skin infections. It can also be used to treat seizures, haemorrhoids and lungs, mouth and throat infections [70]. The effects of oral application of *C. officinalis* flower ethanol extract at dose of 20 and 100 mg/kg body weight have been reported to significantly ($p < 0.01$) promote wound closure and re-epithelialization compared to the control group in excision wound model. In addition, there was significant ($p < 0.05$) increases in hydroxyproline and hexosamine content in the 100 mg/kg extract-treated wounds compared with the untreated animals [71].

6.8. Bignoniaceae

Kigelia africana (Lam.) Benth. is found widespread across tropical Africa including Ghana, Sierra Leone, Gambia, Sudan and Nigeria and also found growing in wet savannah and near river bodies where it occurs in abundance [72]. It is used to treat skin ailments including fungal infections, boils, psoriasis and eczema, leprosy, syphilis, and cancer. The roots, wood and leaves have been found to contain kigelinone, vernolic acid, kigelin, iridoids, luteolin, and 6-hydroxyluteolin [73]. The iridoids have antibacterial property [74]. The methanol stem bark extract of *K. africana* (7.5%, w/w aqueous cream) in rat excision wound model showed significant ($p < 0.05$) wound contraction on day 7 with 72% of wound closure compared to the untreated control group. Wound tissues treated with the extracts showed improved collagenation, re-epitheliazition and rapid granulation formation compared to untreated wound tissues [40].

Spathodea campanulata P. Beauv. is used in folkloric medicine in Ghana and several African countries to treat various forms of wounds [9, 10, 75]. Excision wounds treated with 20% (w/w) *S. campanulata* cream and Cicatrin® cream showed a rapid and comparable decrease ($p < 0.05$) in wound size in rats. In uninfected wounds, both 20% (w/w) *S. campanulata* cream and Cicatrin® cream application resulted in 95% wound closure seen on day 20, and a complete closure seen on day 24. In infected wounds, both 20% (w/w) *S. campanulata* cream and Cicatrin® cream administration led to approximately 91% wound closure on day 24 and a complete wound contraction on day 28 [76].

Tecoma capensis Thumb. Lindl, commonly called Cape honeysuckle, is a shrub which is native of South Africa. The leaf extract of *T. capensis* (5% and 10%, w/w ointment) have been reported to exert significant increase rate wound closure and wound breaking strength in excision and incision wound models, respectively. Again, oral administration of 200 and 400 mg/kg leaf extract significantly increased granuloma breaking strength and hydroxyproline contents in dead space wound model [77].

6.9. Boraginaceae

Heliotropium indicum L. has a pantropical African distribution, but is probably native of tropical America and it is widespread throughout Africa. It is used as an analgesic (rheumatism), diuretic and for treatment of skin problems including yaws, urticaria, scabies, ulcers, eczema, impetigo and wounds [17, 78, 79]. *H. indicum* extracts (petroleum ether, chloroform, methanol and aqueous) promoted wound healing activity. The highest activity was observed with the methanol fraction. Significant increase in the granulation tissue weight, increased hydroxyproline content, and increased activity of superoxide dismutase and catalase level with the animals treated with methanol extract in dead space wound model further augmented the wound healing potential of *H. Indicum* [80].

6.10. Cactaceae

Opuntia ficus-indica (L.), commonly known as cactus or prickly pear, is a tropical and subtropical plant that grows in arid and semi-arid climates with a geographical distribution encompassing Mexico, Latin America, South Africa and Mediterranean countries [81, 82]. It has been used in folklore medicine for the treatment of diseases including inhibition of stomach ulceration [83]. The methanol stems extract of *O. ficus-indica* and its hexane, ethyl acetate, *n*-butanol and aqueous fractions were evaluated for their wound healing activity in rats. The extract and less polar fractions showed significant ($p < 0.05$) wound healing effects compared to the untreated wounds [84]. The wound-healing potential of two lyophilized polysaccharide extracts obtained from *O. ficus-indica* (L.) cladodes applied on large full-thickness wounds in the rat have been reported. When topically applied for 6 days, polysaccharides with a molecular weight >10(4) Da accelerated the re-epithelialization and remodeling phases, also by affecting cell-matrix interactions and by modulating laminin deposition. However, the wound-healing activity is high with polysaccharides with a MW ranging between 10(4) and 10(6) Da than for those with molecular weight >10(6) Da [85].

6.11. Caricaceae

Carica papaya L. is commonly known as pawpaw. The edible part of *C. papaya* is widely used all over the world and is cultivated in most tropical countries. The leaves are used traditionally as a dressing component for wounds [86]. The aqueous leaf extract of *C. papaya* (5% and 10%, w/v extract in vaseline and solcoseryl jelly) accelerated wound healing compared to the wounds treated with blank vaseline [87]. In streptozotocin-induced diabetic rats using excision and dead space wound models, the aqueous extract exhibited 77% reduction in the wound area compared to the controls. The wet and dry granulation tissue weight and hydroxyproline content increased significantly when compared to controls [88]. Carbopol gel containing 1.0% and 2.5% (w/w) of dried papaya latex have been found to accelerate wound closure, increase hydroxyproline content and stimulate epithelialization compared to the control in burn wound model [89].

6.12. Cecropiaceae

Myrianthus arboreus P. Beauv is a dioecious shrub or tree which grows up to 20 m tall. It is found growing in forest zones of tropical Africa including Ghana, Sierra Leone, Sudan, Ethiopia, southern part of DR Congo, Tanzania and Angola. Extracts of the leaves and leafy shoots of *M. arboreus* are used in the treatment of dysentery, diarrhea, wounds, boils, dysmenorrhea and incipient hernia and vomiting. The study revealed that 5% (w/w) methanol leaf extracts of *M. aboreus* cream has potent wound healing capacity with better wound closure ($p < 0.05$) on day 1 and day 9 ($p < 0.001$) compared with untreated wounds in excision wound model. Histological investigations showed enhanced wound tissue proliferation, fibrosis and re-epithelialization compared with the untreated wound tissues [90].

6.13. Combretaceae

Terminalia arjuna (Roxb. Ex DC) Wight and Arn. is native to India and Sri Lanka but it has been planted and naturalized in many African countries. In Mauritius, it is traditionally used in the management of dysentery and rheumatism. The effect of topical application of fractions (fractions I, II and III) obtained from a hydro-alcoholic extract of the stem bark were assessed on the healing of rat dermal wounds. The fractions significantly increased the tensile strength of the incision wounds and degree of re-epithelialization of excision wounds compared to control animals ($p < 0.05$). However, topical treatment with fraction I, consisting mainly of tannins, was found to demonstrate a comparatively high increase in the tensile strength of incision wounds and exhibited the fastest rate of epithelialization and increased hexosamine content [91].

Combretum mucronatum Schum. & Thonn. grows in west Africa in countries such as Ghana Senegal, DR Congo and Gabon. The leaves are traditionally used for treatment of wounds and skin infections. Aqueous leaf extract of *C. mucronatum* has been shown to stimulate viability of human keratinocytes and dermal fibroblasts. The extract stimulated cellular differentiation of primary keratinocytes significantly at 1 and 10 µg/mL. An isolate, procyanidin B2 from *C. mucronatum* at 1 and 10 µM was shown to be responsible for the induction of this cellular differentiation, while epicatechin and procyanidins B5, C1 and D1 also isolated from the extract were inactive [92].

6.14. Crassulaceae

Bryophyllum pinnatum Lam. is a perennial herb that grows in the tropical, subtropical and temperate regions of the world. The plant is well known as an agent for wound healing in folkloric medicine in most part of Asia especially in India. Petroleum ether, alcohol and aqueous leaf extract of *B. pinnatum* at an oral dose of 400 mg/kg showed significant ($p < 0.001$) increase in the breaking strength of incision wound as compared to control group. In the dead space wound healing, granuloma breaking strength and hydroxyproline content of granulation tissue increased significantly ($p < 0.001$) compared to control group. The aqueous extract of *B. pinnatum* also showed significant ($p < 0.001$) increase in wound contraction and formation of scars compared to the control in excision wound model [93].

6.15. Curcubitaceae

Momordica charantia L. also known as bitter gourd or bitter lemon is found in tropical regions including west Africa and it is used in the management of wounds, peptic ulcer, fever, piles and skin infections and parasitic infections [86, 94]. In excision wound model, the methanol leaf extract of *M. charantia* showed significant ($p < 0.05$) wound closure and histological investigation of the wound tissues revealed high fibrosis and collagenation compared to the untreated wound tissues in rats [94].

6.16. Cyperaceae

Cyperus rotundus L. is indigenous to India, but now it is found in tropical, subtropical and temperate regions from Asia, Africa and South America [95]. *C. rotundus* is used in folkloric medicine for the treatment of dyspepsia, fever, pruritis, wounds and pains [64, 96]. An alcoholic extract of tuber parts of *C. rotundus* ointments showed an increase in wound contracting ability, tensile strength and a decrease in wound closure time [97].

6.17. Euphorbiacea

Phyllanthus muellerianus (Kuntze) Exell. is found growing in most tropical region including Africa and Asia and it is used for the treatment of boils, wounds, stomach sores, menstrual disorders, fevers and other skin eruptions. Geraniin is the major phytochemical constituents in the leaves of *P. Mullerianus* [98]. In the excision wound healing, aqueous extract (PLE) of *P. muellerianus* (0.25%, 0.5% and 1%, w/w) and geraniin (0.1%, 0.2% and 0.4%, w/w) significantly ($p < 0.001$) reduced wound area, increased hydroxyproline content and tensile strength compared to the untreated wounds. Histological studies of wound tissues showed high number of fibroblasts and increased collagenation in PLE and geraniin-treated wound tissues. Immunohistochemical investigations revealed high levels of TGF-β_1 in PLE (0.25%, 0.5% and 1%, w/w) and geraniin-treated (0.1%, 0.2% and 0.4%, w/w) wound tissues compared to the untreated wound tissues. Protein band analysis of coomassie stained SDS-PAGE showed significantly ($p < 0.001$) high levels of TGF-β_1 in both PLE (0.25%, 0.5% and 1%, w/w) and geraniin-treated (0.1%, 0.2% and 0.4% ,w/w) wound tissues compared to the untreated wound tissues. SOD activity increased significantly ($p < 0.001$) in both PLE (0.25%, 0.5% and 1%, w/w) and geraniin-treated (0.1%, 0.2% and 0.4%, w/w) wound tissues compared to the untreated wound tissues. SOD, CAT and APx activity increased significantly ($p < 0.01$) in both PLE (0.25%, 0.5% and 1% ,w/w) and geraniin-treated (0.1%, 0.2% and 0.4%, w/w) wound tissues compared to the untreated tissues. However, MPO activity decreased significantly ($p < 0.01$) in PLE (0.25%, 0.5% and 1%, w/w) and 0.2% and 0.4% (w/w) geraniin-treated wound tissues compared to the untreated wound tissues [99]. Hydrophilic extracts from *P. muellerianus* and especially the major isolate, geraniin, exhibited stimulating activity on dermal fibroblasts and keratino-cytes, leading to increased cell proliferation, barrier formation and formation of extracellular matrix proteins [98].

Alchornea cordifolia (Schum. &Thonn.) Muell. Arg. is an evergreen dioecious shrub which grows in the eastern part of Senegal to Kenya and Tanzania and throughout Central Africa to Angola.

The poultice of the leaves is used for the treatment of wounds. The leaves and root bark of *A. cordifolia* are externally applied to treat leprosy and as antidote to snake venom [10, 86]. Aqueous leaf extracts of *A. cordifolia* cream (10%, w/w) in an excision wound model, exhibited potent wound healing capacity with better wound closure ($p < 0.05$) at day 1 and day 9 ($p < 0.001$) compared with untreated wounds. Histological investigations showed enhanced wound tissue proliferation, fibrosis and re-epithelialization compared with the untreated wound tissues [90].

Jatropha curcas L. also called physic nut is a perennial poisonous shrub originated from Central America but has spread to other tropical and subtropical countries and mainly grows in Asia and Africa. The plant has been employed in the management of many ailments including ulcer and sores in some parts of Africa [99, 100]. The leaf and stem bark extracts of *J. curcas* have been found to accelerate the healing process by increasing the skin breaking strength, granulation tissue breaking strength, wound contraction, dry granulation tissue weight and hydroxyproline levels. A marked decrease in epithelialization period was also observed. The histological examination of granulation tissue also showed the presence of more collagen, which has organized to form bundles indicative of advance wound healing [101].

Arabinogalactan protein (JC) from *J. curcas* seed endosperm (mean molecular weight 140 kDa) was isolated by cold water extraction and characterized concerning sugar and amino acid composition. At 10 and 100 µg/mL JC stimulated mitochondrial activity (MTT assay) of HaCaT keratinocytes and dermal fibroblasts and the ATP status of primary keratinocytes. JC did not influence the cellular proliferation, while primary keratinocytes were triggered into differentiation status. Investigations on a potential mode of action of JC were performed on complex organotypic skin equivalents. JC induced HGF, KGF and TGF-β expression, with TGF-β being the main inductor for the differentiation-inducing effect of JC. Also the expression of GM-CSF was stimulated strongly by JC. This *in vitro* activity profile indicated JC to be a potent inductor of cellular differentiation via stimulation of growth hormones and TGF-β-induced cell signaling [102].

Mallotus oppositifolius (Geiseler) Müll. Arg. is found growing in tropical African region regions including Ghana and Nigeria. A leaf or stem bark infusion is applied to cuts and sores as haemostatic and used to treat burns, skin eruptions and rashes [78, 86, 103]. Methanol leaf extract of *M. oppositifolius* showed significant ($p < 0.05$) wound closure, fibrosis and collagenation in excision wound model [94].

Phyllanthus emblica L. also known as *Emblica officinalis* is a native plant from Asia. It is used in folkloric medicine as a wound healing agent either in single formulation or in combination with other medicinal plants. Topical application of ethanol fruit extract (200 µL) of *P. emblica* increases cellular proliferation and cross-linking of collagen at the wound site, which is evidenced by an increase in the activity of extracellular signal-regulated kinase 1/2, along with an increase in DNA, type III collagen, acid-soluble collagen, aldehyde content, shrinkage temperature and tensile strength. Higher levels of tissue ascorbic acid, alpha-tocopherol, reduced glutathione, superoxide dismutase, catalase and glutathione peroxidase support the fact that *P. emblica* promotes antioxidant activity at the wound site in excision wound model [104]. Again, aqueous extract of the fruit of *P. emblica* (0.1 µg/mL) in scratch assay using human umbilical vein endothelial cells (HUVEC) was shown to promote endothelial cell function and wound healing by significantly ($p < 0.05$) promoting NO production, endothelial wound closure, endothelial sprouting, and VEGF mRNA expression which provides further evidence to support the traditional use of *P. emblica* as a wound healing agent [105].

6.18. Fabaceae

Mimosa pudica L. originated in tropical Central and South America and naturalized throughout the tropics including Africa. Its wound healing properties were studied in three different wound models in rats (excision, incision and estimation of biochemical parameter) using both aqueous and methanol root bark extract. Treatment of wounds with ointment containing 2% (w/w) of methanol and aqueous extract exhibited significant ($p < 0.001$) wound healing activity by increasing rate of wound contraction, tensile strength and hydroxyproline content compared to the control. The period for re-epithelialization was reduced compared to the control [106].

Indigofera enneaphylla L. is an under-shrub widely grown throughout India. The plant is used traditionally to treat scurvy, stomach disorders, pain, skin infections and wounds. showed that Ethanol extract of the whole plant extract of *I. enneaphylla* (0.5% and 1%, w/w ointments) significantly increased ($p < 0.001$) rate of wound contraction on day 18 post wounding in excision wound model when compared to the control group. In the incision wound model, both doses of extract also exhibited significant ($p < 0.001$) increase in tensile strength [107].

Tephrosia purpurea L. is an herb which grows in the tropical regions. It is traditionally used in the treatment of bronchitis, boils, bleeding piles, pimples, roots and seeds are used as insecticidal, vermifuge, leprous wound and the juice is used for the eruption on skin. It has found to contain glycosides, rotenoids, isoflavones, flavones, chalcones, flavonoids and sterols. Ethanol aerial parts extract of *T. purpurea* formulated into a 5% (w/w) simple ointment stimulated ($p < 0.05$) wound contraction, tensile strength, hydroxyproline content, protein level in excision, incision and dead space wound models. Histological examination of the wound tissue showed significant ($p < 0.05$) increase in fibroblast cells, collagen fibers and blood vessels formation [104].

6.19. Fagaceae

Quercus infectoria Olivier is a small tree found in Greece, Asia and Iran. The galls of *Q. infectoria* are used traditionally to treat inflammatory diseases including toothache and gingivitis. The wound healing activity of ethanol extract of the galls of *Q. infectoria* was investigated using the incision, dead space and excision wound models in rats. The study revealed a (400 and 800 mg/kg body weight) significantly ($p < 0.05$) increase in tensile strength in extract-treated wound tissues compared to the control group in the incision wound model. In the dead-space wound model the extract significantly ($p < 0.05$) increased dry granuloma weight, granuloma breaking strength and hydroxyproline content compared to the control group. *Q. infectoria* was also identified to significantly ($p < 0.05$) promote wound contraction rate as well as increase levels of superoxide dismutase and catalase activity in wound bed compared to the control in the excision wound model [108].

6.20. Flacourtiaceae

Hydnorcarpus wightiana Blume is widely distributed in India and its neighboring countries. The oil referred to as "chaulmoogra" which is extracted from *H. wightiana* and other species is well known for its anti-leprosy activity. The oil at a dose of 45 mg/kg is also reported to significantly ($p < 0.01$) enhance wound healing by increasing breaking strength and collagen and hydroxyproline contents of wounds compared to the control in incision and dead space wound models, respectively. *H. wightiana* oil administered orally significantly ($p < 0.001$) promoted epithelialization, but not wound contraction rate in excision wound model [109, 110].

6.21. Gentianaceae

Anthocleista nobilis G. Don is used in local medicine in Ghana and other parts of West Africa for curing fever, stomach ache, diarrhea, gonorrhea and also as poultice for sores [72, 111]. Methanol extract of *A. nobilis* at concentration of 33.3% (w/w) significantly ($p < 0.02$) enhanced wound closure and hydroxyproline production compared to the control in the excision wound model in rats. In the incision wound model, the extract significantly increased tensile strength of *A. nobilis* treated-wounds compared to the control. However, the methanol extract of *A. nobilis* had no significant effect on the proliferation of human dermal fibroblast at concentrations as high 50 μg/mL. Doses over 50 μg/mL showed cytotoxic effects on the human dermal fibroblasts [112].

6.22. Ginkgoaceae

Ginkgo biloba L. also known as maiden hair tree is believed to be native of China. The plant has been used in folkloric medicine for its therapeutic purposes especially in mental sicknesses. Bairy and Rao [113] reported that intraperitoneal administration of the 50 mg/kg dried leaf extract of *G. biloba* significantly ($p < 0.01$) promoted the breaking strength and hydroxyproline content of granulation tissue in dead space wounds in rats. However, in excision wounds while it did not affect the wound contraction but epithelization period was significantly ($p < 0.01$) shortened compared to the control.

6.23. Hypericaceae

Hypericum patulum Thumb. is a perennial plant distributed in Southern Africa, Asia and North America. It is used traditionally to treat dog bites and bee sting [114]. Methanol leaf extract of *H. patulum* in the form of an ointment (5% and 10%, w/w) enhanced wound contraction rate, re-epithelialization, tissue granulation and increased tensile strength in rats compared with the control group [115].

Hypericum perforatum L., commonly called St John Worts, Klamath weed, tipton weed, goat weed, and enola weed, is a perennial flowering herb native to Europe, but has spread to temperate locations in Asia, Africa, Australia, Europe and North and South America [116]. Olive oil extracted from the aerial parts of *H. perforatum* is a popular folk remedy for the treatment of wounds in Europe. Aerial parts of *H. perforatum* have been found to possess remarkable wound healing activities. Flavonoids including hyperoside, isoquercitrin, rutin and (–)-epicatechin, and naphthoquinones especially hypericins were found as the active components of *H. perforatum* [117]. The total extract of *H. perforatum* in *in vivo* experimental wound models of linear incision, circular excision and thermal burn showed that topical treatment improve wound contraction rate and period of re-epithelialization [118]. A plant-derived wound dressing containing a mixture of hypericum oil and neem oil (*Azadirachta indica* A. Juss.) in scalp wounds with exposed bone [119] and pediatric burn wounds [120] promoted healing in rats by enhancing granulation tissues formation and re-epithelialization.

6.24. Lamiaceae

Occimum sanctum L. occurs naturally in tropical America, Africa and Asia. It is used tradition-ally in the treatment of diverse ailments like infections and skin diseases [121]. The wound healing parameters were evaluated by using incision, excision and dead space wound models in rats. The alcoholic (400 and 800 mg/kg) and aqueous (400 and 800 mg/kg) extracts of *O. sanctum* significantly ($p < 0.05$) increased wound contraction rate, wound breaking strength, hydroxyproline, hexuronic acid, hexosamines, superoxide dismutase, catalase and reduced glutathione levels. Lipid peroxidation was significantly ($p < 0.05$) reduced when compared with the control group [101]. Goel et al. [122] also reported that 10% *O. sanctum* aqueous leaf extract in petroleum jelly increased rate of wound contraction and re-epithelialization compared to the control in excision model of wound repair in Wistar albino rats.

Occimum gratissimum L. is an aromatic plant found in tropical Africa including Ghana, Nigeria and Kenya among others. The leaves are rubbed between the palms and sniffed as a treatment for blocked nostrils [115]. Leaf extract of *O. gratissimum* promote wound healing by significant wound contraction ($p < 0.05$) on day 10 in extract-treated rats group compared with the control group. Histology of the healed scar showed non-significant ($p > 0.05$) decrease in the mean fibroblast count for the experimental group compared to the control group [123, 124].

Hoslundia opposita Vahl. is used in ethnomedicine to treat sore throats, colds, sores, veneral diseases, herpes and other skin diseases [125], malaria, microbial infections, epilepsy, fever and inflammation [126, 127]. Methanol leaf extract of H. *opposita* at concentration of 33.3% (w/w) significantly ($p < 0.01$) increased wound contraction and hydroxyproline content compared to the control in the excision wound model in rats. In the incision wound model, the extract significantly improved tensile strength of wounds compared to the control. The extract had no significant effect on the growth of human dermal fibroblast up to concentrations of 50 µg/ml and higher concentrations exhibited toxic effects [112].

Hyptis suaveolens (Poit), commonly called bush tea, is a native to tropical America, but it is also widespread in tropical Africa, Asia and Australia. *H. suaveolens* is used in traditional medicine for treatment of various diseases including wounds, skin infections etc. Ethanol leaf extract of *H. suaveolens* (400 and 800 mg/kg body weight) increased skin breaking strength, granuloma breaking strength, wound contraction, hydroxyproline content and dry granuloma weight and decreased the re-epithelialization period in rats. A supportive study made on granuloma tissue to estimate the levels of catalase and superoxide dismutase recorded a significant ($p < 0.05$) increase in the level of these antioxidant enzymes which resulted enhanced collagenation [128]. Shenoy et al. [129] also showed the effect of petroleum ether, alcohol, and aqueous leaf extracts of *H. suaveolens* on excision, incision and dead space wound models using Wistar albino rats. All three extracts at a dose of 500 mg/kg enhanced wound healing by accelerating wound closure and period for re-epithelialization compared to the control. Tensile strength, dry weight granulation tissue, breaking strength of granulation tissue and hydroxyproline content were also increased compared to the control.

Leucas hirta is found in East Africa and India [130, 131]. Decoctions of dry and fresh herbs of *L. hirta* are used for skin diseases and as gargle for the treatment of thrush, respectively. Roots are also used for snake bites [132]. A leaf poultice is used on swelling and boils. The latex of *L. hirta* is applied on lower eyelids to cure eye sores. The wound healing effect of aqueous and methanol leaf extracts of *L. hirta* at a dose of 35 mg/kg was evaluated in excision, incision and dead space wound models in rats. The methanol and aqueous leaf extracts were found to possess significant wound healing activity which was evidenced by decrease in the period of re-epithelialization, increase in the rate of wound contraction, skin breaking strength, granulation tissue dry weight, hydroxyproline content and breaking strength of granulation tissue. Histological study of the granulation tissue showed increased collagenation when compared to the respective control group of animals [133].

6.25. Liliaceae

Allium cepa L. is a biennial herbaceuos plant with edible bulb. It is commonly known as onion. Since ancient times, it has been used traditionally for the treatment of different diseases including various types of wounds, skin problems etc. It contains kampferol, β-sitosterol, ferulic acid, myritic acid, prostaglandins [134]. Shenoy et al. [129] reported that alcohol extract exhibits significant ($p < 0.05$) wound contraction rate, improved tensile strength and increased wound breaking strength, dry weight granuloma and hydroxyproline content compared to the control in excision, incision and dead space wound models in rats.

6.26. Lythraceae

Lawsonia inermis L. is widely distributed throughout Africa. It also occurs in the Middle East. Ethanol leaf extract of *L. inermis* (200 mg/kg/day) demonstrated high rate of wound contraction ($p < 0.001$), a decrease in the period of epithelialization ($p < 0.001$), high skin breaking strength ($p < 0.001$), a significant increase in the granulation tissue weight ($p < 0.001$) and hydroxyproline content ($p < 0.05$). The extract-treated rats showed 71% reduction in the wound area when compared with controls which was 58%. Enhanced wound contraction, increased skin breaking strength, hydroxyproline and histological findings suggest the use of *L. inermis* in the management of wounds in humans may be justified [135].

Punica granatum L., commonly called pomegranate, originated from Iran. It is widely distributed in Mediterranean, Europe, Africa and Asia. Leaf extract of *P. granatum* possess wound healing activity at concentrations of 2.5% and 5% (w/w) in rats. The amount of hydroxyproline increased by twofold in the group treated with 5.0% gel. The extract was found to contain gallic acid and catechin as major compounds [136].

6.27. Malvaceae

Hibiscus rosa sinensis L. is native in the tropics and subtropics [137]. It has been used tradition-ally for the treatment of a variety of diseases as well as to promote wound healing. Ethanol leaf extract (120 mg/kg/day) exhibited an 86% reduction in the wound area compared with controls, which exhibited a 75% reduction in rats. The extract-treated animals showed a significant epithelialization ($p < 0.002$) and had significantly ($p < 0.002$) higher skin-breaking strength than controls. The dry and wet weight of granulation tissue and hydroxyproline content also increased significantly when compared with controls [138]. Bhaskar and Nithya [139] also reported the influence of ethanol flower extract of *H. rosa sinensis* (5% and 10%, w/w) on wound healing in Wistar albino rats using excision, incision and dead space wound model. The extract increased cellular proliferation and collagen synthesis at the wound site, as evidenced by increase in DNA, total protein and total collagen content of granulation tissues. The extract significantly ($p < 0.001$) promoted wound healing which was indicated by improved rates of epithelialization and wound contraction as well as increased wound tensile strength and wet and dry granulation tissue weights compared to the control.

Thespesia populnea (L.) Soland Ex. Corr, also known as Indian Tulip tree, is found growing from West Bengal to South India. It is used locally to treat skin ailments like scabies, psoriasis, wounds and ulcers. Shivakumar et al. [140] reported that ointments containing 5% (w/w) of petroleum ether, alcohol and aqueous leaf extracts *of T. populnea* promote wound contraction and wound breaking strength significantly ($p < 0.01$) when compared to the control groups in excision and incision wound models in rats, respectively.

6.28. Meliaceae

Carapa guianensis Aublet is found in Guiana and Africa. The leaves of *C. guianensis* are used to treat ulcers, skin parasites and skin problems. The ethanol leaf extract of *C. guianensis* exhibited significant reduction ($p < 0.01$) in the wound area when compared to controls with significant decrease in the epithelialization period. Skin breaking strength ($p < 0.001$), wet ($p < 0.002$) and dry ($p < 0.02$) granulation tissue and hydroxyproline content ($p < 0.03$) were significantly higher in extract-treated animals. The increased rate of wound contraction, skin breaking strength and hydroxyproline content may support application of *C. guianensis* for treatment of wounds [141].

Azadirachta indica A. Juss (Neem tree) is a native of Asia but has now naturalized in West Africa. In excision wound model in rats, aqueous leaf extract of *A. indica* significantly in-creased ($p < 0.05$) the rate of wound closure of extract-treated group compared to control group [142]. Methanol leaf extract (5%, w/w ointment) of *A. indica* has also been reported to significantly ($p < 0.05$) promote the wound healing activity in both excision and incision wound models in rats [20]. Pandey et al. [143] reported that *A. indica* oil increases wound tensile strength and wound closure rate in animals using incision and excision wound mod-els, respectively.

6.29. Moraceae

Ficus religiosa L., which is commonly known as bo tree, Pepal tree, Bodhi tree, peepul or sacred fig, is abundantly distributed throughout India, Southeast Asia, Southwest China and the Himalayan foothills. *F. religiosa* is reported to have wound healing, anti-inflammatory, analgesic, antioxidant (lipid peroxidation) properties. Application of simple ointment containing hydro-alcohol leaf extract of *F. reliogiosa* (5% and 10%, w/w) significantly promoted wound contraction rate, epithelization and wound breaking strength in excision and incision wound models, respectively, when compared to the control [144].

6.30. Moringaceae

Moringa oleifera Lam. is commonly known as drumstick and is widely distributed in India, Arabia and cultivated in tropical Africa, tropical America, Sri Lanka, India, Mexico and Malaysia [145]. The whole plant is used in the treatment of psychosis, eye diseases and fever and also as an aphrodisiac. Its leaf poultice is used in the management of wounds [146]. Qualitative phytochemical investigation confirmed the presence of phytosterols, glycosides, tannins, and amino acids in the various leaf extracts of *M. oleifera* whereas its seed extracts showed the presence of phytosterols, glycosides, phenolic compounds, carbohydrates and amino acids. The ethanol and ethyl acetate extracts of the seeds showed significant antipyretic activity in rats, whereas ethyl acetate leaf extract exhibited significant wound healing activity (10%, w/w ointment) on excision, incision and dead space (granuloma) wound models in rats [142].

6.31. Musaceae

Musa sapientum L. originated from native south-western Pacific home and spread to India and to the Islands of the Pacific, then to the West Coast of Africa [147]. It has an ulcer healing activity [148]. Aqueous and methanol extracts (100 mg/kg) have been found to increase wound breaking strength and levels of hydroxyproline, hexuronic acid, hexosamine, superoxide dismutase, reduced glutathione in the granulation tissue and decreased percentage of wound area, scar area and lipid peroxidation when compared with the control group in rats. The wound healing effect of *M. sapientum* may be due to its antioxidant effect and on various wound healing biochemical parameters [149].

6.32. Myrsinaceae

Embelia ribes Burm. is found in the hilly parts of India and grows in southern China, Indonesia and East Africa [150]. Traditionally the seeds are employed as a remedy for toothache, headache and snakebite. The seeds are mainly used for maintaining healthy skin and to support the digestive function [64]. It is also effective in the treatment of fever, abdominal disorders, lung diseases, constipation, fungus infections, mouth ulcer, sore throat, pneumonia, heart disease and obesity [150]. Ethanol leaf extract of *E. ribes* and its isolated quinone compound, embelin, were screened for wound healing activity in rats. In embelin-treated group (4 mg/mL in a 0.2%, w/v sodium alginate gel), re-epithelialization of the incision wound was faster with a high rate of wound contraction. The tensile strength of the incision wound was significantly increased in embelin-treated group than the ethanol extract. In dead space wound model also the weight of the granulation was increased indicating increase in collagenation. The histological examination of the granulation tissue of embelin-treated group showed increased cross-linking of collagen fibers and absence of monocytes [151].

6.33. Oleaceae

Jasminum auriculatum Vahl. is a small, evergreen, climbing shrub widely distributed in Eastern Asia including India, Nepal and Sri Lanka. The leaves are normally used to treat mouth ulcers. Mittal et al. [152] reported that ointment base incorporated with 16% (w/w) of ethanol leaf extract of *J. auriculatum* significantly ($p < 0.05$) decreased the period of re-epithelialization in excision wound model. In the incision wound model, there was significant increase in wound breaking strength and collagen content. Histological examination of wound tissues revealed increased fibroblast proliferation, collagen deposition and neovascularization.

Jasminum grandiflorum L. is an evergreen or deciduous shrub found in East tropical Africa countries including Sudan, Eritrea, Ethiopia, Somalia, Uganda, Kenya, Rwanda as well as in Asia. Traditionally it is used as an aphrodiasic, expectorant, painkiller and also to treat skin diseases including mouth ulcers and skin eruptions. Topical application of ointment *J. grandifolium* leaf extract (2% and 4%, w/w) on excision wounds in rats accelerated the healing process. Tissue growth and collagen synthesis were significantly ($p < 0.05$) higher which was determined by total hydroxyproline, hexosamine, protein and DNA content. The rate of wound healing was faster as determined by wound contraction, tensile strength and other histopathological changes. In addition, the 4% extract-treated wounds showed enhanced ($p < 0.05$) the activity of superoxide dismutase (SOD) and catalase (CAT) with high GSH content and low lipid peroxidation products in wound tissue compared to the control [153].

6.34. Papaveraceae

Argemone mexicana L. is a prickly, glabrous, branching annual herb with yellow juice and showy yellow flowers found in West Indies and Mexico. Traditionally, the plant is used as diuretic, purgative, painkiller, laxative and treatment for skin diseases, wounds and poisons [154]. In excision and incision wound models in rats, methanol, aqueous and chloroform leaf extracts of *A. mexicana* (10%, w/w) ointment significantly ($p < 0.05$) enhanced wound closure, re-epithelialization and breaking strength in wound bed compared to the control group. Histo-logical studies of the extract-treated wound tissues revealed improved collagen deposition and fibroblast proliferation with reduced macrophage infiltration and edema. The methanol extract-treated animals showed significant ($p < 0.01$) increase in dry weight of granulation tissue and hydroxyproline content in dead space wound model. Superoxide dismutase and catalase level in the granulation tissue were significantly increased in methanol extract-treated rats ($p < 0.01$) when compared to the control in dead space wound model. The methanol extract also significantly ($p < 0.05$) improved wound healing in bacterial (*Pseudomonas aeruginosa* and *Staphylococcus aureus*) infected wounds [80].

6.35. Pedaliaceae

Sesamum indicum L. is used in native medicine in Africa and Asia for a variety of diseases. Mucilaginous leaves or leaf sap are used to treat fever, as a remedy for cough and sore eyes, dysentery and gonorrhea. In eastern and southern Africa, the leaves are used for the treatment of ulcers. The seeds of *S. indicum* are used traditionally for the treatment of various kinds of wounds. Seeds and oil treatment (2.5% and 5%, w/w) exhibited significant ($p < 0.05$) decrease in the period of epithelialization and wound contraction, and increased the breaking strength of rat wound tissues compared to the control. Also, the seeds and oil treatment (250 and 500 mg/kg; *po*) in dead space wound model produced a significant increase in the breaking strength, dry weight and hydroxyproline content of the granulation tissue which suggest that the extract and its oil possess wound healing property [155].

6.36. Piperaceae

Piper betel L. is extensively grown in India, Srilanka, Malaysia, Indonesia, Philippines and East African countries [156]. Ointment of white soft paraffin containing 1% of dried residue of aqueous extract of *P. betel* has been reported to possess wound healing activity [157].

6.37. Potulacaceae

Portulaca oleracea L. is a cosmopolitan weed occurring especially in warm areas; it occurs throughout tropical Africa. It is eaten in many African countries including Côte d'Ivoire, Benin, Cameroon, Kenya, Uganda, Angola, South Africa, Sudan and Egypt. It is used for the treatment of ulcers, eczema and dermatitis [158, 159]. Fresh homogenized crude aerial parts of *P. oleracea* accelerated the wound healing process in mice by decreasing the surface area of the wound and increased the tensile strength. The highest rate of contraction was found at dose of 50 mg, followed by 25 mg [160].

6.38. Phyllanthaceae

Bridelia ferruginea Benth. is a common savannah species. Ethnomedicines prepared from the bark, leaves and fruits are used for the treatment of bruises, boils, burns, wounds and skin disease [79]. Ethanol stem bark extract of *B. ferruginea* on wound contraction and epithelization in rats significantly enhanced wound contraction and epithelialization [161] (Udegbunam et al., 2011) and the extract (1–30 µg/mL) has been reported to influence the proliferation of dermal fibroblasts significantly ($p < 0.05$) compared to the untreated cells [162].

6.39. Rubiaceae

Morinda citrifolia L. is one of the most important traditional Polynesian medicinal plants. The primary indigenous use of this plant appears to be of the leaves, as a topical treatment for wound healing. The ethanol leaf extract (150 mg/kg/day, *p.o*) was used to evaluate the wound healing activity in rats, using excision and dead space wound models. The extract exhibited

71% reduction in the wound area when compared with controls which exhibited 57%. The granulation tissue weight and hydroxyproline content in the dead space wounds were also increased significantly in extract-treated animals compared with controls ($p < 0.002$). Enhanced wound contraction, decreased epithelialization time, increased hydroxyproline content and histological characteristics may indicate that noni leaf extract may be beneficial in wound healing [163].

Pentas lanceolata Pentas Benth. originated from East Africa and is commonly called the "Red Egyptian star". The ethanol flowers extract of *P. lanceolata* given by oral route to rats at a dose of 150 mg/kg per day for 10 days was evaluated on its effect on wound healing, using excision wound model. There was significant ($p < 0.05$) increment in granulation tissue weight, tensile strength, hydroxyproline and glycosaminoglycan content. There was marked increment in the wound contraction in extract treated group as compared to that of controls and these effects may be due to increased collagen deposition as well as better alignment and maturation [164].

Rubia cordifolia L. is popular all over the world for its medicinal uses in skin diseases like eczema, dermatitis and skin ulcers. *R. cordifolia* has an extremely large area of distribution, ranging from Africa to tropical Asia, China, Japan and Australia. In Africa, it is found from Sudan and Ethiopia to South Africa. Hydrogel of the alcoholic extract has been found to improve wound contracting ability, wound closure, decrease in surface area of wound, tissue regeneration at the wound site significantly ($p < 0.01$) in treated mice [165].

6.40. Rutaceae

Aegle marmelos L., commonly called Bael in Hindu, is a perennial plant indigenous to dry forests on hills and plains of India, Pakistan, Bangladesh, Sri Lanka, Myanmar, Nepal, Vietnam, Laos, Cambodia and Thailand. The fruits and leaves are used to treat pain, fever, inflammation, respiratory disorders, cardiac disorders, dysentery and diarrhea in folk and Ayuverdic medicine. Jaswanth et al. [166] reported the wound healing effect of methanol root extract of *A. marmelos* (5% and 10%, w/w in simple ointment base) using excision and incision wound models in rats. The extract-treated wounds showed significant ($p < 0.01$) increase in wound contracting ability, reduced wound closure time and increase in the tensile strength compared to the control in excision and incision wound models, respectively. Gautam et al. [167] also reported that rats treated with 200 mg/kg *A. marmelos* ethanol leaf extract significantly ($p < 0.05$) increase wound breaking strength and improved ($p < 0.05$) wound contraction rate in *A. marmelos*-treated wounds compared to the control in excision wound model. This was also supported by histological examination of excised wounds which revealed increased granulation tissues formation and reduced inflammatory cell infiltration in 200 mg/kg treated wound tissues compared to the control. Granulation tissues showed increased ($p < 0.001$) collagen content compared to the control group. Catalase, superoxide dismutase and gluthathionine levels were markedly elevated, whereas lipid peroxidation, myeloperoxidation and nitric oxide levels were markedly ($p < 0.05$) lower in *A. marmelos*-treated wounds compared to the control group.

6.41. Sapotaceae

Mimusops elengi L. is native to India, Sri Lanka, the Andaman Islands, Myanmar and Indo-China, but is commonly planted as an ornamental tree throughout tropical countries including Ghana, Tanzania, Mozambique, Réunion Island and Mauritius. In Asia, the leaves are used medicinally to treat headache, toothache, wounds and sore eyes, and are smoked to cure infections of the nose and mouth. A decoction of the bark mixed with the flowers has been used for treatment of fever, diarrhea, inflammation of the gums, toothache, gonorrhea and wounds. The flowers have been used for the management of diarrhea [161, 168, 169]. Methanol bark extract of *M. elengi* (5%, w/w) exhibited significant ($p < 0.05$) influence on the rate of wound closure, tensile strength and dry granuloma weight. Histological investigation of the wound tissues revealed similar effects consistent with its *in vivo* wound healing properties [170].

6.42. Solanaceae

Datura metel L. is found growing in most tropical countries in Africa and it is used for the treatment of haemorrhoids, boils, sores and skin diseases [171, 172]. The ethanol leaf extract increased cellular proliferation and collagen synthesis at the wound site, as evidenced by increase in synthesis of DNA, total protein and total collagen content of granulation tissues. The extract-treated wounds were found to heal much faster with improved rates of epithelialization and wound contraction and these observations were confirmed by histological examinations of the wound tissues. The leaf extract of *D. metel* significantly ($p < 0.001$) increased the wound breaking strength compared to the controls. Wet and dry granulation tissue weights increased significantly ($p < 0.001$). There was a significant increase in wound closure rate, tensile strength, dry granuloma weight, wet granuloma weight and a decrease in epithelialization period in *D. metel* extract treated group when compared to control and commercial drug treated groups [173].

Solanum xanthocarpum Schrad and Wendl is known as Indian night shade or yellow berried night shade plant. It is more commonly used for the management of diseases like bronchial asthma, cough, worms etc. The fruits facilitate the seminal ejaculation, alleviate worms, itching, and fever and reduce fats [86]. Ethanol leaf extract of *S. xanthocarpum* significantly ($p < 0.01$) improved wound healing via increased re-epithelialization, tensile strength and hydroxyproline content which may be due to the presence of secondary metabolites such as alkaloids, glycosides, saponins, carbohydrates, tannins, phenolic compounds, proteins and fats [174].

6.43. Vitaceae

Cissus quadrangularis L. is a perennial climber popularly known as "Hadjod" in India and is widely distributed in the tropics. Traditionally, it is used to treat gastritis, bone fractures, skin infections, constipations, eye diseases, piles, anemia, asthma, irregular menstruation, burns and wounds. Treatment of wounds with ointment containing 2% (w/w) methanol extract and 2% w/w aqueous extract of *C. quadragularis* significantly ($p < 0.001$) enhanced wound closure and breaking strength compared to the control group in excision and incision wound models, respectively in rats [175].

6.44. Verbenaceae

Clerodendron splendens G. Don is a climbing shrub, mostly found growing on cultivated lands between food crops in Ghana and other West African countries. The plant is used in ethno-medicine in Ghana for the treatment of vaginal thrush, bruises, wounds and various skin infections [72]. The methanol aerial parts extract of *C. splendens* improved wound closure and hydroxyproline biosynthesis compared to the control group in the excision wound model in rats. The extract also increased the tensile strength of wounds compared to the control group [176].

Lantana camara L. occurs widely in the Asia-Pacific region, Australia, New Zealand, Central and South America, West Indies and Africa. It is used in herbal medicine for the treatment of skin itches, wounds, leprosy and scabies [177]. Treatment of the wounds in animals with leaf extract of *L. camara* enhanced the rate of wound contraction, synthesis of collagen and de-creased mean wound healing time [138].

6.45. Zingiberaceae

Curcuma aromatica Salisb. is a medicinal plant cultivated most extensively in India, Bangladesh, China, Thailand, Cambodia, Malaysia, Indonesia, and Philippines. It has been grown in most tropical regions in Africa, America, and Pacific Ocean Islands. Rhizomes of *C. aromatica* are used as a stomachic, carminative and emmenagogue remedies for skin diseases [178] and also for snakebites [179] (Chopra et al., 1941). Report by Santhanam and Nagarajan [157] has shown that ointment of white soft paraffin containing 1% of powdered *C. aromatic* rhizome promotes wound contraction and epithelialization. Kumar et al. [137] also reported that ethanol dried rhizome of *C. aromatica* extract significantly ($p < 0.001$) improved wound contraction in rat excision wound model.

Curcuma longa L., commonly known as tumeric, is a rhizomatous perennial herb native to India. In traditional medicine, it is used to treat skin ailments, wound, worm infestation and as blood purifier. *C. longa* contains three major curcuminoids, namely, curcumin, demethoxycurcumin, and bis-demethoxycurcumin [180]. *C. longa* possesses antibacterial, anti-inflammatory, anti-arthritic, anti-hepatotoxic (liver protective) and anti-allergic properties. Topical application (5% and 10%, w/w simple ointment) of ethanol rhizome extract of *C. longa* promotes significantly ($p < 0.01$) enhanced wound contraction, increased hydroxproline and tensile strength of wounds in excision and incision wound models in rats and rabbits. Histological studies also showed increased collagen, fibroblasts and blood vessels formation [181, 182]. Sidhu et al. [183] reported via immunohistochemical investigations that *C. longa*-treated wounds show highly localized transforming growth factor-β1 in wound bed compared with untreated wounds. There was an increment in the mRNA transcripts of transforming growth factor-β1 and fibronectin in curcumin-treated wounds.

Curcuma purpurascens Blume. is commonly known as "Temu tis" and "Koneng tinggang" in Indonesia. The rhizome of this plant has been reported to have extensive traditional uses in rural communities against different skin ailments and dermatological disorders, especially wounds and burns. Macroscopic evaluation of wounds showed conspicuous elevation in wound contraction ($p < 0.05$) after topical administration of hexane extract of the rhizome of *C. purpurascens* (100 and 200 mg/kg body weight) to wounded rats. Histological analysis revealed enhanced collagen content and fibroblast proliferation and scanty inflammatory cells in the granulation tissues of *C. purpurascens*-treated wounds compared to the control. At the molecular level, *C. purpurascens* facilitated wound-healing process by down-regulating Bax and up-regulating Hsp70 protein at the wound site. In addition, the plant enhanced catalase, glutathione peroxidase, superoxide dismutase activity and reduced malondialdehyde levels in wound tissues compared to the control group [184].

6.46. Zygophyllaceae

Balanites aegyptiaca (L.) Diel is widely distributed in tropical regions of Africa. The plant is used in folk medicine for treatment of circumcision wounds, worm infestation, abdominal and chest pains, and as an abortifacient and contraceptive [177, 185]. Methanol extract of *B. aegyptiaca* at concentration of 33.3% (w/w) significantly ($p < 0.001$) improved wound closure, tensile strength and hydroxyproline production compared to the control in the excision wound model in rats [112].

7. Phenolic compounds with wound healing properties

Though many crude plant extracts have been scientifically demonstrated to have wound healing activities, enriched fractions and isolated compounds from some of these plants have also been shown to possess specific promising wound healing properties. The commonly known effects of the active constituents of plant extracts towards wound healing are known to be through blood clotting, antimicrobial, antioxidant, mitogenic activities and also enhancing the expression of vascular endothelial growth factor thereby improving angiogenesis and blood flow as the tissue repair process advances [179, 186–188]. In chronic wounds, agents inducing differentiation of keratinocytes play an important role.

Plant polyphenols are among the most abundant phytochemicals present in the human diet, and they range from simple molecules such as phenolic acids to highly polymerized compounds, such as condensed tannins [189]. Several plants extracts used in wound healing contain phenolics in the form of procyanidins, flavonoids and phenolic acids [187] as their active ingredients. Tannins and procyanidins are known to actively facilitate wound healing [190].

Resveratrol is a natural polyphenol found predominantly in the skin of red grapes that has been studied extensively for its potential health benefits [191]. Resveratrol is a popular nutritional supplement and ingredient in over-the-counter skin care products. In humans, resveratrol was shown to protect against sun damage to the skin, enhance moisture and elasticity, reduce wrinkle depth and intensity of age spots, and protected keratinocytes from nitrous oxide-induced death [191, 192]. Its positive effect on keratinocytes has beneficial effect on wound healing. Resveratrol administration significantly increased the tensile strength of the abdominal fascia, and increased the hydroxyproline 1 levels *in vivo*. The acute inflammation scores, collagen deposition scores and the neovascularization scores on postoperative days 7 and 14 were found to be significantly higher in the resveratrol treatment group. The amount of granulation tissue and the fibroblast maturation scores were found to be significantly higher on postoperative day 14 in the treatment group when compared to the control group [193].

7.1. Tannins

Tannins are natural polyphenols and in many cases the active constituents in plants in which they are found. Tannins have a wide range of pharmacological activities including antimicrobial, wound healing, antioxidant and anti-inflammatory activities. The physical and chemical properties of tannins suggest that they may act by virtue of their complexation, astringent, antioxidant and radical scavenging activities, and their ability to form complex with proteins [194].

7.2. Ellagitannins

Ellagitannins, namely geraniin and furosin isolated from *Phyllanthus muellerianus*, were demonstrated to stimulate cellular activity, differentiation and collagen synthesis of human skin keratinocytes and dermal fibroblasts. Geraniin and furosin increased the cellular energy status of human skin cells (dermal fibroblasts NHDF, HaCaT keratinocytes) and triggered the cells towards higher proliferation rates. Furosin and geraniin stimulated the biosynthesis of collagen from normal human dermal fibroblasts. Geraniin also significantly stimulated the differentiation in normal human epidermal keratinocytes while furosin had a minor influence on the expression of involucrin and cytokeratins K1 and K10. The study proved that geraniin exhibit stimulating activity on dermal fibroblasts and keratinocytes, leading to increased cell proliferation, barrier formation and formation of extracellular matrix proteins [98].

7.3. Flavanols and proanthocyanidins

Flavanols are a sub-family of flavonoids which are present in plants as aglycones, as oligomers, or esterified with gallic acid and the most common oligomers of procyanidins present in edible plants are derived from epicatechin [189].

Flavanols and procyanidins are chemically able to prevent oxidation, and their administration has been associated with a decrease in oxidative stress markers in humans with improve blood supply to the wounded area to accelerate wound healing. They have been shown to exert a wide range of biological activities including wound healing property. The known biological activities of proanthocyanidins include antioxidant activity, anti-inflammatory activity, antimicrobial activities and wound healing activities [92, 189, 195].

A redox-active grape seed proanthocyanidin extract has been shown to up regulate oxidant and tumor necrosis factor-α inducible VEGF expression in human keratinocytes. Furthermore this grape seed proanthocyanidin extract was shown to accelerate wound contraction and closure *in vivo*, to enhance deposition of connective tissue and to improve histological architecture [186].

Wound healing property of *Camellia sinensis*, also known as green tea, has been linked to the presence of proanthocyanidins which are mainly made up of epicatechin, epigallocatechin, epicatechin-3-gallate and epigallocatechin-3-gallate and these induce differentiation of epidermal keratinocytes and also accelerate epithelial neoformation during wound healing [196].

Similarly, a fraction of the methanol extract of *Persea americana* Mill. seeds, containing high amounts of procyanidins B1 and B2 as well as an A-type trimer, was shown to stimulate proliferation of normal primary keratinocytes and fibroblasts cells but on another hand inhibited the proliferation of HaCaT-keratinocytes [197].

A study conducted on a proanthocyanidins rich fraction from *Hamamelis verginiana* showed that this fraction strongly increased the proliferation of skin cells. This effect was attributed to the tannin fraction, consisting of hydrolysable and condensed tannins, which account to 12% of Hamamelis bark [198].

A study of the wound healing activities of the hydrolyzable tannins from the hydro-alcoholic stem bark extract of *Poincianella pluviosa* enhanced the proliferation of human keratinocytes and dermal fibroblasts, which suggests that epidermal barrier formation can be accelerated by the use of *P. pluviosa* [199]. Treatment of keratinocytes with apple procyanidins has been shown to inhibit apoptosis and promote cell proliferation, migration and survival, necessary for revascularization and re-epithelialization of the wound. *In vivo* studies have shown that apple procyanidins (also known as procyanidins B1, B2 and C1) not only stimulate angiogenesis but also cause epithelial cells to grow mimicking keratinocyte re-epithelialization [200].

Epicatechin also blocks radiation-induced apoptosis via down-regulation Jun N-terminal kinase and p-38 in the HaCaT cells [201]. Epicatechin and procyanidins dimers are known to inhibit NADPH-oxidase and the subsequent superoxide production by directly binding to the enzyme or regulating calcium influx, or potentially inhibiting the binding of ligands that trigger NADPH-oxidase activation to their receptors (e.g. TNF-α). These functions are means by which epicatechin may provide cytoprotection to the cell. Both epicatechin and the respective procyanidin dimers can interact with the DNA-binding site of the nuclear factor kappa B (NF-κB) proteins, preventing the interaction of NF-κB with κB sites in gene promoters, thus inhibiting gene transcription [189]. The reduced NF-κB activation results in the suppression of inflammatory cytokines [200].

Procyanidins are known to induce the differentiation of keratinocytes. It has been reported that epigallocatechin-3-gallate induces differentiation of human epidermal keratinocytes [202]. In comparison to epigallocatechin-3-gallate, procyanidin B2 is more inductive to differentiation at lower concentrations [92].

Procyanidin B2 is also known to have beneficial effects in pathologies with pro-inflammatory components by inhibiting NF-κB-driven gene expression, including various cytokines and anti-apoptotic prote [203, 204]. It has been reported that several selective protein kinase C inhibitors, including procyanidin B-2, promote hair epithelial cell growth [205]. This presupposes that procyanidin B2 could be useful for aesthetic purposes during wound healing by stimulating the regrowth of skin appendages in the wounded area.

Procyanidin C1 inhibits nitric oxide production and the release of pro-inflammatory cytokines (IL-6 and TNF-α). Additionally, the potent anti-inflammatory effect of procyanidin C1 occurs through inhibition of mitogen-activated protein kinase and NF-κB signaling pathways. These two factors play a major role in controlling inflammation in the wounds [206]. In wound healing, procyanidin C1 activity presents a novel and effective means of inflammation control. Procyanidin dimers and trimers extracted from grape seeds are also known to exhibit higher growth-promoting activity than the monomer on hair epithelial cells *in vivo* [207].

7.4. Flavonoids

Flavonoids are a chemically defined group of polyphenols that have a basic structure of two aromatic rings (A and B) linked through three carbons that usually form an oxygenated heterocycle (C ring). The chemical characteristics of the C ring define the various subgroups of flavonoids by providing different arrangements of hydroxy, methoxy, and glycosidic groups, and the bonding with other monomers [208].

An important effect of flavonoids is the scavenging of oxygen-derived free radicals, reduction of liquid peroxidation, anti-inflammatory and wound healing activities. A drug that inhibits lipid peroxidation is believed to increase the viability and strength of collagen fibers and prevents cell damage by promoting DNA synthesis Flavonoids prevent or delay the onset of cell necrosis and also improve vascularity to the wounded area [179].

Several flavonoids, including quercetin, result in a reduction in ischemia-reperfusion injury through the activity of constitutive nitric-oxide synthase which is important in maintaining the dilation of blood vessels [209]. Quercetin, in particular, inhibits both cyclooxygenase and lipoxygenase activities, thus diminishing the formation of their inflammatory metabolites [210, 211].

Certain flavonoids, notably diosmin and hesperidin, have been used routinely in Europe for many years to treat varicose veins, hemorrhoids, and the edema that accompanies chronic venous insufficiency. These flavonoids have now been employed in the treatment of wounds. Purified micronized flavonoid fraction, comprising 90% diosmin and 10% hesperidin, is basically used as a phelebotonic and vasculoprotector agent. It also has anti-inflammatory and anti-edematous actions. In a clinical study, groups with infected wounds that were orally and topically treatment, accelerated wound healing when compared to the untreated control group. This was confirmed with surface area measurements and histopathological evaluation. This study showed that oral or topical administration of micronized flavonoid fraction in infected wounds is beneficial [212].

A flavonoid rich fraction of *Martynia annua* L. has also been shown to induce mature collagen fibers and promote fibroblasts with improved angiogenesis in an *in vivo* model [213]. Isovitexin and vitexin are the major flavonoid constituents of *Jatropha multifida* L. which is used commonly for the treatment of infected wounds and skin [214].

Flavonoids from *Vernonia arborea* and *Pentas lanceolata* have been reported to promote wound healing by their astringent and antimicrobial properties, which seems to be responsible for wound contraction and increased rate of epithelialization [215].

Martynia annua L. is a plant that has tannins, phenols, flavonoids, carbohydrates and antho-cyanins as its constituents [216]. A flavonoid rich fraction and luteolin isolated from *M. annua* was shown to improve wound healing in streptozotocin induced diabetic rats. The results showed that, percent wound contraction were significantly greater for the flavonoid rich fraction and luteolin-treated groups. Presence of matured collagen fibers and fibroblast with better angiogenesis were observed histopathologically in these groups [213].

8. Fats and oils with wound healing properties

Several unsaturated fatty acids such as oleic, linoleic, eicosapentanoic and arachidonic acids are among the natural ligands for perosisome proliferative activator receptors (PPAR) which are involved in wound healing. These PPAR are nuclear hormone receptors and are up regulated in keratinocytes after injury and have been found to be important regulators of re-epithelialization [217, 218]. Also ω-3 polyunsaturated fatty acids (PUFA) eicosapentaenoic acid (EPA) and docosahexaenoic acid (DHA) affect the synthesis and activity of proinflammatory cytokines which to a large extent initiate the inflammatory stage of wound healing [219, 220]. It can therefore be said that the presence of these fatty acids in plant extracts and other compounds could contribute to the survival and differentiation of keratinocytes through the activation of PPAR. Also they may promote the recovery of the epidermal barrier, skin homeostasis and anti-inflammatory activity to the skin during the wound healing process.

8.1. Eucalyptus oil (Dinkum oil)

This oil is obtained by steam distillation of fresh leaves of *Eucalyptus globules* which belongs to the family Myrtaceae. It is indigenous to Australia and Tasmania. It is cultivated in United States, Spain, Portugal and India. It contains eucalyptol, pinene, camphene, phellandrene, citronellal and geranyl acetates. In skin care, it is used to treat burns, blisters, herpes, cuts, wounds, skin infections and insect bites [221].

8.2. Aroeira (*Schinus terebinthifoliu*) oil

The aroeira tree (*Schinus terebinthifolius* Raddi.) belongs to the family Anacardiaceae and it is popularly known as Brazilian pepper, Florida Holly, rose pepper and Christmas berry. It is used to treat wounds and ulcers of skin and mucous membranes, against infections of the respiratory system, digestive system, genito-urinary tract, hemoptysis and metrorrhagia [222]. The essential oil of *S. terebinthifoliu* is obtained by hydro-distillation of crushed fresh leaves. Aroeira oil is reported to accelerate the healing process of wounds by significantly ($p < 0.01$) increasing contraction of oil-treated wounds in rats [223].

8.3. Virgin coconut oil

Cocos nucifera L. (Arecaceae), commonly known as coconut, is a palm, which thrives within the tropical zone. Its fresh kernel is consumed by people all over the world. Oil of *C. nucifera* which is extracted from the dried inner flesh of coconut [224] predominantly contains medium chain triglycerides, with 86.5% saturated fatty acids, 5.8% monounsaturated fatty acids, and 1.8% polyunsaturated fatty acids. Virgin coconut oil is also known to have antibacterial and antifungal properties [225, 226]. Excised wounds treated with virgin coconut oil healed much faster, as indicated by a decreased time of complete epithelization and increased in pepsin-soluble collagen, as well as an increase in fibroblast proliferation and neovascularization [227]. Also in burn wounds, there was improvement in wound contraction and decreased period of epithelialization when treated with coconut oil [224].

8.4. *Vitis vinifera* (grape) oil

Oil extracted from the seeds of grapes *Vitis vinifera* (Family Vitaceae) has been found to exhibit wound healing activity. In the excision wound model, grape oil-treated animals had increased wound area contraction and hydroxyproline content. Also histological analysis of the grape oil-treated wound tissue showed increased well organized collagen band [228].

8.5. *Vaccinium macrocarpon* (cranberry) oil

Vaccinium macrocarpon (family Ericaceae) is an evergreen creeping shrub native to North America [229]. Excision wounds on animals treated with cranberry oil showed faster rates of wound area contraction with higher hydroxyproline content. The cranberry oil-treated wound tissue had well organized bands of collagen [228].

8.6. *Melaleuca alternifolia* (Tea tree) oil

The essential oil derived from steam distillation of the leaves and terminal branches of *Melaleuca alternifolia* (family Myrtaceae) commonly known as tea tree [230], is composed of a mixture of monoterpenes, 1-terpinen-4-ol, cineole and other hydrocarbons. Tea tree oil possesses antimicrobial, anti-inflammatory and analgesic properties [231]. Tea tree oil has been reported to aid in healing of bacterial infected wounds, including diabetic wounds, character-ized by reduced healing time, rapid reduction in inflammation, pain and wound odor [232, 233].

8.7. *Vitellaria paradoxa* (Shea tree) oil

Vitellaria paradoxa (family Sapotaceae) commonly known as shea butter is an indigenous species of Sub-Saharan African [234]. The nuts and seeds are a very rich source of fats and oils, from which shea butter is derived. Shea butter is known to accelerate healing after circumcision [235]. The healing effect of shea butter may be attributed to the presence of allantoin, since it is a substance known to stimulate the growth of healthy tissues in ulcerous wounds [236].

8.8. Virgin fatty oil of *Pistacia lentiscus*

Pistacia lentiscus L. (Anacardiaceae) is a dioecious sclerophyllous evergreen species widely distributed along the Mediterranean basin. The essential oil of *P. lentiscus* obtained by hydro-distillation of leaves, fruits or trunk exudates called mastic gum [229] contains 73% unsaturated fatty acids (oleic and linoleic) and 25.8% saturated fatty acids (palmitic and stearic) and has been proven to exhibit antimicrobial, antioxidant, anti-inflammatory and antiatherogenic activities [237, 238]. The virgin fatty oil of *P. lentiscus* exhibited wound healing property in burn wound model in rabbits. *P. lentiscus* oil treated wounds showed higher wound contraction and faster time of healing as compared to the untreated wounds. *P. lentiscus* virgin fatty oil promoted significantly ($p < 0.05$) wound contraction and reduces epithelization period in rabbit model [239].

9. Miscellaneous substances

9.1. Wound healing properties of honey

Honey is a collection of nectar processed by honey bees [240]. It is rich in nutrients and defined substances such as glucose, fructose, sucrose, minerals, vitamins, antioxidants, amino acids and many other products, which may be responsible for its numerous therapeutic roles and potency [241]. Its therapeutic properties include antimicrobial activity which may be attributed to its osmotic effect, a naturally low pH, and the production of hydrogen peroxide [242, 243]. Honey attacks antibiotic-resistant strains of bacteria and prevents bacterial growth even when wounds are heavily infected [244]. Again, honey has been reported to exhibit antioxidant activity [245, 246]. In wound care, honey has been used extensively as wound healing agent for almost all kinds of wounds. It has been assessed for the treatment of venous leg ulcers, burns, chronic leg ulcers, pressure ulcers, as well as diabetic wound [247], with scarless healing in cavity wounds, less edema, fewer polymorphonuclear and mononuclear cell infiltrations, less necrosis, better wound contraction, improved epithelialization, lower glycosaminoglycan and proteoglycan concentrations, increased granulation tissue formation and tissue growth, collagen synthesis and development of new blood vessels in the bed of wounds [241].

10. Conclusion

Most of these medicinal plants and natural products traditionally used for the treatment and management of these various types of wounds had their wound healing properties, including wound contraction, tensile strength, antioxidant and antimicrobial activities, hydroxyproline content assay and histological investigations namely re-epithelization, collagen synthesis, granulation, proliferation and differentiation of fibroblasts and keratinocytes, assessed and evaluated through *in vitro* and *in vivo* model studies. Hence there is a need to subject these products to both primary and advanced clinical studies with specific types of wounds to ascertain or confirm the reported wound healing properties. These trials must be done after safety profiles of these products have been determined.

Author details

Christian Agyare[1*], Emelia Oppong Bekoe[2], Yaw Duah Boakye[1], Susanna Oteng Dapaah[1], Theresa Appiah[1] and Samuel Oppong Bekoe[3]

*Address all correspondence to: cagyare.pharm@knust.edu.gh; chrisagyare@yahoo.com

1 Department of Pharmaceutics, Faculty of Pharmacy and Pharmaceutical Sciences, Kwame Nkrumah University of Science and Technology, Kumasi, Ghana

2 Department of Pharmaceutics and Pharmaceutical Microbiology, School of Pharmacy, University of Ghana, Legon, Accra, Ghana

3 Department of Pharmaceutical Chemistry, Faculty of Pharmacy and Pharmaceutical Sciences, Kwame Nkrumah University of Science and Technology, Kumasi, Ghana

References

[1] Ramzi SC, Vinay K, Stanley R. Pathologic Basis of Diseases, 5th ed., WB Saunders Company, Philadelphia; 1994. p. 86.

[2] Strodtbeck F. Physiology of wound healing. Newborn Infant Nurs Rev. 2001; 1: 43–45.

[3] Mathieu D, Linke JC, Wattel F. Non-healing wounds. In: Handbook on hyperbaric medicine, Mathieu DE (ed). Netherlands: Springer; 2006; p. 812.

[4] Menke NB, Ward KR, Witten TM, Bonchev DG, Diegelmann RF. Impaired wound healing. Clin Dermatol. 2007; 25: 19–25.

[5] Nelzen O, Bergqvist D, Lindhagen A. The prevalence of chronic lower-limb ulceration has been underestimated: results of a validated population questionnaire. Br J Surg. 1996; 83: 255–258.

[6] Baranoski S, Ayello EA. Wound dressings: an evolving art and science. Adv Skin Wound Care. 2012; 25: 87–92.

[7] Benbow M. Debridement: wound bed preparation. J Community Nurs. 2011; 25: 18–23.

[8] MacDonald J. Global initiative for wounds and lymphedema. J Lymphedema. 2009; 4: 92–95.

[9] Houghton PJ, Hylands PJ, Mensah AY, Hensel A, Deters A. *In vitro* tests and ethnopharmacological investigations: wound healing as an example. J Ethnopharmacol. 2005; 100: 100–107.

[10] Agyare C, Asase A, Lechtenberg M, Niehues M, Deters A, Hensel A. An ethnopharmacological survey and *in vitro* confirmation of ethnopharmacological use of medicinal

plants used for wound healing in Bosomtwi-Atwima-Kwanwoma area, Ghana. J Ethnopharmacol. 2009; 125: 393–403.

[11] Davidson JM. Animal models for wound repair. Archives Derm Res. 1998; 290: 1–11.

[12] Dorsett-Martin WA, Wysocki AB. Rat models of skin wound healing. In: Source Book of Models for Biomedical Research, Humana Press; 2008. p. 778.

[13] Gal P, Kilik R, Mokry M, Vidinsky B, Vasilenko T, Mozes S, Lenhardt L. Simple method of open skin wound healing model in corticosteroid-treated and diabetic rats: standardization of semi-quantitative and quantitative histological assessments. Vet Med. 2008; 53: 652–659.

[14] Gottrup F, Argen MS, Karlsmark T. Models for use in wound healing research: a survey focusing on *in vitro* and *in vivo* adult soft tissue. Wound Repair Regen. 2000; 8: 83–96.

[15] Tarnuzzer RW, Schultz GS. Biochemical analysis of acute and chronic wound environments. Wound Repair Regen. 1996; 4: 321–325.

[16] Agyare C, Bempah SB, Boakye YD, Ayande PG, Adarkwa-Yiadom M, Mensah KB. Evaluation of antimicrobial and wound healing potential of *Justicia flava* and *Lannea welwitschii*. Evid Based Complement Altern. 2013. Article ID 632927, 10 pp.

[17] Burkill HM. 1985. The Useful Plants of Tropical West Africa. Royal Kew Botanical Gardens K, London, UK; 1985; pp. 293–295.

[18] Shubhashini S, Kantha DA. Investigations on the phytochemica activities and wound healing properties of *Adhatoda vasica* leave in Swiss albino mice. Afr J Plant Sci.2011; 5(2): 133–145.

[19] Fikru A ME, Eguale T, Debella A, Mekonnen GA. Evaluation of *in vivo* wound healing activity of methanol extract of *Achyranthes aspera* L. J Ethnopharmacol. 2012; 143: 469–474.

[20] Barua CC, Talakdar A, Barua AG, Chakraborty A, Sarma RK, Bora RS. Evaluation of the wound healing activity of methanolic extract of *Azadirachta Indica* (Neem) and *Tinospora cordifolia* (Guduchi) in rats. Pharmacologyonline. 2010; 1: 70–77.

[21] Hossain AI, Faisal M, Rahman S, Jahan R, Rahmatullah M. A preliminary evaluation of antihyperglycemic and analgesic activity of *Alternanthera sessilis* aerial parts. BMC Complement Altern Med. 2014; 14: 169.

[22] Jalalpure SS, Arawal N, Patil MB, Chimkode R, Tripathi A. Antimicrobial and wound healing activities of leaves of *Alternanthera sessilis* Linn. Int J Green Pharm. 2008; 2: 141–144.

[23] Ullah MO, Haque M, Urmi KF, Zulfiker AH, Anita ES, Begum M, Hamid K, Uddin SJ. Anti-bacterial activity and brine shrimp lethality bioassay of methanolic extracts of

fourteen different edible vege's from Bangladesh. Asian Pac J Trop Biomed. 2013; 3: 1–7.

[24] Neeharika V, Fatima H, Reddy BM. Evaluation of antinociceptive and antipyretic effect of Pupalia lappacea Juss. Int Curr Pharm J. 2013; 2: 23–28.

[25] Apenteng JA, Agyare C, Adu F, Ayande PG, Boakye YD. Evaluation of wound healing potential of different leaf extracts of *Pupalia lappacea*. Afr J Pharm Pharmacol. 2014; 8: 1039–1048.

[26] Udegbunam SO, Udegunam RI, Muogbo CC, Ayamwu MV, Nwaehugor CO.Wound healing and antibacterial properties of methanolic extract of *Pupulia lappacea* Juss in rats. BMC Complement Altern Med. 2014; 14: 157.

[27] Siddiqui MZ, Chowhury, Prasad N, Thomas M. Buchanania lanzan: a species of enormous potentials. World J Pharm Sci. 2014; 2: 374–379.

[28] Pattnaik A, Sarkar R, Sharma A, Yadav KK, Kumar A, Roy P, Sen T. Pharmacological studies on Buchanania lanzan Spreng.-A focus on wound healing with particular reference to anti-biofilm properties. Asian Pac J Trop Biomed. 2013; 3: 967–974.

[29] Chitra V, Dharabu PP, Pavan KK, Alla NR. Wound healing activity of alcoholic extract of *Buchanania lanzan* in Albino rats. Int J ChemTech Res. 2009; 1: 1026–1031.

[30] Jamil SS, Nizami Q, Salam M. Centella asiatica (Linn.) Urban: a review. Nat Prod Radiance. 2007; 6: 158–170.

[31] Bylka W, Znajdek-Awiżeń P, Studzińska-Sroka E, Brzezińska M. *Centella asiatica* in cosmetology. Postepy Dermatol Alergol. 2013; 30: 46–49.

[32] Bylka W, Znajdek-Awiżeń P, Studzińska-Sroka E, Dańczak-Pazdrowska A, Brzezińska M. Centella asiatica in dermatology: an overview. Phytother Res. 2014; 28: 1117–1124.

[33] Shukla A, Rasik AM, Jain GK, Shankar R, Kulshrestha DK, Dhawan BN. *In vitro* and *in vivo* wound healing activity of asiaticoside isolated from *Centella asiatica*. J Ethnopharmacol. 1999; 65: 1–11.

[34] Rechinger KH. Flora Iranica, Apiaceae. Academische Druck-U-Verganstalt. Graz: Austria. 1981; 162: 140–142.

[35] Mozaffarian V. A Dictionary of Iranian Plant Names. Tehran: Farhang Moaser Publisher; 1996. p. 739.

[36] Gohari AR, Saeidnia SA. Review on Phytochemistry of *Cuminum cyminum* seeds and its standards from field to market. Pharmacognosy J. 2011; 3: 1–5.

[37] Patil DN KA, Shahapurkar AA, Hatappakki BC. Natural cumin seeds for wound healing activity in albino rats. Int J Biol Chem. 2009; 3: 148–152.

[38] Nayak BS, Pinto-Pereira ML. Catharanthus roseus flower extract has wound-healing activity in Sprague Dawley rats. BMC Compliment Altern Med. 2006; 6: 41–39.

[39] Krasner DL RG, Sibbald RG. Chronic wound care: A Clinical source book for health professionals, HMP Communications, Malvern, Ala, USA, 4th ed.; 1990.

[40] Agyare C, Dwobeng AS, Agyepong N, Boakye YD, Mensah KB, Ayande PG, Adarkwa-Yiadom M. Antimicrobial, antioxidant, and wound healing properties of *Kigelia africana* (Lam.) Beneth. and *Strophanthus hispidus* DC. Adv Pharmacol Sci. 2013. Article ID 692613, 10 pp.

[41] Singh VP, Sharma SK, Kare VS. Medicinal plants from Ujjain District Madhya Pradesh, Indian Drugs. 1980; 17: 7–12.

[42] Shah GL, Gopal GV. Ethnomedical notes from the tribal inhabitants of the north Gujarat (India). J Ecotoxicol Bot. 1988; 6: 193–221.

[43] Joshi MC, Patel MB, Mehta PJ. Some folk medicines of Dangs, Gujarat State. Bull Med Ethnobot Res. 1980; 1: 8–24.

[44] Veerapur VP, Palkar MB, Srinivasa H, Kumar MS, Patra S, Rao PGM, Srinivasan KK. The effect of ethanol extract of *Wrightia tinctoria* bark on wound healing in rats. J Nat Prod. 2004; 4: 155–159.

[45] Omale J, Ubimago UOTG. In-vitro anthelmintic activity of *Saba florida* (Benth) extracts against Nigerian adult earth worm (*Terrestris lumbricoides*). Am J Phytomed Clin Ther. 2014; 2(6), 758–766.

[46] Omale J, Victoria IA. Excision and incision wound healing potential of *Saba florida* (Benth) leaf extract in *Rattus novergicus*. Int J Pharm Biomed Res. 2010; 1: 101–107.

[47] Ahmed KKM, Rana AC, Dixit VK. *Calotropis* species (Ascelpediaceae) – A comprehensive review. Pharmacog Mag. 2005; 1: 48–52.

[48] Chitme HR, GhobadiR, Chandra M, Kaushik S. Studies on anti-diarrhoeal activity of *Calotropis gigantea* R. Br. in experimental animals. J Pharm Pharm. Sci. 2004; 7: 70–75.

[49] Argal A, Pathak AK. Antidiarrhoeal activity of *Calotropis gigantea* flowers. Indian J Nat Prod. 2005; 21: 42–44.

[50] Deshmukh PT, Fernandes J, Atul A, Toppo E. Wound healing activity of *Calotropis gigantea* root bark in rats. J Ethnopharmacol. 2009; 125; 178–181.

[51] Parsons WT, Cuthbertson EG. Noxious weeds of Australia. CSIRO Publishing; 2001. 712.

[52] Rasik MA, Raghubir R, Gupta A, Shukla A, Dubey MP, Srivastava S, Jain HK, Kulshrestha KD. Healing potential of *Calotropis procera* on dermal wounds in guinea pigs. J Ethnopharmacol. 1999; 68: 261–266.

[53] Akkol EK, Koca U, Pesin I, Yilmazer D. Evaluation of the wound healing potential of *Achillea biebersteinii* Afan.(Asteraceae) by *in vivo* excision and incision models. Evid-Based Complement Altern Med. 2011. Article ID 474026, 7 pp., 2011.

[54] Almagboul AZ, Farroq AA, Tyagi BR. Antimicrobial properties of certain Sudanese plants used in folk medicine: screening for antibacterial activity part 2. Fitoterapia. 1985; 56: 103–109.

[55] Ekundayo OS, Sharma S, Rao EV. Essential oils of *Ageratum conyzoides*. Linn Planta Med. 1987; 54: 55–57.

[56] Borthakur N, Baruah AKS. Search for precocenes in *Ageratum conyzoides* L. of Northeast India. J India Chem Soc. 1987; 64: 580–581.

[57] Watt JM, Breyer-Brandwijk MG. The medicinal and poisonous plants of South and Eastern Africa.197–8. 2nd Edn. London. E&S Livingstone Ltd., London, UK; 1962. 1457.

[58] Oladejo OW, Imosemi IO, Osuagwu FC, Oluwadara OO, Aiku A, Adewoyin O, Ekpo OE, Oyedele OO, Akang EEU. Enhancement of cutaneous wound healing by methanolic extracts of *Ageratum conyzoides* in the Wistar rat. Afr J Biomed Res. 2003; 6: 27–31.

[59] De Rouw DEA. The fallow period as weed-break in shifting cultivation (tropical wet forests). Agric Ecosys Environ. 1995; 54: 31–43.

[60] Olaoye SOA. *Chromolaena odorata* in the tropics and its control in Nigeria. In: Moody K. (Ed.) Weed control in tropical crops. Volume II. Weed Science Society of the Los Banos, Philippines, 1986, pp. 279–293.

[61] Phan T, Wang Lee, See P, Grayer JR, Chan S, Lee ST. Phenolic compounds of *Chromolaena odorata* protect cultured skin cells from oxidative damage: implication for cutaneous wound healing. Biol Pharm Bull. 2001; 24: 1373–1379.

[62] Koca U, Suntar PI, Keles H, Yesilada E, Akkol EK. *In vivo* anti-inflammatory and wound healing activities of *Centaurea iberica* Trev. ex Spreng. J Ethnopharmacol. 2009; 126: 551–556.

[63] Nadkarni AK. Indian Materia Medica. Popular Prakashan Private Limited. Bombay: 3rd ed; 2007. 1163.

[64] Chopra RN, Nayar SL., Chopra IC. Glossary of Indian Medicinal Plants, Publications and Information Directorate, CSIR, New Delhi; 1956. 88–89.

[65] Kirtikar KR, Basu BD. Dehra Dun: International Book Distributors. Indian Medicinal Plants; 1999; 1347.

[66] Sadaf F, Saleem R, Ahmed M, Ahmad SI. Healing potential of cream containing extract of *Sphaeranthus indicus* on dermal wounds in guinea pigs. J Ethnopharmacol. 2006, 107: 161–163.

[67] Udupa AL, Kulkarni DR, Udupa SL. Effect of *Tridax Procumbens* on wound healing. Pharm Biol. 1995; 33: 37–40.

[68] Yaduvanshi B, Mathur R, Mathur SR, Velpandian T. Evaluation of wound healing potential of topical formulation of leaf juice of *Tridax procumbens* L. in mice. Indian J Pharm Sci. 2011; 73: 303–306.

[69] Yogesh PT, Biswaddeep D, Tania P, Deeali YT, Kishori GA, Pradeep BP. Evaluation of wound healing potential of aqueous and ethanolic extracts of *Tridax procubens* Linn. in Wistar Rat. Asian J Pharm Clin Res. 2012; 5: 4, 141–145.

[70] Leach MJ. Calendula officinalis and wound healing: A Systematic review. Wounds. 2008; 20: 236–243.

[71] Preethi KC, Kuttan R. Wound healing activity of flower extract of *Calendula offlcinalis*. J Basic Clin Physiol Pharmacol. 2009; 20: 73–80.

[72] Irvine FR. Woody Plants of Ghana. Oxford University Press, Oxford, UK 1961. 868.

[73] Houghton PJ. Tesausage tree (*Kigelia pinnata*): Ethnobotany and recent scientific work. S Afr J Bot. 2002; 68: 14–20.

[74] Picerno P AG, Marzocco S, Meloni M, Sanogo R, Aquino RP. Anti-inflammatory activity of verminoside from *Kigelia africana* and evaluation of cutaneous irritation in cell cultures and reconstituted human epidermis. J Nat Prod. 2005; 68: 1610–1614.

[75] Mensah AY, Fleischer TC, Adu F, Agyare C, Ameade AE. Antimicrobial and antioxidant properties of two Ghanaian plants used traditionally for wound healing. J Pharm Pharmacol. 2003; 55: S-4.

[76] Ofori-Kwakye K KA, Bayor MT. Wound healing potential of methanol extract of *Spathodea campanulata* stem bark formulated into a topical preparation. Afr J Trad Complement Altern Med. 2011; 8: 218–223.

[77] Saini NK SM, Srivastava B. Evaluation of wound healing activity of *Tecomaria capensis* leaves. Chin J Nat Med. 2012; 10: 138–141.

[78] Iwu MM. Handbook of African medicinal plants. CRC Press BR, Florida, United States; 1993. p. 464.

[79] Sofowora A. Medicinal plants and traditional medicines in Africa. New York CJ, Wiley & Sons, UK; 1993. p. 320.

[80] Dash GK, Murthy PN. Evaluation of *Argemone mexicana* L. leaves for wound healing activity. J Nat Prod Plant Res. 2011; 1: 46–56.

[81] Butera D, Tosoriere L, Di Gaudio F, Bongiorno A, Allegra M, Pintaudi AM, Kohen R, Livrea M. A. Antioxidant activities of sicilian prickly pear (*Opuntia ficus indica*) fruit extracts and reducing properties of its betalains: Betanin and indicaxanthin. J Agric Food Chem. 2002; 50: 6895–6901.

[82] Hassan F, El-RazekA, Hassan AA. Nutritional value and hypoglycemic effect of prickly cactus pear (*Opuntia Ficus-Indica*) fruit juice in alloxan-induced diabetic rats. Aust J Basic Appl Sci. 2012; 5: 356–377.

[83] Galati EM, Mondello MR, Giufferida D, Dugo G, Miceli N, Pergolizzi S, Taviano MF. Chemical characterization and biological effects of Sicilian *Opuntia ficus indica* (L.) Mill. Fruit juice: antioxidant and antiulcerogenic activity. J Agric Food Chem. 2003; 51: 4903–4908.

[84] Park EH, Chun MJ. Wound healing activity of *Opuntia ficus indica*. J Ethnopharmacol. 2001; 72: 165–167.

[85] Trombetta D, Puglia C, Perri D, Licata A, Pergolizzi S, Lauriano ER, Bonina FP. Effect of polysaccharides from *Opuntia ficus-indica* (L.) cladodes on the healing of dermal wounds in the rat. Phytomedicine. 2006; 13: 352–358.

[86] Burkill HM. The Useful Plants of West Tropical Africa ne, vol 3:11, Royal Kew Botanical Gardens, Kew, London, UK; 1995. 868p.

[87] Mahmood AA, Sidik K, Salmah I. Wound healing activity of *Carica papaya* L. aqueous leaf extract in rats. Int J Mol Med Adv Sci. 2005; 1: 398–401.

[88] Nayak BS, Pereira LP, Maharaj D. Wound healing activity of *Carica papaya* L. in experimentally induced diabetic rats. Indian J Exp Biol. 2007; 45: 739.

[89] Gurung S, Škalko-Basnet N. Wound healing properties of *Carica papaya* latex: in vivo evaluation in mice burn model. J Ethnopharmacol. 2009; 121: 338–341.

[90] Agyare C, Ansah AO, Ossei PPS, Apenteng JA, Boakye YD. Wound healing and anti-infective properties of *Myrianthus arboreus* and *Alchornea cordifolia*. Med Chem. 2014; 4: 533–539.

[91] Chaudhari M, Mengi S. Evaluation of phytoconstituents of *Terminalia arjuna* for wound healing activity in rats. Phytother Res. 2006; 20: 799–805.

[92] Kisseih E, Lechtenber M, Petereit F, Sendker J, Brandt S, Agyare C, Hensel A. Phyto-chemical characterization and in vitro wound healing activity of leaf extracts from *Combretum mucronatum* Schum. & Thonn.: Oligomeric procyanidins as strong inductors of cellular differentiation. J Ethnopharmacol. 2015; 174: 628–636.

[93] Khan M, Patil PA, Shobha JC. Influence of *Bryophyllum pinnatum* (Lim.) leaf extract on wound healing in albino rats. J Nat Remedies. 2004; 4: 41–46.

[94] Agyare C, Amuah E, Adarkwa-Yiadom M, Osei-Asante S, Ossei SPP. Medicinal plants used for the treatment of wounds and skin infections: assessment of wound healing and antimicrobial properties of *Mallotus oppositifolius* and *Momordica charantia*. Int J Phytomedicine. 2014; 6: 50–58.

[95] Gordon-Gray KD. Cyperaceae in Natal. National Botanical Institute P, South Africa; 1995. p. 218.

[96] Chopra RN, Chopra IC, Varma BS. Glossary of Indian Medicinal Plants, CSIR, New Delhi; 1969. p. 119.

[97] Puratchikody A, Devi CN, Nagalakshmi G. Wound healing activity of *Cyperus rotundus* Linn Indian J Pharm Sci. 2006; 68: 97–101.

[98] Agyare C, Lechntenberg M, Deters A, Petereit F, Hensel A. Ellagitannins from Phyllanthus muellerianus (Kuntze) Exell.: Geraniin and furosin stimulate cellular activity, differentiation and collagen synthesis of human skin keratinocytes and dermal fibroblasts. Phytomedicine. 2011; 18: 617–624.

[99] Gonasekera MM, Gunawardan VK, Mohammed SG, Balasubramania S. Pregnancy terminating effects of *Jatropha curcas* in rats. J Ethnopharmacol. 1995; 47: 117–123.

[100] Igoli JO, Ogaji D. Tor-Anyim TA, Igoli NP.Traditional Medicine practice among the Igede people of Nigeria. Afr J Trad Compliment Altern Med. 2005; 2: 134–152.

[101] Shetty S, Udupa L. Evaluation of antioxidant and wound healing effects of alcoholic and aqueous extract of *Ocimum sanctum* Linn in rats. Evid-Based Complement Altern Med. 2008; 5: 95–101.

[102] Zippel J, Wells T, Hensel A. Arabinogalactan protein from Jatropha curcas L. seeds as TGFβ1-mediated inductor of keratinocyte in vitro differentiation and stimulation of GM-CSF, HGF, KGF and in organotypic skin equivalents. Fitoterapia. 2010; 81: 772–778.

[103] Kabran FA, Maciuk A, Okpekon TA, Leblanc K, Seon-Meniel B, Bories C, Champy P, Djakouré L A, Figadère B. Phytochemical and biological analysis of *Mallotus oppositifolius* (Euphorbiaceae). Planta Med. 2012; 78: 1381.

[104] Lodhi S, Pawar RS, Jain AP, Singhai AK. Wound healing potential of *Tephrosia purpurea* (Linn.) Pers. in rats. J Ethnopharmacol. 2006; 108: 204–210.

[105] Chularojmontri L, Suwatronnakorn M, Wattanapitayakul SK. *Phyllanthus emblica* L. enhances human umbilical vein endothelial wound healing and sprouting. Evid-Based Complement Altern Med. 2013. Article ID 720728, 9 pp., 2013.

[106] Kokane DD, More YR, Kale BM, Nehete NM, Mehendale CP, Gadgol HC. Evaluation of wound healing activity of root of *Mimosa pudica*. J Ethnopharmacol. 2009; 124: 311–315.

[107] Sivagamy M, Jeganathan, Manavalan R, Senthamarai R. Wound healing activity of *Indigofera enneaphylla* Linn. Int J Adv Pharm Chem Biol. 2012; 1: 211–214.

[108] Umachigi SP, Jayaveera KN, Kumar CA, Kumar GS, Kumar DK. Studies on wound healing properties of *Quercus infectoria*. Trop J Pharm Res. 2008; 7: 913–919.

[109] Oommen ST, Rao M, Raju CVN. Effect of oil of Hydnocarpus on wound healing1. Int J Lepr Other Mycobact Dis. 1999; 67: 154.

[110] Oommen ST. The effect of oil of hydnocarpus on excision wounds. Int J Lepr Other Mycobact Dis. 2000; 68: 69–70.

[111] Dokosi OB. Herbs of Ghana. Ghana Universities Press; 1998. p. 765.

[112] Annan K, Dickson R. Evaluation of wound healing actions of *Hoslundia opposita* Vahl, *Anthocleista nobilis* G. Don. and *Balanites aegyptiaca* L. J Sci Tech (Ghana), 2008; 28(2): 26–35.

[113] Bairy KL, Rao CM. Wound healing profiles of *Ginkgo biloba*. J Nat Remedies. 2001; 1: 25–27.

[114] Baruah A, Sarma D, Saud J, Singh RS. In vitro regeneration of *Hypericum patulum* Thunb.-A medicinal plant. Indian J Experiment Biol. 2001; 39: 947–949.

[115] Mukherjee KP, Verpoorte R, Suresh B. Evaluation of *in-vivo* wound healing activity of *Hypericum patulum* (Family: Hypericaceae) leaf extract on different wound model in rats. J Ethnopharmacol. 2000; 70: 315–321.

[116] Gleason HA, Cronquist A. Manual of Vascular Plants of Northeastern United States and Adjacent Canada. 2nd ed. Bronx, NY: The New York Botanical Garden; 1991. 810.

[117] Süntar IP, Akkol EK, Yılmazer D, Baykal T, Kırmızıbekmez H, Alper M, Yeşilada E. Investigations on the in vivo wound healing potential of *Hypericum perforatum* L. J Ethnopharmacol. 2010; 127: 468–477.

[118] Prisăcaru AI, Andritoiu CV, Andriescu C, Hăvârneanu EC, Popa M, Motoc AGM, Sava A. Evaluation of the wound-healing effect of a novel *Hypericum perforatum* ointment in skin injury. Rom J Morphol Embryol. 2013; 54: 1053–1059.

[119] Laeuchli S, Vannotti S, Hafner J, Hunziker T, French L. A Plant-derived wound therapeutic for cost-effective treatment of post-surgical scalp wounds with exposed one. Res Complement Med. 2014; 21: 88–93.

[120] Mainetti S, Carnevali F. An experience with pediatric burn wounds treated with a plant-derived wound therapeutic. J Wound Care. 2013; 22: 681–689.

[121] Godhwani S, Godhwani JL, Vyas DS. *Ocimum sanctum* – a preliminary study evaluating its immunoregulatory profile in albino rats. J Ethnopharmacol. 1988; 24: 193–198.

[122] Goel A, Kumar S, Singh DK, Bhatia AK. Wound healing potential of *Ocimum sanctum* Linn. with induction of tumor necrosis factor-alpha. Indian J. Exp. Biol. 2010; 48: 402–406.

[123] Osuagwu FC, Oladepo OW, Imosemi IO, Adewoyin BA, Adewoyin OO, Ekpe OE, Olumadara OO. Wound healing activities of methanolic extracts of *Ocimum gratissum* leaf in Wistar rats – a preliminary study. Afr J Med Sci. 2004; 33: 23–26.

[124] Chah KF, Eze CA, Emuelosi CE, Esimone CO. Antibacterial and wound healing properties of methanolic extracts of some Nigerian medicinal plants. J Ethnopharmacol. 2006; 104: 164–167.

[125] Abbiw DK. Useful plants of Ghana: West African uses of wild and cultivated plants. Intermediate Technology Publications and The Royal Botanic Gardens; Kew, UK 1990. p. 337.

[126] Olajide OA, Oladiran OO, Awo SO, Makinde JM. Pharmacological evaluation of *Hoslundia opposita*. Phytother. Res. 1998; 12: 364–366.

[127] Moshi MJ, Kagashe GA, Mwambo ZH. Plants used to treat epilepsy in Tanzanian tradition. J Ethnopharmacol. 2005; 97: 327–336.

[128] Shirwaikar A, Shenoy R, Udupa AL, Udupa SL, Shetty S. Wound healing property of ethanolic extract of leaves of *Hyptis suaveolens* with supportive role of antioxidant enzymes. Indian J Exp Biol. 2003; 41: 238–241.

[129] Shenoy C, Patil MB, Kumar R, Patil S. Preliminary phytochemical investigation and wound healing activity of *Allium cepa* Linn. (Liliaceae). Int J Pharm Pharm Sci. 2009; 2: 167–175.

[130] Mukerjee SK. *A revision of the Labiatae of the Indian Empire* (Doctoral dissertation), University of Edinburgh.

[131] Ryding O. Phylogeny of the Leucas Group (Lamiaceae). Syst Botany. 1998; 23: 235–247.

[132] Williamson EM. Major herbs of Ayurveda L, Churchill Livingstone, UK; 2002. p. 361.

[133] Manjunatha BK, Vidya SM, Krishna V, Mankani KL. Wound healing activity of *Leucas hirta*. Indian J Pharm Sci. 2006; 68: 380–384.

[134] Dahanukar SA, Kulkarni RA, Rege NN. Pharmacology of medicinal plants and natural products. Indian J Pharmacol. 2000; 32: S81–S118.

[135] Nayak BS, Isitor G, Davis EM, Pillai GK. The evidence based wound healing activity of *Lawsonia inermis* Linn. Phytother Res. 2007; 21(9): 827–831.

[136] Chidambara MKN, Vittal KR, Jyothi MV, Uma DM. Study on wound healing activity of *Punica granatum* peel. J Med Food. 2004; 7: 256–259.

[137] Kumar A, Singh A. Review on Hibiscus Rosa sinensis. Int J Res Pharm Biomed Sci., 2012; 3: 534–538.

[138] Nayak BS, Raju SS, Eversley M, Ramsubhag A. Evaluation of wound healing activity of *Lantana camara* L. – a preclinical study. Phytother Res. 2009; 23: 241–245.

[139] Bhaskar A, Nithya V. Evaluation of the wound-healing activity of *Hibiscus rosa sinensis* L. (Malvaceae) in Wistar albino rats. Indian J Pharmacol. 2012; 44: 694–698.

[140] Shivakumar H, Prakash T, Rao RN, Swamy BJ, Nagappa AN. Wound healing activity of the leaves of *Thespesia populnea*. J Nat Remedies. 2007; 7: 120–124.

[141] Nayak SB KJ, Milne MD, Pinto-Pereira L, Swanston HW. Extract of *Carapa guianensis* L. Leaf for its wound healing activity using three wound models. Evid-Based Complement Altern Med. 2011, Article ID 419612, 6 pp.

[142] Hukkeri VI, Nagathan CV, Karadi RV, Patil BS. Antipyretic and wound healing activities of *Moringa oleifera* Lam. in rats. Indian J Pharm Sci. 2006; 68:124–126.

[143] Pandey IP, Ahmed SF, Chhimwal S, Pandey S. Chemical composition and wound healing activity of volatile oil of leaves of *Azadirachta indica* A. Juss. Adv Pure Appl Chem. 2012; 1: 62–66.

[144] Roy K, Shivakumar, Sarkar S. Wound healing potential of leaf extracts of *Ficus religiosa* on Wistar albino strain rats. Int J Pharm Tech Res, 2009; 1: 506–508.

[145] Kirtikar KR, Basu BD. In; Indian Medicinal Plants, 1st edn. Vol. III, International Book Publishers, Dehradun; 1980; 676.

[146] Chopra RN. In: Indigenous Drugs of India, 2nd edn., Vol. I. Academic Publishers, Kolkata; 1993; 792.

[147] Rahman MM. Bangladesh: (IUCN) International Union for Conservation of Nature. Invasive plants of Sundarbans. Interim report under SBCP Project; 2003. p.132.

[148] Goel RK KSA-udfisweoMs, Tamrab hasma, *Asparagus racemosus* and *Zingiber officinale*. Indian J Pharmacol. 2002; 34: 100–110.

[149] Agarwal PK, Singh A, Gaurav K, Goel S, Khanna HD, Goel RK. Evaluation of wound healing activity of extracts of plantain banana (*Musa sapientum* var. *paradisiaca*) in rats. Indian J Exp Biol. 2009; 47:32–34.

[150] Lal B, Mishra N. Importance of *Embelia ribes*: An update. Int J Pharm Sci Res. 2013; 4: 3823–3838.

[151] Kumara SHM, Krishna V, Shankarmurthy K, Abdul RB, Mankani KL, Mahadevan KM, Harish BG, Raja NH. Wound healing activity of embelin isolated from the ethanol extract of leaves of *Embelia ribes* Burm. J Ethnopharmacol. 2007; 109: 529–534.

[152] Mittal A, Satish SS, Anima P. Evaluation of wound healing, antioxidant and antimicrobial efficacy of *Jasminum auriculatum* Vahl. leaves. Avicenna J Phytomed. 2015: 1–11.

[153] Chaturvedi AP, Kumar M, Tripathi YB. Efficacy of *Jasminum grandiflorum* L. leaf extract on dermal wound healing in rats. Int Wound J. 2013; 10: 675–682.

[154] Rajvaidhya S, Nagori BP, Singh GK, Dubey BK, Desai P, Jain S. A review on *Argemone mexicana* Linn.-an Indian medicinal plant. Int J Pharm Sci Res. 2012; 3: 2494–2504.

[155] Kiran K, Asad M. Wound healing activity of *Sesamum indicum* L. seed and oil in rats. Ind. J Exp Bio. 2008; 46: 777–782.

[156] Parmer VS JS, Bisht KS. Phytochemistry of genus *Piper*, Phytochemistry. 1997; 46: 597–673.

[157] Santhanam G, Nagarajan S. Wound healing activity of *Curcuma aromatica* and *Piper betle*. Fitoterapia. 1990; 61: 458–459.

[158] Rubatzky VE, Yamaguchi M. World vegetables: principles, production and nutritive values. 2nd edn. Chapman & Hall, New York, United States; 1997. p. 843.

[159] P Phillips SM. Portulacaceae. In: Beentje, H.J. (Ed). Flora of Tropical East Africa. A.A. Balkema, Rotterdam, Netherlands; 2002; p. 40.

[160] Rashed NA, Afifi UF, Disi AM. Simple evaluation of the wound healing activity of a crude extract of *Portulaca oleracea* L. (growing in Jordan) in *Mus musculus* JVI-1. J Ethnopharmacol. 2003; 88:131–136.

[161] Pennington TD. The genera of Sapotaceae. Royal Botanic Gardens K, Richmond, United Kingdom and the New York Botanical Garden, New York, United States; 1991. p. 307.

[162] Adetutu A, Morgan WA, Corcoran O. Ethnopharmacological survey and *in vitro* evaluation of wound-healing plants used in South-western Nigerian. J Ethnopharmacol. 2011; 137: 50–56.

[163] Nayak BS, Sandiford S, Maxwell A. Evaluation of the wound-healing activity of ethanolic extract of *Morinda citrifolia* L. Leaf. Evid-Based Complement Altern Med. 2009; 6: 351–356.

[164] Nayak SB, Vinuta B, Geetha B, Sudha B. Experimental evaluation of *Pentas lanceolata* flowers for wound healing activity in rats. Fitoterapia. 2005; 76: 671–675.

[165] Karodi, Jadhav M, Rub R, Bafna A. Evaluation of the wound healing activity of a crude extract of *Rubia cordifolia* L. (Indian madder) in mice. Int J Appl Res Nat Prod. 2009; 2: 12–18.

[166] Jaswanth A, Sathya S, Ramu S, Puratchikody A, Ruckmani K. Effect of root extract of *Aegle marmelos* on dermal wound healing in rats. Anc Sci life. 2001; 20: 111.

[167] Gautam MK, Purohit V, Agarwal M, Singh A, Goel RK. In vivo healing potential of *Aegle marmelos* in excision, incision, and dead space wound models. Sci World J. 2014. Article ID 740107, 9 pp.

[168] Lemmens RHMJ. *Mimusops elengi* L. In: Louppe D, Oteng-Amoako, A. A., Brink, M. (Editors). Prota 7(1): Timbers/Bois d'œuvre 1 [CD-Rom]. PROTA, Wageningen, Netherlands; 2005.

[169] Shah PJ, Gandhi MS, Shah MB, Goswami SS, Santani D. Study of *Mimusops elengi* bark in experimental gastric ulcers. J Ethnopharmacol. 2003; 89: 305–311.

[170] Gupta N, Jain UK. Investigation of wound healing activity of methanolic extract of stem bark of *Mimusops elengi* Linn. Afr J Tradit Complement Altern Med. 2011; 8: 98–103.

[171] Ratsch C. The Encyclopedia of Psychoactive Plants: Ethnopharmacology and its Applications. Rochester: Park Street Press 1998: p. 944.

[172] Avery AG. "Historical Review." In Blakeslee – the Genus Datura, New York: Ronald Press; 1959: 3–15.

[173] Nithya V. Evaluation of the wound healing activity of Datura metel L. in Wistar albino rats. Inventi Rapid: Ethnopharmacol. 2011; 4.

[174] Dewangan II BM, Jaiswal V, Verma VK. Potential wound healing activity of the ethanolic extract of Solanum xanthocarpum Schrad and Wendl leaves. Pak J Pharm Sci. 2012; 25: 189–194.

[175] Bharti M, Bias M, Singhasiya A. Evaluation of wound healing activity of Cissus quadrangularis. World J Pharm Pharm Sci. 2014; 3: 822–834.

[176] Gbedema SY, Kisseih E, Adu F, Annan K, Woode E. Wound healing properties and kill kinetics of Clerodendron splendens G. Don, a Ghanaian wound healing plant. Pharmacog Res. 2001; 2:63–68.

[177] Liu HW, Nakanishi K. The structure of balanitins; potent molluscicides isolated from Balanites aegyptiaca. Tetrahedron. 1982; 38:513–519.

[178] Kojima H, Yanai T, Toyota A. Essential oil constituents from Japanese and Indian Curcuma aromatica rhizomes. Planta Med. 1998; 64: 380–381.

[179] Arun MSS, Anima P. Herbal boon for wounds. Int J Pharmacy Pharm Sci. 2013; 5, 1–12.

[180] Bhagavathula N, Warner RL, DaSilva M, McClintock SD, Barron A, Aslam MN, Varani J. A combination of curcumin and ginger extract improves abrasion wound healing in corticosteroid-impaired hairless rat skin. Wound Repair and Regen. 2009; 17: 360–366.

[181] Pawar RS, Toppo FA, Mandloi AS, Shaikh S. Exploring the role of curcumin containing ethanolic extract obtained from Curcuma longa (rhizomes) against retardation of wound healing process by aspirin. Indian J Pharmacol. 2015; 47:160–166.

[182] Kundu S, Biswas TK, Das P, Kumar S, De DK. Turmeric (Curcuma longa) rhizome paste and honey show similar wound healing potential: a preclinical study in rabbits. The Int J Lower Extre Wounds. 2005; 4: 205–213.

[183] Sidhu GS, Singh AK, Thaloor D, Banaudha KK, Patnaik GK, Srimal RC, Maheshwari RK. Enhancement of wound healing by curcumin in animals. Wound Repair Regen. 1998; 6: 167–177.

[184] Rouhollahi E, Moghadamtousi SZ, Hajiaghaalipour F, Zahedifard M, Tayeby F, Awang K, Mohamed Z. Curcuma purpurascens Bi. rhizome accelerates rat excisional wound healing: involvement of hsp70/Bax proteins, antioxidant defense, and angiogenesis activity. Drug Des Dev Ther. 2015; 9: 5805–5813.

[185] Kamel MS, Ontani K, Kurokawa T, Assaf HM, El-Shannawany MA. Studies on *Balanites aegyptiaca* fruits, an antidiabetic Egyptian folk medicine. Phytochemistry. 1991; 31: 3565–3569.

[186] Khanna S, Venojarvi M, Roy S, Sharma N, Trikha P, Bagchi D, Bagchi M, Sen CK. Dermal wound healing properties of redox-active grape seed proanthocyanidins. Free Rad Biol Med 2002; 33: 1089–1096.

[187] Ghosh P, Gaba A. Phyto-extracts in Wound healing. J Pharm Sci. 2013; 16: 760–820.

[188] Thakur R, Jain N, Pathak R, Sandhu SS. Practices in wound healing studies of plants. Evid-Based Complement Alternat Med. 2011; 17. Article ID 438056.

[189] Fraga CG, Oteiza PI. Dietary flavonoids: role of (−)-epicatechin and related procyanidins in cell signaling. Free Rad Biol Med 2011; 51: 813–823.

[190] Fakhim SA, Babaei H, Nia AK, Ashrafi J. Wound healing effect of topical grape seed extract (*Vitis Vinifera*) on rat palatal mucosa. Int J Curr Res Aca Rev. 2015; 3(6):477–489.

[191] Shirley D, McHale C, Gomez G. Resveratrol preferentially inhibits IgE-dependent PGD2 biosynthesis but enhances TNF production from human skin mast cells. Bioch Bioph Acta 2016; 1860: 678–685

[192] Novelle MG, Wahl D, Diéguez C, Bernier M, de Cabo R. Resveratrol supplementation: Patel, H. H., and Insel, P. A. Lipid rafts and caveolae and their role in compartmentation of redox signaling. Antioxidant and Redox Signaling 2009; 11: 1357–1372.

[193] Yaman I DH, Kara C, Kamer E, Diniz G, Ortac R, Sayin O. Effects of resveratrol on incisional wound healing in rats. Surg Today. 2013; 43(12): 1433–1438.

[194] Haslam, E. Natural polyphenols (vegetable tannins) as drugs: possible modes of action. J Nat Prod. 1996; 59: 205–215.

[195] Aerts RJ, Barry TN and McNabb WC. (Polyphenols and agriculture: beneficial effects of proanthocyanidins in forages. Agric Ecosys Environ. 1999; 75: 1–12.

[196] Neves ALA, Komesu MC, Di Matteo, MA. Effects of green tea use on wound healing. Int J Morphol. 2010; 28: 905–910.

[197] Ramos-Jerz MDR, Villanueva S, Jerz G, Winterhalter P, Deters AM. *Persea americana* Mill. Seed: Fractionation, characterization, and effects on human keratinocytes and fibroblasts. Evid-Based Complement Alternat Med. 2013; 2013: 391247.

[198] Deters A, Dauer A, Schnetz E, Fartasch M, Hensel, A. High molecular compounds (polysaccharides and proanthocyanidins) from *Hamamelis virginiana* bark: Influence on human skin keratinocyte proliferation and differentiation and influence on irritated skin. Phytochemistry. 2001; 58: 949–958.

[199] Bueno FG, Panizzon GP, Souza EV, Mello DL, Lechtenberg M, Petereit F, João Carlos J, de Mello P, Hensel A. Hydrolyzable tannins from hydroalcoholic extract from *Poincianella pluviosa* stem bark and its wound-healing properties: phytochemical investiga-

tions and influence on in vitro cell physiology of human keratinocytes and dermal fibroblasts. Fitoterapia. 2014; 99: 252–260.

[200] McKelvey K, Xue M, Whitmont K, Shen K, Cooper A, Jackson C. Potential anti-inflammatory treatments for chronic wounds. Wound Pract Res. 2012; 20: 86–89.

[201] Shin YS, Shin HA, Kang SU, Kim JH, Oh YT, Park KH, Kim CH. Effect of epicatechin against radiation-induced oral mucositis: *In vitro* and *in vivo* study. PLoS ONE 2013; 8: e69151.

[202] Balasubramanian S, Efimova T, Eckert RL. Green tea polyphenol stimulates Ras, MEKK1, MEK3 and p38 cascade to increase activator protein 1 factor-dependent involucrin gene expression in normal human keratinocytes. J Biol Chem. 2002; 277: 1828–1836.

[203] Mackenzie GG, Adamo AM, Decker NP, Oteiza PI. Dimeric procyanidin B2 inhibits constitutively active NF-kappa B in Hodgkin's lymphoma cells independently of the presence of Ikappa B mutations. Biochem Pharmacol. 2008; 75: 1461–1471.

[204] Mackenzie GG, Delfino JM, Keen CL, Fraga CG, Oteiza PI. Dimeric procyanidins are inhibitors of NF-kappa B-DNA binding. J Biol Chem. 2002; 277: 1828–1836.

[205] Kamimura A, Takahashi T. Procyanidn B-2 extracted from apples, promotes hair growth: a laboratory study. Brit J Dermatol. 2002; 146: 41–51.

[206] Byun EB, Sung NY, Byun EH, Song DS, Kim JK, Park JH, Song BS, Park SH, Lee JW, Byun MW and Kim JH. The procyanidin trimer C1 inhibits LPS-induced MAPK and NF-κB signaling through TLR4 in macrophages. Int J Immunopharmacol. 2013; 15: 450–456.

[207] Takahashi T, Kamiya T, Hasegawa A, Yokoo Y. Procyanidin oligomers selectively and intensively promote proliferation of mouse hair epithelial cells *in vitro* and activate hair follicle growth *in vivo*. J Invest Dermatol. 1999; 112: 310–316.

[208] Crozier A, Jaganath IB, Clifford MN., Deters A, Dauer A, Schnetz E, Fartasch M, Hensel, A. High molecular compounds (polysaccharides and proanthocyanidins) from *Hamamelis virginiana* bark: influence on human skin keratinocyte proliferation and differentiation and influence on irritated skin. Phytochemistry. 2001; 58: 949–958.

[209] Nijveldt RJ, van Nood E, van Hoorn DE, Boelens PG, van Norren K, van Leeuwen PA. Flavonoids: a review of probable mechanisms of action and potential applications. Am J Clin Nutr. 2001; 74 (4): 418–425.

[210] Robak J, Gryglewski RJ. Bioactivity of flavonoids. Pol J Pharmacol 1996; 48: 555.

[211] Ferrandiz ML, Nair AG, Alcaraz MJ. Inhibition of sheep platelet arachidonate metabolism by flavonoids from Spanish and Indian medicinal herbs. Pharmazie 1990; 45: 206–208.

[212] Hasanoglu A, Ara C, Ozen S, Kali K, Senol M, Ertas E. Efficacy of micronized flavonoid fraction in healing of clean and infected wounds. Int J Angiol. 2001; 10(1): 41–44.

[213] Lodhi S, Singhai KK. Wound healing effect of flavonoid rich fraction and luteolin isolated from *Martynia annua* Linn. on streptozotocin induced diabetic rats. Asian Pac J Trop Med. 2013; 6: 253–259.

[214] Hirota BCK, Miyazaki CMS, Mercali CA, Verdan MC, Kalegari M, Gemin C, Lordello AL, Miguel MD, Miguel OG. C-glycosyl flavones and a comparative study of the antioxidant, hemolytic and toxic potential of *Jatropha multifida* leaves and bark. Int J Phytomedicine 2012; 4: 1–5.

[215] Ambigas S, Narayanan R, Gowri D, Sukumar D, Madhavan S. Evaluation of wound healing activity of flavonoids from *Ipomea carnea* Jacq. Ancient Sci Life 2007; 26: 45–51.

[216] Mali PC, Ansari AS, Chaturvedi M. Antifertility effect of chronically administered *Martynia annua* root extract on male rats. J Ethnopharmacol. 2002; 82(3): 61–67.

[217] Goldstein JT, Dobrzyn A, Clagett-Dame M, Pike JW, DeLuca HF. Isolation and characterization of unsaturated fatty acids as natural ligands for the retinoid-X receptor. Arch Biochem Biophys. 2003; 420(1): 185–193.

[218] Michalik L, Wahli W. Peroxisome proliferator-activated receptors (PPARs) in skin health, repair and disease. Biochim Biophys Acta (BBA)-Mol Cell Biol Lipids. 2007; 1771 (8): 991–998.

[219] Efron PA, Moldawer LL. Cytokines and wound healing: the role of cytokine and anticytokine therapy in the repair response. J Burn Care Res. 2004; 25(2): 149–160.

[220] Calder PC. n–3 Polyunsaturated fatty acids and inflammation: from molecular biology to the clinic. Lipids. 2003; 38(4): 343–352.

[221] Hukkeri VI, Karadi R V, Akki KS, et al. Wound healing property of Eucalyptus globulus L. leaf extract'. Indian Drugs. 2002; 39(9): 481–483.

[222] Medal JC, Vitorino MD, Habeck DH, Gillmore JL, Pedrosa JH, De Sousa LP. Host specificity of *Heteroperreyia hubrichi* Malaise (Hymenoptera: Pergidae), a potential biological control agent of Brazilian peppertree (*Schinus terebinthifolius* Raddi). Biol Control. 1999; 14(1): 60–65.

[223] Estevão LRM, Mendonca FDS, Baratella-Evêncio L, et al. Effects of aroeira (*Schinus terebinthifoliu* Raddi) oil on cutaneous wound healing in rats. Acta Cir Bras. 2013; 28(3): 202–209.

[224] Srivastava P, Durgaprasad S. Burn wound healing property of *Cocos nucifera*: an appraisal. Indian J Pharmacol. 2008; 40(4): 144–146.

[225] Bergsson G, Arnfinnsson J, Steingrimsson Ó, Thormar H. Killing of Gram-positive cocci by fatty acids and monoglycerides. Note Apmis. 2001; 109 (10): 670–678.

[226] Chadeganipour M, Haims A. Antifungal activities of pelargonic and capric acid on *Microsporum gypseum*. Mycoses. 2001; 44(3–4):109–112.

[227] Nevin KG, Rajamohan T. Effect of topical application of virgin coconut oil on skin components and antioxidant status during dermal wound healing in young rats. Skin Pharmacol Physiol. 2010; 23(6): 290–297.

[228] Shivananda NB, Dan Ramdatg D, Marshall JR, Isitor G, Xue S, Shi J. Wound-healing properties of the oils of *Vitis vinifera* and *Vaccinium macrocarpon*. Phyther Res. 2011; 25(8): 1201–1208.

[229] Castola V, Bighelli A, Casanova J. Intraspecific chemical variability of the essential oil of *Pistacia lentiscus* L. from Corsica. Biochem Syst Ecol. 2000; 28(1): 79–88.

[230] Carson CF, Riley T V. Antimicrobial activity of the essential oil of *Melaleuca alternifolia*. Lett Appl Microbiol. 1993; 16(2): 49–55.

[231] Carson CF HK, Riley TV. *Melaleuca alternifolia* (tea tree) oil: a review of antimicrobial and other medicinal properties. Clin Microbiol Rev. 2006; 19(1): 50–62.

[232] Halcón L, Milkus K. *Staphylococcus aureus* and wounds: a review of tea tree oil as a promising antimicrobial. Am J Infect Control. 2004; 32(7): 402–408.

[233] Edmondson M, Newall N, Carville K, Smith J, Riley T V, Carson CF. Uncontrolled, open-label, pilot study of tea tree (*Melaleuca alternifolia*) oil solution in the decolonisation of methicillin-resistant *Staphylococcus aureus* positive wounds and its influence on wound healing. Int Wound J. 2011; 8 (4): 375–384.

[234] Carette C, Malotaux M, van Leeuwen M, Tolkamp M. Shea nut and butter in Ghana: opportunities and constraints for local processing. Rep Proj Oppor Shea Nuts North Ghana. 2009. pp. 1–88.

[235] Goreja WG. Shea Butter: The Nourishing Properties of Africa's Best-Kept Natural Beauty Secret. TNC International Inc; Stone Mountain, Georgia 2004.

[236] Wallace-Bruce S, Appleton H. Shea Butter Extraction in Ghana. Intermediate Technology Publications Ltd (ITP); London, UK 1995.

[237] Benhammou N, Bekkara FA, Panovska TK. Antioxidant and antimicrobial activities of the *Pistacia lentiscus* and *Pistacia atlantica* extracts. Afri J Pharm Pharmacol. 2008; 2(2): 22–28.

[238] Dedoussis GVZ, Kaliora AC, Psarras S, et al. Antiatherogenic effect of *Pistacia lentiscus* via GSH restoration and downregulation of CD36 mRNA expression. Atherosclerosis. 2004; 174(2): 293–303.

[239] Djerrou J, Maameri Z, Hamdo-Pacha Y, et al. Effect of virgin fatty oil of Pistacia lentiscus on experimental burn wound's healing in rabbits. Afri J Trad Complement Altern Med. 2010; 7(3): 258–263.

[240] El-Soud A, Helmy N. Honey between traditional uses and recent medicine. Maced J Med Sci. 2012; 5(2): 205–214.

[241] Al-Waili N SK, Al-Ghamdi AA. Honey for wound healing, ulcers, and burns; data supporting its use in clinical practice. Sci World J. 2011; 11: 766–787.

[242] Bang LM, Buntting C, Molan P. The effect of dilution on the rate of hydrogen peroxide production in honey and its implications for wound healing. J Altern Complement Med. 2003; 9(2): 267–273.

[243] Subrahmanyam M, Sahapure AG, Nagane NS, Bhagwat VR, Ganu J V. Effects of topical application of honey on burn wound healing. Ann Burns Fire Disasters. 2001; 14(3): 143–145.

[244] Maeda Y, Loughrey A, Earle JAP, et al. Antibacterial activity of honey against community-associated methicillin-resistant *Staphylococcus aureus* (CA-MRSA). Complement Ther Clin Pract. 2008; 14(2): 77–82.

[245] Islam A, Khalil I, Islam N, et al. Physicochemical and antioxidant properties of Bangladeshi honeys stored for more than one year. BMC Complement Altern Med. 2012; 12(1): 1.

[246] Al-Mamary M, Al-Meeri A, Al-Habori M. Antioxidant activities and total phenolics of different types of honey. Nutr Res. 2002; 22(9): 1041–1047.

[247] Alam F, Islam MA, Gan SH, Khalil MI. Honey: a potential therapeutic agent for managing diabetic wounds. Evid-Based Complement Altern Med. 2014; 2014: 16

5

Pressure Ulcers

Jill M. Monfre

Abstract

Pressure ulcers or pressure injuries occur in all health care settings and are considered a quality care indicator. Individuals in every health care setting must routinely be assessed for factors that place them at risk for development of pressure ulcers and have routine skin assessments to assess for the presence of pressure ulcers. If risks for pressure ulcer development or actual pressure ulcers are identified, it is crucial that a prevention and treatment plan be developed and implemented to address the risks and treat the wounds. For a prevention and treatment plan to be comprehensive and effective, it must be evidence based and multidisciplinary. The plan needs to address the risk factors or wound concerns specific to the individual and include education for the providers, caregivers and individuals at risk for pressure ulcer development and/or with pressure ulcers. Expert consensus panels concur that despite evidence-based multidisciplinary comprehensive pressure ulcer prevention plans, there are clinical situations in which pressure ulcers are deemed unavoidable.

Keywords: Pressure, Ulcer, pressure injury, decubitus, bed sore, prevention, treatment

1. Introduction

Pressure ulcers, also referred to as decubitus ulcers, pressure sores or bed sores and recently referred to as pressure injures by the National Pressure Ulcer Advisory Panel (NPUAP) [1], are a common occurrence in all health care settings, including acute care hospitals, long-term care facilities, rehabilitation centers and subacute care centers [2]. Pressure ulcers have a significant impact on patients, families and health care facilities. These wounds can cause pain and suffering to individuals, produce emotional distress for families and significant others, increase the length of a hospital stay and increase the costs to facilities. The incidence of a pressure ulcer can also lead health care providers to feel as though they have failed to deliver quality care to those who have been entrusted to their care [3]. It is important to identify individuals who are at risk for pressure ulcer development or those who have developed a pressure ulcer, in order to implement preventative or treatment measures; these individuals also require close monitoring.

2. Definition

The National Pressure Ulcer Advisory Panel (NPUAP), an organization comprised of leading experts in health care dedicated to the prevention and management of pressure ulcers, during a consensus conference held in the spring of 2016 replaced the term pressure ulcer with pressure injury to more accurately reflect injuries related to pressure in both intact and ulcerated skin [1]. The NPUAP also revised their definition of a pressure injury as *localized damaged to the skin and/or underlying soft tissue usually over a bony prominence or related to a medical or other device. The injury can present as intact skin or an open ulcer and may be painful. The injury occurs as a result of intense and/or prolonged pressure or pressure in combination with shear. The tolerance of soft tissue for pressure and shear may also be affected by microclimate, nutrition, perfusion, comorbidities and condition of the soft tissue* [1]. The European Pressure Ulcer Advisory Panel (EPUAP), also a leading organization of wound care experts, continues to use the term pressure ulcer as well as the definition originally developed in conjunction with the NPUAP, which states a pressure ulcer is a *localized injury to the skin and/or underlying tissue usually over a bony prominence, as a result of pressure, or pressure in combination with shear* [4].

3. Etiology

Pressure ulcers, the term that will be used throughout this chapter, occur across all health care settings with the most common setting for the occurrence of pressure ulcers being acute care hospitals followed by long-term care facilities then equally in occurrence in an individual's home and nursing facilities [5]. Pressure ulcers usually occur on the lower half of the body with two-thirds occurring in the pelvic region such as the sacrum, coccyx or hip areas and one-third occurring on the lower extremities. The occurrence of pressure ulcers on the heels is increasing. **Table 1** indicates bony prominences of the body, the location where pressure ulcers occur most often [6].

Approximately 10% of pressure ulcers are device related [7]. Multiple medical devices or pieces of medical equipment can lead to pressure ulcer development. Items such as endotracheal tubes, feeding tubes, cervical collars, tracheostomy tubes and positive pressure airway masks all have the potential for creating pressure ulcers due to pressure points created by the device. Transfer boards or slide boards place an individual at risk for shear injuries due to sliding over the firm surface.

The most common age group for the incidence of pressure ulcers is the elderly, especially those 70 and older. The occurrence of a pressure ulcer in an elderly individual increases their mortality rate fivefold. In hospital, when a patient has developed a pressure ulcer, mortality increases by 25% in the over 70 age group [5].

Prone position (lying on stomach)

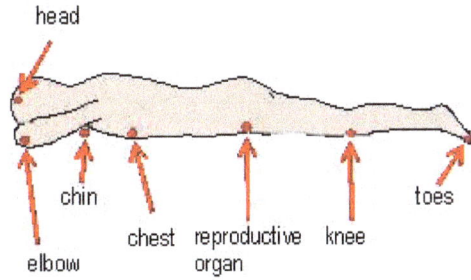

Supine position (lying on back)

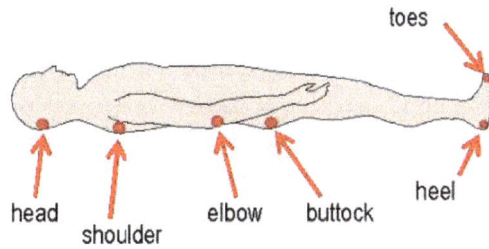

Lateral position (lying on side)

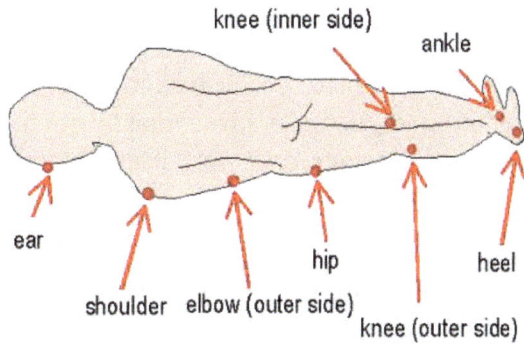

Sitting position

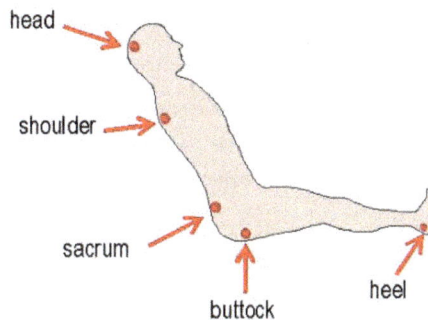

Table 1. Pressure ulcer pressure points.

4. Pathogenesis

The development of a pressure ulcer is not solely dependent upon pressure [8]. Multiple factors that modify the effect of pressure on tissues play a role in the development of pressure ulcers. The tolerance tissues have to external load depends on the duration of the exerted load. High loads can be tolerated for short periods of time, while relatively low loads can be tolerated for longer periods of time. The internal load in the tissues, as a result of the external load, causes cell deformation, occlusion of blood and lymphatic vessels and ischemia. If the internal load could be measured a risk for pressure ulcer, development could potentially be quantified [8].

A pressure ulcer results from sustained compression of soft tissues [5]. This compression occurs most often between a bony prominence and an external surface. Blood flow supplies oxygen and nutrients to the tissues. If pressure is sustained, the blood supply to the tissues is interrupted. When the blood flow is interrupted, oxygen and nutrients are not delivered to the tissues. Without oxygen and nutrients, the tissue will be damaged and eventually die [5].

Not all types of pressure are equally damaging to tissues [9]. Hydrostatic pressure, the pressure exerted by a liquid, as is endured by divers for long periods of time does not result in pressure ulcer formation. Yet localized pressure, as is exerted on the sacrum of a bedbound patient in the supine position for an extended period of time, often causes tissue distortion and blockage of the blood vessels resulting in much more damage. Studies related to localized pressure have found that pressure applied over a bony prominence resulted in more damage to the muscle than to the skin causing the study team to conclude that the muscle is more sensitive to pressure than is the skin or subcutaneous tissue [9].

Further studies identified specific factors associated with the development of a pressure ulcer including; interface pressure, shear, moisture and friction [4]. The NPUAP, after investigating shear and friction which have long been associated with pressure ulcer development, has eliminated friction from its definition of a pressure ulcer the explanation of which will be discussed below [10].

Interface pressure contributes to pressure ulcer development, as it is the pressure that develops between the skin and a surface upon which an individual is sitting or lying. Interface pressure is a measure commonly used to evaluate the effectiveness of a support surface [11]. Pressure mapping measures interface pressures and helps to determine appropriate positioning [8].

Not all localized pressure results in a pressure ulcer. When the pressure of short duration is relieved, blood flow returns to the area. This occurrence is known as reactive hyperemia, blood vessels in the area of pressure dilate in an attempt to overcome the ischemia that occurs with the pressure. Reactive hyperemia is transient and is also described as blanchable erythema — an area that becomes white when pressed with a finger and returns to erythema when the compression is removed [11].

Pressure that is not relieved and is of longer duration leads to further decreased capillary blood flow, occlusion of lymphatic vessels and tissue ischemia. Over a bony prominence, pressure of 20 mmHg can increase to as much as 300 mmHg. If this pressure is sustained, destruction of deep tissues can occur including destruction of muscle, subcutaneous tissue, dermis and epidermis [11].

When capillaries are occluded metabolic waste begins to accumulate in the surrounding tissues due to the lack of oxygen and nutrients. Capillaries that are damaged become more permeable and leak fluid into the interstitial space-causing edema. Perfusion is slowed through the edematous tissue; therefore, hypoxia worsens. Hypoxia increases cell death that results in an increased metabolic waste released into the surrounding tissues [11]. The ensuing edema further compresses small vessels causing increased edema and ischemia. Local tissue death occurs, which results in a pressure ulcer [7].

Shear is an applied force that causes an opposite yet parallel sliding motion such as when an individual slides in a bed or chair. The individual's skeletal structure slides in one direction yet the skin layer is restrained in the original position secondary to friction forces. In these situations, when shear is involved, multiple studies have found the pressure needed to occlude the blood vessels is much less than in an area where shear force is not involved [5, 8]. Elderly individuals are at higher risk for the effects of shear due to the decreased amount of elastin in their skin which is a normal consequence of aging [5].

Moisture, another factor associated with the development of pressure ulcers, alters the resiliency of the epidermis to external forces [11]. The effects of friction and shear are increased in the presence of moisture. Increased moisture is often associated with incontinence, perspiration or wound exudate [5].

Friction was originally determined to be a causative factor in the development of pressure ulcers after a study by Sidney Dinsdale was published in 1974 [10]. The results of this study showed that significantly less pressure was needed to stimulate the development of a full or partial thickness wound when the pressure was applied in conjunction with friction.

There are several forms of friction as they relate to the development of pressure ulcers. Friction, as a general term, is the rubbing of two body parts together. It is also a force that resists the motion of two bodies and/or material elements sliding against each other. In relation to skin breakdown, the type of friction, that is of concern is dry friction, of which there are two types, namely static and kinetic. Static friction is the force that resists the motion between two bodies when there is no sliding. There are multiple aspects that impact the amount of static friction at the skin surface including an individual's hydration level and what the individual is in contact with, for example bed linen. Moisture is an important factor relative to static friction as humidity and liquid moisture increases the friction and may cause an individual to adhere to a surface. Dynamic friction, also known as kinetic friction, is the force between two bodies relative to one another as they are sliding. Dynamic friction occurs when an individual slides downward in bed or rubs a foot in a shoe causing a blister. Such a blister may be misdiagnosed as a pressure ulcer.

In relation to the Dinsdale study, the type of friction applied during the study was not noted. The results of this study showed that the blood flow to the epidermis in a given area was not significantly different when pressure and friction were applied together and when pressure was applied alone. Investigators concluded that increased susceptibility of lesions with friction was not due to ischemia in the epidermis. Three decades later, it has been hypothesized that the friction used in Dinsdale's study was creating shear strain or deformation in deeper layers of tissue. Current hypothesis is that friction causes mechanically damaging shear strain of superficial tissue cells and tissue damage results directly from excessive deformation not ischemia as previously thought.

Friction is an important factor as it leads to shear stress and strain yet does not alone lead to the development of a pressure ulcer. Friction contributes to the development of a pressure ulcer due to the shear forces it can create. In other words, friction causes the shear forces in the tissue, which can increase the risk of tissue breakdown and lead to the development of a pressure ulcer. Therefore, shear remains in the current NPUAP definition of a pressure ulcer yet friction is eliminated. Including friction would be redundant as friction is now thought to be a cause of shear. Also, eliminating friction may decrease the number of wounds that are misdiagnosed as pressure ulcers when they are caused solely by friction [10].

5. Pressure ulcer stages

Pressure ulcers are classified by the amount of visible tissue loss [4]. Depth of tissue loss is important, as it determines a treatment plan of care and can impact payment. Once a wound is determined to be a pressure ulcer, it is assigned a pressure ulcer-specific stage or category. No other wound utilizes this same staging/categorizing system. A stage or category is assigned after careful and thorough assessment of the pressure ulcer to determine the extent of tissue destruction. To complete this assessment, one must have a competent understanding of the anatomy of the tissue layers involved and of the physiology of pressure ulcer development.

The NPUAP has defined the stages or categories of pressure ulcers as follows (**Table 2**):

EPUAP staging guideline	
Stage I	Nonblanchable erythema—Intact skin with nonblanchable redness of a localized area usually over a bony prominence. Darkly pigmented skin may not have visible blanching; its color may differ from the surrounding area. The area may be painful, firm, soft, warmer or cooler as compared to adjacent tissue. Category I may be difficult to detect in individuals with dark skin tones. May indicate "at-risk" persons.
Stage II	Partial thickness skin loss—partial thickness loss of dermis presenting as a shallow open ulcer with a red pink wound bed, without slough. May also present as an intact or open/ruptured serum-filled or sero-sanguinous-filled blister. Presents as a shiny or dry shallow ulcer without slough or bruising. This category should not be used to describe skin tears, tape burns, incontinence-associated dermatitis, maceration or excoriation
Stage III	Full-thickness skin loss—Full-thickness tissue loss. Subcutaneous fat may be visible but bone, tendon or muscles are not exposed. Slough may be present but does not obscure the depth of tissue loss. May

	include undermining and tunneling. The depth of a category/stage III pressure ulcer varies by anatomical location. The bridge of the nose, ear, occiput and malleolus do not have (adipose) subcutaneous tissue and category/stage III ulcer can be shallow. In contrast, areas of significant adiposity can develop extremely deep category/stage III pressure ulcers. Bone/tendon is not visible or directly palpable.
Stage IV	Full-thickness tissue loss—Full-thickness tissue loss with exposed bone, tendon or muscle. Slough or eschar may be present. Often includes undermining and tunneling. The depth of a category/stage IV pressure ulcer varies by anatomical location. The bridge of the nose, ear, occiput and malleolus do not have (adipose) subcutaneous tissue and these ulcers can be shallow. Category/stage IV ulcers can extend into muscle and/or supporting structures (e.g., fascia, tendon or joint capsule) making osteomyelitis or osteitis likely to occur. Exposed bone/muscle is visible or directly palpable.
Unstageable	Full-thickness skin or tissue loss—depth unknown—Full-thickness tissue loss in which actual depth of the ulcer is completely obscured by slough (yellow, tan, gray, green or brown) and/or eschar (tan, brown or black) in the wound bed. Until enough slough and/or eschar are removed to expose the base of the wound, the true depth cannot be determined, but it will be either a category/stage III or IV. Stable (dry, adherent, intact without erythema or fluctuance) eschar on the heels service as "the body's natural (biological) cover" and should not be removed
Suspected deep tissue injury (sDTI)	SDTI depth unknown—Purple- or maroon-localized area of discolored intact skin or blood-filled blister due to damage of underlying soft tissue from pressure and/or shear. The area may be preceded by tissue that is painful, firm, mushy, boggy, warmer or cooler as compared to adjacent tissue. Deep tissue injury may be difficult to detect in individuals with dark skin tomes. Evolution may include a thin blister over a dark wound bed. The may further evolve and become covered with thin eschar. Evolution may be rapid exposing additional layers of tissue even with optimal treatment.

Table 2. Pressure ulcer staging [4].

An illustration of the pressure ulcer stages/categories is seen in **Table 3** [1].

As pressure ulcers heal, the lost muscle, subcutaneous fat or dermis are not replaced with like tissue before they re-epithelialize [12]. A pressure ulcer fills in with scar tissue, which is composed primarily of endothelial cells, fibroblasts, collagen and extracellular matrix. Therefore, a stage-III pressure ulcer, for example, cannot, as the wound heals, become a stage-II pressure ulcer and progress on to a stage-I pressure ulcer because the term stage I would not accurately reflect the structures that are now present under the newly re-epithelialized tissue. Referring to a healing stage-III pressure ulcer as a stage II, then a stage-I pressure ulcer is known as reverse staging or down staging and is not acceptable. The stage needs to reflect the scar tissue that has developed. Therefore, the stage for this healing pressure ulcer is "healing stage-III pressure ulcer" and when the pressure ulcer has healed, the stage is a "healed stage-III pressure ulcer," indicating the pressure ulcer is now filled with granulation or scar tissue and resurfaced with epithelium [12].

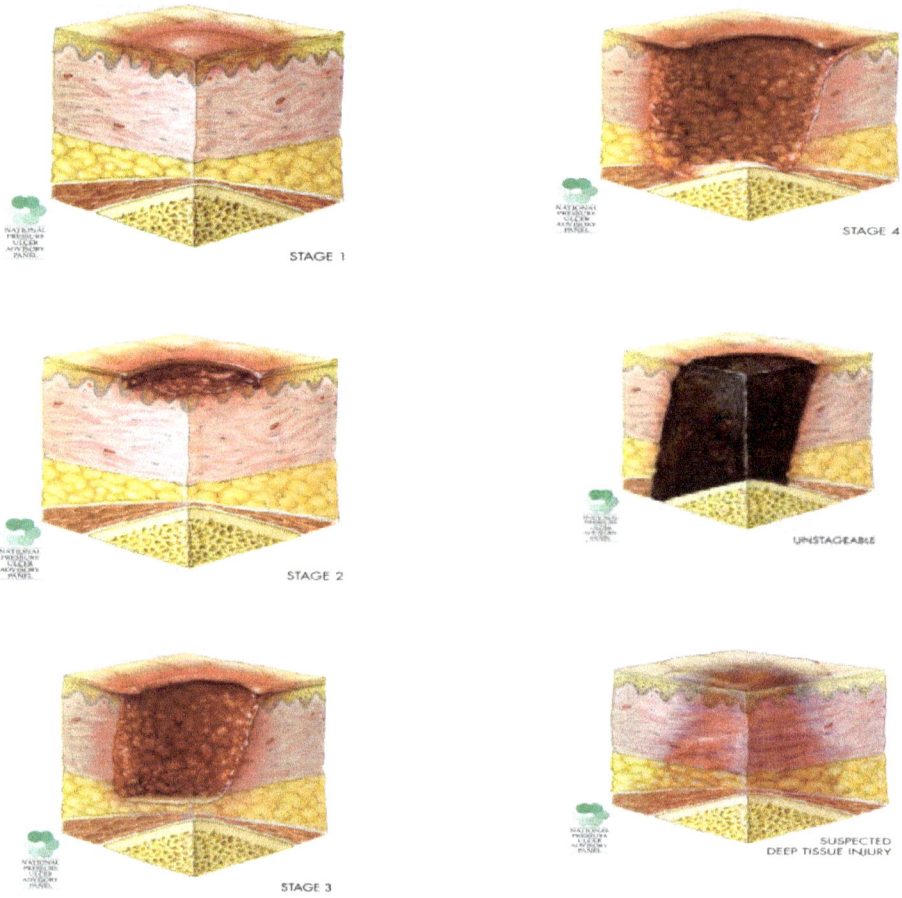

STAGE 1

STAGE 4

STAGE 2

UNSTAGEABLE

STAGE 3

SUSPECTED
DEEP TISSUE INJURY

Table 3. Pressure ulcer injury/ulcer stages/categories.

Mucosal pressure injuries are *pressure injuries found on mucous membranes with a history of a medical device in use at the location of the ulcer* [1]. A mucous membrane is the moist lining of a body cavity, such as the gastrointestinal tract, nasal passages, urinary tract and vaginal canal, that communicates with the exterior. When pressure is applied to a mucous membrane, ischemia can result that can lead to a pressure ulcer. Mucous membranes are vulnerable to pressure especially related to medical devices such as oxygen tubing, feeding tubes, urinary catheters and fecal containment devices [13].

The anatomy of mucous membranes impacts the staging or categorizing of a mucous membrane pressure injury [13]. There are two types of mucous membrane tissue; nonkeratinized stratified squamous epithelium and an underlying connective tissue layer, the lamina propria. These layers are similar to the epidermis and dermis and are connected via rete pegs. At the interface of the two layers is a basal laminal layer. The epithelial layer is continuously renewed through migration of lower layers of epithelium to the surface. The epithelium of the mucosa, although is not keratinized like the epithelium of the skin. The lamina propria generally contains blood vessels, elastin and collagen fibers [13].

Injured mucosa heals similarly as skin with the exception of scar formation [13]. There is an increasing evidence that the fibroblasts in mucosa resembles fetal fibroblasts. Most mucosal injuries heal without scar formation [13].

The staging or categorizing of pressure ulcers that is used for the skin cannot be used to stage mucosal pressure injuries [13]. Nonblanchable erythema cannot be seen in mucous membranes, as superficial tissue losses of the nonkeratinized epithelium are so shallow they cannot be differentiated from deeper, full thickness injuries. The coagulum seen on a mucous membrane pressure injury resembles slough yet it is actually soft blood clot. Muscle is seldom seen in a mucous membrane pressure injury and bone is not present in these tissues. Therefore, pressure injuries located on a mucous membrane are referred to as mucous membrane pressure injuries [13].

6. Pressure ulcer prevention

There are several factors that have been associated with the development of pressure ulcers. Many of these factors affect an individual's ability to withstand episodes of pressure and shear as well as decrease the length of time or amount of pressure necessary to cause tissue damage. Risk factors that can lead to pressure ulcer development include age, immobility, nutritional deficiencies, skin moisture and incontinence, vasopressor use, chronic diseases such as diabetes or stroke, smoking, behavioral issues leading to noncompliance, poor general health and sensory loss [14, 15]. No single factor can explain all pressure ulcers rather it is a complex interaction among factors which increases the probability of pressure ulcer development

Braden scale	Norton scale	Waterlow scale	Jackson Cubbin scale
Sensory perception	Physical condition	Sex	Age
Moisture	Mental status	Age	Weight
Activity	Activity	Appetite	Skin condition
Mobility	Mobility	Nurses' visual assessment of skin	Mental status
Nutrition status	Continence	condition	Mobility
Friction/shear		Mobility	Nutrition
		Continence	Respiration
		Factors contributing to tissue Malnutrition	Continence
		Neurologic deficits	Hygiene
		Major surgery or trauma	Hemodynamic status
		Medication	

Table 4. Pressure ulcer risk assessment tools.

Prevention begins with identifying those individuals at risk for pressure ulcer development. A pressure ulcer risk assessment instrument that has been validated for use in the specific age group should be utilized. In the Unites States, the most common adult risk assessment instruments are The Braden and Norton scales that have been tested for validity in predicting pressure ulcer development risk [7, 16]. In Britain, the most common scales are the Braden and the Waterlow. The Jackson Cubbin Scale is specific to European critical care (**Table 4**).

These scales will identify specific factors related to assessment categories that place an individual at risk for pressure ulcer development. Once specific factors are identified, a prevention plan to address those factors can be implemented to reduce or eliminate the risk of pressure ulcer development [3, 16]. With the implementation of an evidence-based pressure ulcer prevention plan, pressure reduction can occur which will preserve the microcirculation and prevent the development of pressure ulcers [17]. A pressure ulcer prevention plan is multifaceted. Factors related to prevention and discussed further in treatment, as these factors are also included in a treatment plan, include; mobility, moisture and continence care, nutrition and hydration, support surfaces, documentation and education. No single intervention has been found that will consistently, reliably and completely reduce pressure ulcer development. Pressure ulcer prevention involves multiple interventions and a multidisciplinary team to affect the identified factors and reduce the risk of pressure ulcer development.

7. Pressure ulcer treatment

The treatment of pressure ulcers is based on the physiology of wound healing. Wound healing is a complex process that changes with the health status of the individual [17]. A health care provider needs to have a basic knowledge of the phases of wound healing including; hemostasis, inflammation, proliferation and maturation. Once a provider understands wound healing, one has a significant piece of the knowledge necessary to develop a pressure ulcer treatment plan [18].

7.1. Phases of wound healing

The first phase of wound healing is hemostasis. Briefly, in this phase, damaged blood vessels are sealed when platelets form a stable clot to seal the blood vessel. The platelets also stimulate the clotting cascade through the production of thrombin that initiates the production of fibrin. The fibrin mesh ultimately strengthens the platelet aggregate into a hemostatic plug. Hemostasis occurs within minutes of injury unless the injured individual has underlying clotting disorders [18].

In the second phase of wound healing, the inflammation phase, the erythema, swelling and warmth that occur are often associated with pain. This phase of wound healing usually lasts up to 4 days after injury. During this phase, neutrophils or PMN's (polymorphonucleocytes) and plasma are leaked from the blood vessels into the surrounding tissue. These factors clean debris from the surrounding tissue and provide the first line of defence against infection. Macrophages are also active in the second phase of wound healing acting to destroy bacteria and secreting growth factors which direct the third phase of wound healing.

Chronic wounds, wounds that take longer than 12 weeks to heal, often remain in the inflammatory stage longer than occurs with acute wounds. Cellular and molecular abnormalities within a wound bed prevent progression through the stages of healing [19]. Chronic wounds contain elevated inflammatory cytokines and proteases. Chronic wounds do not respond to growth factors in the same manner in which acute wounds do. Specifically related to pressure ulcers, the volume of exudate is often times increased in chronic wounds. Secondary to infection, the exudate may be more purulent. If protein levels are low, the exudate may appear thinner [19]. Chronic wounds often have inadequate blood supply that also contributes to delayed healing and the formation of unhealthy granulation tissue.

The third phase of wound healing, the proliferation phase, begins approximately 4 days after injury and usually lasts until day 21 postinjury. The activity during this phase is replacement of dermal tissue and possibly subdermal tissue and contraction of the wound. Fibroblasts secrete collagen, which is the framework upon which new dermal regeneration, can occur. Angiogenesis, development of new capillaries, also occurs during this phase of wound healing. Keratinocytes differentiate to form the protective outer layer.

In the final phase of wound healing, maturation, remodeling of the dermal layer occurs to produce greater tensile strength. The cells that are involved in this process are fibroblasts. This process can take up to 2 years to complete [18].

7.2. Principles of wound healing

In addition to knowledge of wound healing, a provider must also be aware of the principles of wound treatment and intervention. For a wound to progress to healing, the wound bed must be well vascularized, free of devitalized tissue, free of infection and moist. Continual evaluation of a wound is necessary as the wound progresses through the stages of wound healing.

7.3. Dressings

No one dressing is appropriate for all wounds. There are multiple factors that will affect the dressing selected for a particular wound **Table 5**.

Knowledge of the properties of available wound dressings and an understanding that a treatment plan may need to change as the wound progresses through the stages of healing is vital. Wounds that do not advance through the process of healing in a reasonable or expected time frame must be assessed for issues that have not been previously identified or wound changes that have occurred and the treatment plan re-evaluated **Table 6**.

The principles in selecting dressings for pressure ulcer treatment include eliminate dead space, control exudate, prevent bacterial overgrowth, ensure proper moisture balance, cost-efficiency, and manageability for the individual, caregiver and providers.

Several adjuvant therapies/advanced dressings have been used to treat pressure ulcers. These therapies include (a) platelet-derived growth factor (PDGF) applied to the wound bed, which will stimulate the growth of cells involved in wound healing and granulation tissue formation; (b) negative pressure wound therapy (NPWT), which utilizes subatmospheric pressure applied to a wound via a sealed dressing to promote wound healing, the applied suction removes drainage and increases blood flow to the wound; and (c) hyperbaric oxygen therapy, delivered in multiple modes—total body, body part or mask—exposes the body to 100% oxygen at a higher pressure than normally experienced, this therapy provides oxygen necessary to stimulate wound healing and combats infection by enhancing leukocyte and macrophage activity [20]. PDGR and hyperbaric oxygen, although supported for use, have less support than does NPWT in studies conducted on individuals with pressure ulcers [20].

Wound depth	Partial thickness
	Full thickness
Wound description	Necrotic
	Slough
	Granulating
	Epithelializing
Wound characteristics	Dry
	Moist
	Heavily exudating
	Malodorous
	Excessively painful
	Difficult to dress
Bacterial description	Colonized
	Infected

Table 5. Wound description.

Alginate	Highly absorbent, useful for wounds with copious exudate. Alginate rope is particularly useful to pack exudate cavities or tracts
Hydrofiber	Absorbent dressing used for exudative wounds
Debriding agents	Useful for necrotic wounds, often used as an adjunct to surgical debridement
Foam	Useful for clean granulating wounds with minimal exudate
Hydrocolloid	Useful for dry necrotic wounds, wounds with minimal exudate or clean granulating wounds
Hydrogel	Useful for dry, sloughy, necrotic wounds
Transparent film	Useful for clean, dry wounds with minimal exudate, protect high friction areas
Negative pressure wound therapy	Conforms to the wound bed by suction and stimulates wound contraction while removing exudate

Table 6. Dressings [17].

There is limited evidence, although moderate strength, indicating support for the use of radiant heat dressings to improve pressure ulcer healing. Radiant heat dressings are noncontact dressings attached to a heating element. These dressings provide warmth to the wound and have been found to increase capillary blood flow to the area and thus increase wound healing. Also with limited yet moderate strength of evidence is the use of electrical stimulation, which provides a direct electrical current through the wound bed using electrodes on the surface of the wound. One hour daily session has been shown to be most effective. Caution has been noted not to use electrical stimulation on individuals with cancer as the treatment could stimulate the cancerous cells. The American College of Physicians specifically notes electrical stimulation in its guidelines [15].

7.4. Treatment plan

Prior to the development of a comprehensive pressure ulcer treatment plan, consideration should be given to an individual's psychological, behavioral and cognitive status. The individual's goals and prognosis need to be determined as well as the resources an individual has available, both financially and as caregivers.

A multidisciplinary team is needed to develop a comprehensive pressure ulcer prevention and treatment plan, as numerous factors are addressed. The team may include the individual's primary care provider, a wound care specialist, nurses or medical assistants who will provide wound care or education, social workers who will assist the individual and family members with resources and emotional concerns, a physical therapist who will provide assistance with mobility therapy and any other necessary consultants.

Within the plan, the following needs may need to be addressed.

Debridement of necrotic tissue within an acute wound may be necessary to be able to completely assess the wound. Necrotic tissue may obscure underlying fluid collections that need to be identified. Necrotic tissue also promotes bacterial growth that impairs wound healing and therefore should be debrided [17]. However, debridement is not recommended for stable dry eschar on heel wounds with no edema, erythema or fluctuance. Debridement can be achieved by multiple methods including sharp debridement, mechanical, enzymatic or autolytic debridement. Most sharp debridement can be completed at bedside, yet if more extensive sharp debridement is needed it may need to be performed in an operating room [17].

Mobilization of an individual is an important component to a pressure ulcer treatment plan. Since, by definition, a pressure ulcer is caused, in part, by pressure, if an individual begins to mobilize pressure will be relieved individuals who cannot ambulate redistributing pressure on a support surface needs to be investigated.

Moisture management, controlling incontinence and excess perspiration by wicking moisture away from the skin, will impact the effect of moisture. Managing moisture will increase the ability of the epidermis to return to its original state after being exposed to pressure. Shear and friction also will not be as detrimental to the skin when moisture is not allowed to be in contact with the skin for prolonged periods of time.

Nutrition studies indicated weak evidence that nutritional interventions provide benefits in the prevention or treatment of pressure ulcers [15]. A guideline presented by the American College of Physicians in 2015 cited moderate quality evidence supporting protein supplements in treating pressure ulcers. A Cochrane review in 2014 concluded that there is no evidence to support nutritional interventions, including protein, provide any benefits in preventing or treating pressure ulcers. A study regarding vitamin C supplements concluded that there was no change in wound healing. No results were noted related to zinc due to insufficient evidence. Although, evidence supports that providing adequate nutrition is important. Oral nutrition is preferred, yet if not possible; provide nutrition by the most appropriate route.

Oxygenation and perfusion must be ensured. A primary reason for inadequate tissue oxygenation is vasoconstriction as a result of sympathetic over activity. Blood volume deficit, pain and hypothermia are common causes of sympathetic overactivity for which the end result could be increased risk for pressure ulcer development.

Infection is usually determined clinically [15]. All open wounds contain some degree of bacteria. Healing is most often not impaired until bacteria reach a high colony count. If a wound culture needed, evidence indicates the Levine technique should be used. This technique involves rotating a swab over a 1 cm^2 patch of wound with enough pressure to express fluid from the wound for 5 s. A tissue or bone biopsy is the preferred method of identification of osteomyelitis, although biopsies of this nature are not always feasible. Magnetic resonance imaging (MRI) and nuclear medicine tests are more sensitive and specific than conventional plain radiography in identifying osteomyelitis. When bone is exposed in a pressure ulcer, osteomyelitis is often presumed.

An individual with increasing pain may be exhibiting a sign of a wound infection. Other signs of an acute wound infection include erythema around the ulcer's edges, induration, warmth and purulent drainage, no progression toward healing for 2 weeks, friable granulation tissue, foul odor, new necrotic tissue or lack of even spread of granulation tissue across the base of the wound. An individual may also exhibit systemic symptoms of a wound infection including fever, delirium and confusion [15].

Repositioning is replacing the term turning. The aim of repositioning individuals at risk for pressure ulcer development is to relieve pressure and/or redistribute pressure. It has been found that a slight change in position can be adequate to aid in relieving pressure. A turn of 30°, as previously encouraged for an individual in bed, for pressure relief, is not always needed to relieve pressure from bony prominences.

There is no research to support repositioning individuals every 2 h will aid in preventing the development of pressure ulcers; this recommendation is based on expert opinion [15]. The frequency of repositioning will, in part, be determined by an individual's tissue tolerance or the ability of both the individual's skin and its underlying structures to withstand pressure without an adverse effect.

As a provider or caregiver, when an individual at risk for pressure ulcer development is in bed, avoid positions with the head of the bed elevated to the point in which excess pressure and shear are applied to the sacrum and coccyx. This is most often any point beyond 30°.

In the seated position, the greatest exposure to pressure is to the ischial tuberosities. The area of the ischial tuberosities is relatively small; therefore, the pressure will be high. Without pressure relief, a pressure ulcer will develop quickly.

If a patient has a reddened area as a result of a previous episode of pressure loading, it is not advisable to position the individual on the same body surface. The reddened area indicates the body has not recovered from the previous position on the body surface and continues to require relief from the pressure load.

If heels are left in contact with a surface for a prolonged period of time, it is not unusual for heel pressure ulcers to develop due to the significant volume of bony structure in relation to the soft tissue in the heel. For the protection of the heels or treatment of heel, pressure ulcers assure that heels are elevated off any surface. Heels should be elevated so as to distribute the weight of the leg along the calf without putting pressure on the Achilles tendon. To avoid obstruction of the popliteal vein, which begins behind the knee, which may lead to a deep vein thrombosis, care must be taken to not hyperextend the knee.

Physical conditions of certain populations require additional care in positioning. These populations include those with spinal cord injuries, those that are insensate, older adults, individuals that have sustained hip fractures or those that do not maintain a healthy lifestyle.

Support surface use has been validated in studies for the prevention of pressure ulcers in high-risk individuals and for the treatment of individuals with pressure ulcers. A support surface reduces pressure by spreading the tissue load over a larger area, thus decreasing the load over bony prominences. A support surface also manages the microclimate including moisture and temperature.

Support surface selection is based on mobility, comfort and circumstances of care. In a home setting, consideration is given to the structure of the home including width of doors, power supply and available ventilation for heat from the motor as these factors relate to the support surface to be utilized. If a spouse or significant, other will share the bed consideration should be given to his or her comfort also.

Regular foam does not distribute patient weight uniformly and may worsen or cause pressure ulcers. A higher specification foam mattress is more effective in preventing pressure ulcers

When an individual is placed on a low-air loss, surface consideration must be given to the linens and pads used on the surface. Linens and pads should not be of materials that will block the air flow.

An issue that can negatively impact an individual at risk for pressure ulcer development or with a pressure ulcer that is related to any support surface is bottoming out. Bottoming out occurs when an individual's pelvic region or buttocks sink down and the support surface no longer provides adequate redistribution of pressure. An assessment for bottoming out can be performed with a hand check. Place a hand, palm side up under the support surface directly below the individual's buttocks region. If the individual can feel your hand or if less than an inch of support material is evident, the individual has bottomed out and the surface should be replaced [16].

Physician consults are generally part of a comprehensive treatment plan for individuals with pressure ulcers. Specialists may be consulted to debride wounds or with more complex wounds to perform flap procedures. Infectious disease physicians may be consulted to provide input or to monitor infected wounds especially if osteomyelitis is suspected or confirmed.

Education of providers, caregivers and individuals with pressure ulcers is a vital component to any prevention or treatment plan. Without adequate education, failure of a plan is probable. Education of providers should include how to complete a comprehensive skin and wound assessment as well as documentation of the assessments. Providers also require education on the facilities process for wound care treatment, including the principles of wound care and the products available on the wound care formulary.

Caregivers or the individual with a pressure ulcer need to be educated on the cause of the pressure ulcer, the contributing factors, prevention measures, proper nutrition, appropriate wound treatment and appropriate times to contact a provider. Education should include materials in a format understandable for the caregivers and individuals. For individuals with chronic conditions, such as spinal cord injuries, there are often times formal education programs in rehabilitation centers. It is also common to request a caregiver to receive education in the hospital prior to a patient being discharged. Education is crucial to an effective prevention and treatment plan.

8. Unavoidable pressure ulcers

In 2014, the NPUAP hosted a multidisciplinary international conference to explore the issue of unavoidable pressure ulcers. This conference brought experts together to explore, within the context of organ systems, the issue of unavoidable pressure ulcers [14]. At a previous conference in 2010, also hosted by the NPUAP, an unavoidable PU was defined *as one that may occur even though providers have evaluated the individual's clinical condition and PU risk factors have been evaluated and defined and interventions have been implemented that are consistent with individual needs, goals and recognized standards of practice.*

It was agreed upon by those in attendance at the 2014 conference that unavoidable pressure ulcers do occur. This conference also established consensus on risk factors that have in some situations been shown to increase the likelihood of the development of unavoidable pressure ulcers. In summary, the organ systems which were identified that may in some situations contribute to the development of unavoidable pressure ulcers included; (a) impaired tissue oxygenation/cardiopulmonary dysfunction—an individual cannot be repositioned due to the potential for a fatal event related to hemodynamic status, (b) hypovolemia—an individual is hemodynamically unstable which often leads to an inability to reposition an individual, (c) body edema/anasarca–leads to decrease pressure-loading tolerance and increased risk of pressure ulcer development, (d) peripheral vascular disease, lower extremity arterial and venous disease—compromised circulation that contributes to ischemia which leaves tissues more vulnerable to pressure ulcer development. Within this category, other subcategories were identified including chronic kidney disease, whereas the change in tissue tolerance may increase the likelihood of pressure ulcer development, hepatic injury which results in hypo-albuminemia that leads to edema and anasarca, sensory impairment, skin issues related to extremes in age, multiorgan dysfunction syndrome, critical status and burns all which leave patients prone to pressure ulcer development, (e) body habitus—obesity compromises an individual's ability to prevent shear injury during movement, pressure ulcer development related to moisture due to increased diaphoresis and inability to redistribute pressure over bony prominences and (f) immobility—associated with vascular congestion, dependent edema, compromised lung aeration, decreased red blood cell mass, dyspnea and activity tolerance leading to increased risk for unavoidable pressure ulcer development. The consensus panel also agreed that further research is necessary to examine the issue of unavoidable pressure ulcers [21].

9. Summary

A pressure ulcer rate is considered a quality care indicator in most health care settings and being an international health care concern. Most pressure ulcers are preventable. With a thorough assessment, including an assessment of an individual's skin and an assessment of pressure ulcer development risk, a comprehensive prevention and treatment plan can be developed and implemented to enhance positive outcomes.

Author details

Jill M. Monfre

Address all correspondence to: jmonfre@uwhealth.org

University Hospital, University of Wisconsin, Madison, Wisconsin, USA

References

[1] National Pressure Ulcer Advisory Panel. NPUAP Pressure Injury Stages [Internet]. April 13, 2016. Available from: http://www.npuap.org/resources/educational-and-clinical-resources/npuap-pressure-injury [Accessed: April 27, 2016]

[2] Lyder C. H. Pressure ulcer prevention and management. JAMA. 2003;289(2):223–226.

[3] Satekova L., Ziakova K. Validity of pressure ulcer risk assessment scales: review. Central European Journal of Nursing and Midwifery. 2014;5(2):85–92.

[4] National Pressure Ulcer Advisory Panel. NPUAP Pressure Ulcer Stages/Categories [Internet]. 2014. Available from: http://www.npuap.org/resources/educational-and-clinical-resources [Accessed: February 18, 2016]

[5] Grey J. E., Enoch S., Harding K. G. ABC of wound healing: pressure ulcers. BMJ. 2006;332(25):472–475.

[6] Images of Imgarcade. [Internet]. April 2015, Available from: http://www.Imgarcade.com [accessed February 13, 2016]

[7] Cooper K. L. Evidence-based prevention of pressure ulcers in the intensive care unit. Critical Care Nurse. 2013;33(6):57–66.

[8] Reenalda J., Jannink M., Nederhand M., Ijzerman M. Clinical use of interface pressure to predict pressure ulcer development: a systematic review. Assistive Technology. 2009;21:76–85.

[9]   Loerakker, S. Aetiology of pressure ulcers [thesis]. Eindhoven, Netherlands: Eindhoven University of Technology; 2007. 24 p.

[10]   National Pressure Ulcer Advisory Panel. Friction Induced Skin Injuries-Are They Pressure Ulcers? A National Pressure Ulcer Advisory Panel White Paper [Internet]. November 20, 2012. Available from: http://NPUAP.org [Accessed: February 14, 2016]

[11]   Pieper B. Mechanical forces: pressure, shear and friction. In: Ruth A. Bryant, editor. Acute & Chronic Wound Nursing Management. 2nd ed. St. Louis: Mosby; 2000. pp. 221–264.

[12]   National Pressure Ulcer Advisory Panel. The Facts about Reverse Staging in 2000. The NPUAP Position Statement [Internet]. 2000. Available from: http://www.NPUAP.org [Accessed: February 26, 2016]

[13]   National Pressure Ulcer Advisory Panel. Mucosal Pressure Ulcers [Internet]. August 2008. Available from: http://www.NPUAP.org [Accessed: February 23, 2016]

[14]   Edsberg L. E., Langemo D., Baharestani M. M., Posthauer M. E., Goldberg M. Unavoidable pressure injury. J Wound Ostomy Continence Nurs. 2014;41(4):313–334.

[15]   Raetz J., Wick K. Common questions about pressure ulcers. American Family Physician. 2015;92(10):888–894.

[16]   Ratliff C. R. Pressure ulcer prevention. Advance for NP's and PA's. 2016;18(6):24–29.

[17]   Bluestein D., Javaheri A. Pressure ulcers: prevention, evaluation, and management. American Family Physician. 2008;78(10):1186–1194.

[18]   The Canadian Association of Wound Care. The Basic Principles of Wound Healing [Internet]. Available from: http://cawc.nwt [Accessed: February 24, 2016]

[19]   Ousey, K. Chronic wounds-an overview. Journal of Community Nursing 2009;23(7):20–24.

[20]   National Pressure Ulcer Advisory Panel, European Pressure Ulcer Advisory Panel, PAN Pacific Pressure Ulcer Injury Alliance, editors, London England. Prevention and Treatment of Pressure Ulcers: Clinical Practice Guideline. 2nd ed. Australia: Cambridge Media; 2014. 308 p.

[21]   Black J. M., Edsberg L., Baharestani M. M., Langemo D., Goldberg M., McNichol L., Cuddigan J. Pressure ulcers: avoidable or unavoidable? results of the national pressure ulcer advisory panel consensus conference. Ostomy Wound Management. 2011;57(2): 24–36.

6

How Plasma Membrane and Cytoskeletal Dynamics Influence Single-Cell Wound Healing: Mechanotransduction, Tension and Tensegrity

Eric Boucher, Tatsuya Kato and Craig A. Mandato

Abstract

Organisms are able to recover from injuries by replacing damaged tissues, which recover by replacing damaged cells and extracellular structures. Similarly, a cell recovers from injuries by replacing damaged components of its structural integrity: its plasma membrane and cytoskeletal structures. Cells can be thought of as tensegral structures, their structural integrity relying on the interplay between tensile forces generated within and without the cell, and the compressive elements that counteracts them. As such, direct or indirect insults to the plasma membrane or cytoskeleton of a cell may not only result in the temporary loss of structural integrity, but also directly impact its ability to respond to its environment. This chapter will focus on the various aspects linking tensile forces and single-cell wound healing: where and how are they generated, how does the cell counteract them and how does the cell return to its previous tensegrity state? These questions will be explored using ubiquitous and cell-type specific examples of single-cell repair processes. Special attention will be given to changes in plasma membrane composition and area to cytoskeletal dynamics, and how these factor each other to influence and effect single-cell repair.

Keywords: single-cell wound healing, tensegrity, plasmalemma dynamics, cytoskeleton dynamics, mechanotransduction

1. Introduction

Cells are neither amorphous blobs nor rigid, unchanging structures. They are able to sense, react and most of the time recover from many types of physical insults ranging from pores created by osmotic shock or bacterial toxins to mechanical damages of various origins and intensity. Whatever the origin, the loss of barrier function provided by the plasmalemma leads to many potentially harmful effects including, but not limited to, the loss of intracellular content, the uncontrolled entry of Ca^{2+} and exposure of the intracellular milieu to reactive oxygen species (ROS), all of which may lead to a broad range of diminished cellular function, or even cell death. The negative effects of cellular injury are not limited to biochemical processes, they also directly affect the cell's structural integrity. As such, single-cell repair is as much a return to normal cell function as it is a return to structural integrity.

While they share common general steps of wound stabilization, resealing of plasmalemma damage and cytoskeletal remodeling, wound-healing mechanisms have been shown to vary widely according to the types of injury and cell-types. This chapter, using ubiquitous and injury- and cell-specific examples, aims to present an overview of the different mechanisms proposed for wound healing. Particular focus is put on how mechanotransduction, tension and tensegrity influences single-cell wound healing.

2. Background

2.1. Cells are tensegral structures

In eukaryotic cells, structural integrity is achieved and maintained through tensegrity [1], a term originally coined by the architect R. Buckminster Fuller as a portmanteau of "tensile integrity." Tensegrity describes stable structures achieved through prestress and the interaction of opposing stretch and compression elements [2]. In the cell, cytoskeletal actin filaments act as the main stretch-generating elements and microtubules are the main compression-bearing elements [3]. The role of intermediate filaments is not as well defined, as vimentin has been suggested to act principally as a major component that allows chondrocytes to withstand compressive loading, its contribution to the regulation of cytoskeletal tension and elastic modulus being relatively minor [4, 5]. While tensegrity is mainly achieved through these cytoskeletal elements, the plasma membrane has also been shown to play a key role in the cell's tensegrity [6]. Indeed, the composition and shape of the plasma membrane [7, 8], its intrinsic in-plane tension and membrane-to-cortex attachments (MCAs) [6] and the various external forces that may act on a cell's plasma membrane [9–11] have all been suggested to contribute to cellular tensegrity. The terminology surrounding these forces can be somewhat opaque and as such are defined in greater detail in **Figure 1**.

2.2. Plasma membrane disruptions, tensegrity and spontaneous repair

Early observations of lipid bilayers [12], liposomes [13] and erythrocyte ghosts [14] have shown that resealing of small lesions (<1 nm) are thermodynamically favored events [14]. Disruption of lipid membranes leads to the loss of barrier function of the plasma membrane, which may lead to uncontrolled changes in osmolality and hydrostatic pressure. These changes may be sufficient to alter the wounded cell's apparent membrane tension and thus its tensegrity state [11].

Apparent membrane tension

The force required to effectively deform liposomal membranes has historically been referred simply as "membrane tension". The plasma membrane of cells also contains relatively high amounts of proteins that specifically or non-specifically link them to cytoskeletal structures and therefore require higher amounts of energy to deform than lipid vesicles. As such, it is more accurate to use "apparent membrane tension" in the case of cells since it is the sum of the tensile forces produced by the intrinsic in-plane tension and the membrane-to-cortex attachments (MCAs).

a.   In-plane tension of the plasma membrane

In-plane tension of the plasma membrane is generated by the osmotically controlled difference in hydrostatic pressures between the cytosol and extracellular fluid directly acting on the plasmalemma [11, 12] and on the attached cytoskeleton [13]. In-plane tension is thus a factor of the mechanical and viscoelastic properties of the plasmalemma and can be influenced by variations in plasmalemma area [12, 14], shape [7, 8, 15] and composition [7, 16].

b.   Membrane-to-cortex attachments (MCAs).

In eukaryotic cells, adhesion between the plasma membrane and the relatively stiffer cortical cytoskeleton significantly contributes to a cell's apparent membrane tension [17]. Whereas in-plane tension is usually considered to be uniform across the membrane, MCA is able to vary across the cell surface, thereby creating areas of high and low apparent membrane tension in polarized cells [18], as well as membrane blebs in areas of low MCA. The specifics of MCA regulations are still unclear, but involves several membrane associated proteins such as filamin, spectrin, ankyrin, and affixin, as well as involving inner leaflet PIP2, as it is known to bind to or affects a great number of actin binding and remodeling proteins such as MARCKS, cofilin, profilin, gelsolin, vinculin, talin, α-actinin, WASP, Arp2/3, and the Rho family of GTPases (reviewed in [19]).

c.   Focal adhesions and Stress-fibers

External parameters such as the forces generated via cell-matrix adhesion are partly mediated by integrins, a group of heterodimeric transmembrane proteins that bind a variety of extra-cellular matrix (ECM) proteins. Integrins connect to the actin cytoskeleton via numerous intracellular linker proteins such as talin and vinculin. Uneven distribution of these adhesion complexes into "focal adhesions" can therefore influence cytoskeletal and apparent membrane tension, but their assembly and disassembly can also induce variations in apparent membrane tension. Indeed, focal adhesions [20, 21] and stress fibers [22] can act as mechanosensors and induce actin depolymerization through a variety of processes including mechanosensitive ion channels, RhoA signaling or directly via F-actin and cofilin (reviewed in [20]).

Figure 1. Tensile forces in the unwounded cell.

Immediately following its disruption, the plasma membrane also loses its asymmetry [15] and individual membrane phospholipids become disordered around the wound edge, which creates edge tension [16]. Indeed, plasma membrane damage directly alters the membrane composition, shape, and its physical properties. Mechanical damage also exposes hydrophobic domains of phospholipid molecules to the comparatively aqueous environment of the newly formed wound edge, which in turn creates a difference in chemical potential between the phospholipids of the wound edge and those of the planar membrane [13]. It is this so-called edge tension [16] that along with the line tension [17] present on the wound edge, provides the driving force necessary for the lateral movement of phospholipids [18, 19] and spontaneous resealing of phospholipid membranes. Rates of spontaneous resealing of these relatively simple systems have been shown to depend on a variety of factors that also affect single-cell wound healing: bilayer composition [19], Ca^{2+} concentration [20] and disruption radius [13]. On the contrary, liposomes, erythrocytes and erythrocyte ghosts membranes are associated with a variety of proteins such as spectrin, which diminish overall phospholipid lateral movement and lead to high tension at the wound edge [21]. As such, neither large liposomes, nor erythrocyte ghosts possess the machinery necessary to actively respond to the dramatic loss of tensegrity and changes in localized tensions that are created by large membrane disruption. Consequently, large erythrocyte ghosts' wounds do not spontaneously reseal under physiological conditions [14]. This has been attributed to a number of factors, including the presence of strong MCAs [19] and the lack of endomembranes [22] (**Figure 1**).

Finally, plasma membrane disruption also exposes the cell to high levels of ROS and Ca^{2+} ions, either of which can be detrimental to normal cell function. Numerous pathways involving membrane dynamics such as the capacitation [23] and acrosomal reaction [24] steps of sperm maturation (reviewed in [25]) involve Ca^{2+}-dependent signaling. Exocytosis events, such as surfactant secretion [26–28], as well as neuroendocrine [29], synapses [30–32] and auditory cells exocytosis [33, 34], are similarly Ca^{2+} dependent. These events are mediated by a variety of Ca^{2+}-binding proteins such as calpains, annexins and synaptotagmins. Unsurprisingly, the uncontrolled Ca^{2+} entry that accompanies plasma membrane damage has been shown to activate the same families of Ca^{2+}-binding proteins (reviewed in [35]). The downstream effects of Ca^{2+} entry will eventually lead to an overall diminution of apparent membrane tension.

3. Early events of single-cell wound healing are mechanically driven processes

Single-cell repair proper is an active process, requiring dynamic and concerted manipulations of the cell's membrane and cytoskeletal compartments. Most of these processes, however, take place relatively late following injury or are dependent on preliminary disruption of cytoskeletal structures. In this subchapter, we present the principal wound mitigation events that are activated in the moments immediately following injury and facilitate the subsequent exocytosis-, endocytosis- or membrane-shedding-mediated wound-healing processes.

3.1. Caveolae-mediated decrease of in-plane membrane tension

Caveolae are plasma membrane invaginations with a diameter of 50–80 nm and specific flask-like morphology [36]. Caveolae have long been known to flatten in response to mechanically induced membrane deformation stretch [37]. Indeed, the preincubation of cells with methyl-β-cyclodextrin diminishes the time to cell lysis upon hypotonic challenge [38]. Methyl-β-cyclodextrin is a cholesterol-depleting compound that has also been shown to severely reduce the number of caveolae at the cell surface [39], probably by limiting the recruitment of caveolin oligomers to the plasma membrane. Caveolae can thus be viewed as a "membrane buffer" that limits injury-induced increases in apparent membrane tension by diminishing the in-plane tension without the need of additional membrane components from Ca^{2+}-dependent exocytosis (**Figure 1**). Instead, additional membrane area is produced by the rapid flattening and disassembling of caveolae upon mechanical stress, which are rapidly reassembled upon mechanical stress release [40].

The exact molecular events leading to caveolae assembly and disassembly is still somewhat unclear, the specifics of which go beyond the scope of this chapter. Briefly, their assembly is initiated by the clustering and further recruitment of phosphatidylinositol 4,5-bisphosphate (PIP_2), phosphatidylserine (PS) and cholesterol with caveolin oligomers. Recruitment of various cavins oligomers will further increase the local concentration of negatively charged lipid, which in turn nucleates membrane curvature and formation of caveolae structure by the way of electrostatic cavins-cavins or cavins-membrane interactions (reviewed in [41, 42]).

While caveolin-3-deficient mice exhibit robust muscular degeneration [43], the relative contribution of caveolae in protection against stretch-induced mechanical deformation is therefore difficult to judge. An attractive, albeit speculative, hypothesis is that caveolae are involved in both wound prevention and healing. Firstly, they can act as a membrane reserve that buffers the cell against local or global increases in in-plane membrane tension. Secondly, they can passively potentiate plasma membrane repair by releasing apparent membrane tension near the wound edge, a site of initial high membrane tension because of both high line tension and MCA-related tether forces. Finally, caveolae are also known to play central roles in dysferlin-mediated exocytosis (see Section 4.1.3.1) and the endocytic removal of bacterial pores ([44, 45]; see Section 4.2.1) and small mechanical lesions ([45]; see Section 4.1.3.2).

3.2. Protein array-mediated wound site stabilization

Most of the wound-healing mechanisms described to date (see Section 4) require a substantial lowering of apparent membrane tension. This is achieved in a number of ways, including the disruptions of MCAs through both Ca^{2+}-dependent and Ca^{2+}-independent membrane repair mechanisms (see Section 4). These Ca^{2+}- and mechanosensor-mediated disruption of the MCAs and cytoskeletons have been shown to occur in large areas surrounding the wounds or throughout the cell and therefore only help to stabilize the wound indirectly.

The annexins form a large family of Ca^{2+}-sensitive, negatively charged phospholipid-binding proteins (reviewed in [46]). Upon wounding, annexin V translocate to the internal leaflet of the damaged membrane where it binds to the newly exposed phosphatidylserine residues on the wound edge and self-assembles into two-dimensional (2D) arrays [47]. These arrays have been shown to be able to cluster phospholipids, thereby reducing the lateral diffusion of phospholipids [48]. As such, these arrays may help stabilize the wound site until the apparent membrane tension has sufficiently been lowered by other wound-healing mechanisms (reviewed in [35]; see Section 3.1) Indeed, laser ablation experiments performed on murine perivascular cells have shown that the formation of annexin V arrays was necessary for normal wound healing and cell survival [49]. Similar wound stabilization arrays have also been proposed to involve mitsugumin 53 (MG53) oligomers, mini-dysferlinC72 and caveolins [50].

3.3. Cytoskeletal and MCA dynamics and wound healing

The cytoskeleton constitutes a substantial component of apparent membrane tension in eukaryotic cells through MCAs (**Figure 1**). Consequently, cortical cytoskeleton dynamics can also reduce apparent membrane tension and constitutes an important preliminary step of single-cell wound healing. Indeed, actin destabilization has been demonstrated to enhance active membrane resealing in a variety of cell types, including 3T3 fibroblasts [51], septal neurons [52] and RGM1 gastric epithelial cells [53].

3.3.1. Direct and indirect regulation of single-cell injury by cytoskeleton dynamics

Considering actin's importance for wound healing, it is not surprising that cellular injury affects actin dynamics in several ways. Changes of tensegrity experienced by damaged cells may lead to cytoskeletal remodeling either directly or through mechanotransductive signals. Indeed, sonoporation experiments showed that disruptions of existent plasmalemmal and adjacent cytoskeletal structures were enough to elicit a sustained and broad secondary disruption of the actin cytoskeleton [54]. As previously stated, actin filament bundles are the main providers of tensile forces necessary for a cell's tensegrity ([1]; **Figure 1**). Cells usually respond to external changes in tensile forces by modulating the sizes, numbers and distributions of F-actin and stress fibers in order to preserve mechanical homeostasis (reviewed in [55]). This is exemplified by experiments performed on endothelial cells [56] and osteoblasts [57] in which compression-induced stress fiber collapse through buckling, followed by actin disassembly events [56, 58]. Computer-assisted modeling strongly suggests that the loss of tensile force within the actin fiber upon its buckling is sufficient to induce actin disassembly [59, 60]. Whether a similar phenomenon contributes to actin fiber disassembly following mechanical damage is intriguing, as it would mean that actin filaments are able to act as their own mechanosensor. Indeed, a series of experiments showed that the tension state of individual actin filaments were inversely proportional to the binding affinity and actin filament-severing activity of cofilin [61–63]. Cofilin is an actin-binding protein that is known to accelerate actin depolymerization at the pointed end, which is also able to sever F-actin [64, 65]. This type of mechanosensing is especially attractive in the context of single-cell wound healing, as it is more sensitive and could induce downstream signals much faster than other traditional mechanosensors such as mechanosensitive ion channels [66], integrins, talin, or other F-actin-localized mechanosensors (reviewed in [62]).

Aside from mechanically related disruptions, cortical and cytoskeletal actin filaments are also disrupted in a variety of Ca^{2+}-dependent manners. Indeed, permeabilization of cells by bacterial pores, such as streptolysin O (SLO), leads to an increase in intracellular Ca^{2+} without substantial direct damage to the plasmalemma or subjacent actin cytoskeleton and also incites actin depolymerization [67]. While Ca^{2+} is able to disrupt actin filaments on its own [68, 69], the effect of Ca^{2+} on the disruption of normal cytoskeletal architecture is probably best exemplified by its activation of calpains. Calpains are Ca^{2+}-dependent, intracellular cysteine proteases that are known for their relative specificity [70]. Among others, calpains have been shown to cleave talin [71] into a large globular head domain that directly binds integrins, PIP_2 and focal adhesion kinases, and a rod domain that binds vinculin and actin. Its degradation by calpains upon wounding would therefore be compatible with the cytoskeletal remodeling that follows membrane disruptions.

3.3.2. Cytoskeletal dynamics is at the center of single-cell wound healing processes

Aside from its role in reducing apparent membrane tension, cytoskeleton remodeling is further required for single-cell wound healing as several plasma-resealing processes involve exocytosis of various vesicles such as lysosomes, MG53-positive vesicles and AHNAK-positive vesicles (reviewed in [35]; see Sections 4.1.2 and 4.1.3.1). As such, these intracellular vesicles must undergo actin- or microtubule-mediated transport to the wound site. An intact cortical cytoskeleton would therefore hinder not only transport and fusion of these vesicles, but also the subsequent removal of the damaged portions of the plasma membrane through endocytosis, blebbing or membrane-shedding processes. However, it should be noted that active repair mechanisms, such as exocytosis, cannot occur with just a minimal actin structure [67]. Reorganization of the cytoskeleton needs to be balanced in such a way that vesicles from intracellular pools are able to cross the actin barrier layer [53], then undergo docking to the wound site facilitated by remaining actin filaments [72] and the kinesin and myosin motor proteins [73].

4. Archetypes of single-cell repair: influence of injury type and cell type

As previously stated, disruptions of the plasma membrane or cytoskeletal structures may lead to local or global increases in apparent membrane tension that prohibits spontaneous resealing to occur. Furthermore, plasma membrane damage can be accompanied by direct or indirect disruptions of the cytoskeleton, which worsen the damaged cell structural integrity. In contrast, plasma membrane disruptions generated by pore-forming toxins (PFTs) have little to no immediate impact on local in-plane membrane tension. As such, Ca^{2+}-mediated exocytosis (see Section 4.1.2) and cytoskeletal remodeling (see Section 3.3) and cell-type (**Table 1**) may have profoundly different impacts depending on the type and size of the injury and may determine the healing pathway that is available to the cell (**Figure 2**) (reviewed in [35, 74]). Indeed, while uncontrolled entry of Ca^{2+} is a hallmark of all injury types, its intensity and distribution, together with the nature and size of the wound, as well as tissular context may control how the wound is repaired (**Figure 2**). The following section aims to present each wound-healing processes in the cellular context of which they were first identified. As it will become apparent in the next subsection, some processes, such as exocytosis, are quasi-ubiquitous, albeit with slight variations in vesicle species or molecular players involved. On the other hand, other processes, such as ESCRT-mediated membrane shedding (see Section 4.2.2) seem to be heavily dependent on wound size.

Cell type	Repair mechanism	Experimental wound type(s)	Major molecular players	Reference(s)
Germ cells				
Oocytes	"Membrane patch" formation	Mechanical wounding; laser wounding	Yolk granules; syntaxins; SNAP-25	[22, 75]

Cell type	Repair mechanism	Experimental wound type(s)	Major molecular players	Reference(s)
	Synaptotagmin-mediated exocytosis and "vertex fusion"	Mechanical wounding; laser wounding	Yolk granules; synaptobrevin; synaptotagmin VII; SNAP-25	[76–82]
	Actomyosin contractile ring	Mechanical wounding; laser wounding	RhoA; Cdc42; F-actin; myosin II; microtubules	[83–89]
Somatic cells				
Neuronal cells	Synaptotagmin-mediated exocytosis	Axon transection	Lysosomes; synaptotagmin I; syntaxin I;	[90, 91]
	Calpain-mediated vesicle fusion	Axon transection	Calpains	[52, 92–94]
Fibroblasts	Synaptotagmin-mediated exocytosis	Mechanical wounding	Lysosomes; synaptotagmin I; Synaptotagmin VII; VAMP-7; Syntaxin-4; SNAP-23	[76, 77, 95]
	Facilitated resealing	Laser wounding	Predocked TGN-vesicles; myosin IIA; PKC	[51, 96–98]
	Potentiated resealing	Laser wounding	PKG; CREB	[99]
Muscle cells	"Membrane patch" formation; Dysferlin-mediated exocytosis	Mechanical wounding; laser wounding	Lysosomes; calpains; mini-dysferlinC72; MG53; KIF5B; AHNAK; S100A10; Annexin II	[50, 100–107]
	Caveolae-mediated endocytic repair	Mechanical wounding	ASM[2]; Caveolin-3; annexin I	[108–113]
Epithelial cells	Caveolae-mediated endocytosis	PFTs[1]	ASM; Caveolin-3; annexin I	[45, 108, 110]
	ESCRT-mediated shedding	PFTs	ALG-2; ESCRT-III; ALIX; Vps4	[74, 114]

PFTs: Pore-forming toxins; ASM: Acid Sphingomyelinase

Table 1. Wound healing mechanisms according to cell-type.

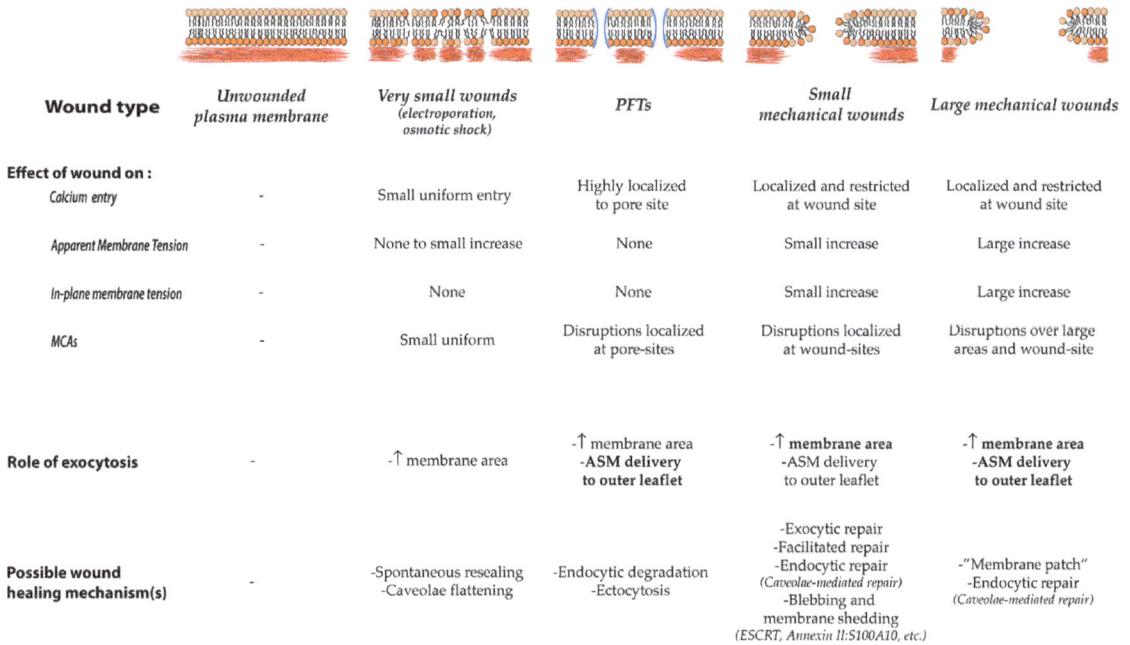

Wound type	Unwounded plasma membrane	Very small wounds (electroporation, osmotic shock)	PFTs	Small mechanical wounds	Large mechanical wounds
Effect of wound on :					
Calcium entry	-	Small uniform entry	Highly localized to pore site	Localized and restricted at wound site	Localized and restricted at wound site
Apparent Membrane Tension	-	None to small increase	None	Small increase	Large increase
In-plane membrane tension	-	None	None	Small increase	Large increase
MCAs	-	Small uniform	Disruptions localized at pore-sites	Disruptions localized at wound-sites	Disruptions over large areas and wound-site
Role of exocytosis	-	-↑ membrane area	-↑ membrane area -ASM delivery to outer leaflet	-↑ membrane area -ASM delivery to outer leaflet	-↑ membrane area -ASM delivery to outer leaflet
Possible wound healing mechanism(s)	-	-Spontaneous resealing -Caveolae flattening	-Endocytic degradation -Ectocytosis	-Exocytic repair -Facilitated repair -Endocytic repair (Caveolae-mediated repair) -Blebbing and membrane shedding (ESCRT, Annexin II:S100A10, etc.)	-"Membrane patch" -Endocytic repair (Caveolae-mediated repair)

Figure 2. Schematic (top) depicts lateral sections of the plasma membrane before and after different types of wounding (individual phospholipids represented as orange and beige heads with hairpin-like tails; cortical actin network represented as red lines; toxic pores represented in blue). Table (bottom) lists changes to wound-type-dependent factors of Ca^{2+} influx and tension, role of exocytosis and possible wound healing mechanisms upon different types of wounding. MCAs: membrane-to-cortex attachments; PFTs: pore-forming toxins.

4.1. Large wounds: exocytic repair, membrane patches and endocytic repair

4.1.1. Oocytes

Oocytes of *Xenopus laevis* and sea urchins are large, easily accessible and manipulable cells. While their size and lack of adhesive and cell-cell contact-derived tension distinguish them from mammalian somatic cells, these characteristics also provide a simpler platform which helped to elaborate the first models of single-cell wound healing. Oocytes have been observed to recover form very large mechanical disruptions of both the plasma membrane and cytoskeleton (>1000 μm^2) [75].

4.1.1.1. "Membrane patch"-mediated resealing

In addition to providing essential amino acids and other nutrients for oocyte development, yolk platelets also act as vesicle reservoirs upon plasma membrane injury of oocytes in a variety of species [22, 75]. Upon wounding, there is a rapid influx of Ca^{2+} from the extracellular milieu to the intracellular space, which favors rapid homotypic fusions of yolk granules [75]. These homotypic vesicular fusogenic events lead to the formation of a large "membrane patch" that eventually covers the gap present at the wound site [75–77]. It is perhaps best to think of the "membrane patch" model of wound healing as a somewhat oocyte-specific process. Indeed, this model relies almost entirely on homotypic fusions [75], and yolk granules offer a pool of readily available vesicle reserves that is incomparable with those available to somatic cells [78]. Also, while the "membrane patch" model of single-cell repair has also initially been proposed for the repair of large wounds in somatic cells [79, 80], it now appears that large somatic cell membrane disruptions are directly removed by endocytosis, which heavily relies on exocytosis and heterotypic fusion events (reviewed in [35, 81]; see Section 4.1.3.2). Whether these apparent differences are an intrinsic property of oocytes, a direct consequence of the wound size involved, larger wounds exposing larger areas of the intracellular space to Ca^{2+}, or of the higher density of available vesicles in oocytes, remains open for interpretation.

While the mechanism behind membrane patch formation is sufficient to block unregulated exchanges between extra- and intracellular spaces, it does not technically reseal the membrane, or restore membrane continuity or normal plasma membrane composition and shape. The way this resealing is achieved is still somewhat unclear and is the subject of two alternate but compatible models. The first states that heterotypic fusion events between intracellular vesicles, the membrane patch and the borders of the wounded plasma membrane first restore membrane continuity, after which contraction of an actomyosin ring restores normal plasma membrane composition and shape ([82]; see Section 4.1.1.2). The so-called "vertex fusion" model relies on the same heterotypic fusion events but states that multiple fusion pores would form around the periphery of the wounded region. Expansion of these fusion pores may cause shedding of a membrane fragment containing both wound residual portions of the patch vesicle, in a mechanism reminiscent of the one observed for yeast vacuoles ([83, 84]; reviewed in [81]).

4.1.1.2. Actomyosin contractile ring

As previously discussed, disruptions of the plasma membrane may be accompanied by, as well as induce direct and indirect cytoskeletal disruptions. Restoration of the local cytoskeleton is primarily driven by the contraction of a purse-string structure primarily assembled from F-actin and myosin II [82]. This actomyosin ring is anchored to the plasma membrane at frequent points along its border [82], and its closure has been shown to restore normal membrane composition and shape [82].

Formation of the actomyosin array is controlled by the Ca^{2+}-dependent recruitment and activation of Rho family GTPase proteins [85]. In *Xenopus* oocytes, activated Rho GTPases Ras homolog family member A (RhoA) and cell division control protein 42 homolog (Cdc42) localize to exclusive, concentric zones around the wound [86, 87]. These GTPases influence the activities of, among many other downstream targets, myosin light-chain kinase (MLCK) and myosin phosphatase [88, 89]. Through the above effectors, RhoA indirectly regulate the phosphorylation levels of myosin II light chains, mediating the assembly and contraction of the actomyosin ring (reviewed in [85]). As for Cdc42, its interactions with neural Wiskott-Aldrich syndrome protein (N-WASP) and actin-related protein 2/3 (Arp2/3) [90–92] induce construction of highly dynamic, branched F-actin networks [86]. Binding of Arp2/3 with the C terminus of N-WASP, which is activated by Cdc42, stimulates Arp2/3's actin nucleation activity [91], accelerating production of actin networks critically involved in actomyosin ring assembly. The formation of contractile arrays has been demonstrated to also be regulated by an underlying "signaling treadmill" [93] in which gradients of Rho GTPase activities influence F-actin turnover. RhoA is preferentially activated and maintains its zone of high activity at the leading edge of the wound [93], while active Cdc42 encircles the inner RhoA zone [86]. The processes leading to the establishment of these concentric zones is still somewhat unclear, but a recent study by Vaughan et al. [94] has led to some interesting insights. They observed that wounding induced the formation of micrometer-scale PIP_2-, phosphatidylinositol 3,4,5-trisphosphate (PIP_3)- and phosphatidylserine (PS)-, phosphatidic acid (PA)- and diacylglycerol (DAG)-enriched domains. This is of particular interest as PS moved to a zone closest to the wound edge, near to an area of high RhoA activity, whereas PIP_2 and PIP_3 were observed to be associated with the so-called Cdc42 zone. As for DAG and PA, both of them were shown to immediately segregate in a zone overlapping that of which of RhoA and Cdc42 activity. Since DAG is known to be able to recruit PKCβ and PKCη [95], the authors suggested that generation of DAG at the wound site could therefore act as an upstream signal for the regulation of RhoA and Cdc42. Whether a similar signal cascade exist for somatic cells is still unclear, but cell-lifting experiments done of primary epithelial cells induced phospholipase D (PLD) activation was transient, consistent with a possible role in membrane repair and PLD inhibitors inhibited membrane resealing upon laser injury [96].

Whether such a contractile ring can form in the smaller wounds associated with somatic cells is unclear, but the formation of strikingly similar concentric zones of Rho1, Cdc42 and Rac have been shown to form in *Drosophila* syncytial embryos following plasma membrane wounding (reviewed in [97]).

4.1.2. Neuronal cells and fibroblasts: insights into exocytic repair

Neuronal cells have markedly polarized membranes, with extreme distances between axons and the cell soma. The elongated morphology of axons make them particularly susceptible to shear stress injury and offering a challenge to vesicle trafficking. Fibroblasts, on the other hand, offer a relatively simpler platform for the study of single-cell wound healing.

While the repair of oocytes relies on homotypic fusion of abundant yolk granules (see Section 4.1.1.1), repair of mammalian cells has long been observed to depend on the Ca^{2+}-dependent exocytosis of intracellular vesicles [98]. Conventional lysosomes are not only the major vesicles responsible for Ca^{2+}-dependent exocytosis in non-neuronal and non-secretory cells [99], but also occupy a central role in the exocytic [100] and endocytic models of single-cell repair (see Section 4.1.3.2). The lysosomes involved in plasmalemma repair can be defined as lysosomal-associated membrane protein 1 (LAMP-1)-positive [100], acid sphingomyelinase (ASM)-containing intracellular vesicles [101].

Exocytosis-mediated repair attracted considerable interest when Steinhardt et al. [98] specified the mechanistic similarities with Ca^{2+}-triggered synaptic exocytosis, both of which are dependent on Ca^{2+} [102, 103] and actin cytoskeleton dynamics [104–106]. Ca^{2+}-triggered synaptic exocytosis involves the interaction of synaptotagmin I, a C2 domains-containing protein present in exocytic vesicles and the soluble N-ethylmaleimide-sensitive factor (NSF) attachment protein receptor (SNARE) complexes of the synaptic membrane (reviewed in [107]). Interestingly, neurotransmission inhibitors botulinum neurotoxin A and B also negatively affected or completely blocked membrane healing in sea urchin embryos and Swiss 3T3 fibroblasts [98]. Similarly, treatment with an antibody targeting the active synaptotagmin I C2A domain was observed to prevent membrane resealing of squid and crayfish giant axons [108], 3T3 fibroblasts [100] and rat PC12 cells [109]. In contrast to the neuron-specific synaptotagmin I [110], synaptotagmin VII is ubiquitously expressed and has been found to also influence exocytic membrane repair of other cell types such as sea urchin embryos [98, 103], Chinese hamster ovary cells [100], Swiss 3T3 fibroblasts [98, 100, 111], mouse embryonic fibroblasts [112] and epithelial cells [113–115]. Indeed, embryonic fibroblasts of synaptotagmin VII-deficient mice were observed to have defects in lysosome exocytosis and wound resealing [112]. The mechanism involves the Ca^{2+}-dependent activation and recruitment of synaptotagmin VIII-positive vesicles [111], which are then transported to the wound site via microtubule-dependent trafficking [116]. Once at the plasma membrane, lysosome-bound synaptotagmin VII interacts with the SNARE formed by vesicle-associated membrane protein 7 (VAMP-7), syntaxin-4 and synaptosomal-associated proteins (SNAPs), such as SNAP-23, which leads to heterologous fusion of the lysosome with the plasma membrane [115].

As opposed to the "membrane-patch" model that relies on predominantly homotypic fusions, the exocytic model of single-cell repair assumes the predominance of heterotypic fusion events with the plasma membrane. Indeed, early microneedle-wounding experiments clearly showed a punctate distribution of lysosomal marker LAMP-1 around the wound site [100]. These heterotypic fusion events were initially thought to promote resealing by increasing plasma membrane surface area [100, 117], thereby lowering in-plane membrane tension (see Section 3.1), which could theoretically favor spontaneous resealing events between the two wound edges of with nearby vesicles [118]. Indeed, inhibiting the lowering of in-plane membrane tension via actin stabilization, or by inhibiting exocytosis via neurotoxins A and B ([51, 118] inhibits successful cell repair but is rescued by artificially reducing in-plane tension via the addition of surface active Pluronic F68 NF [51]).

As previously stated, the in-plane tension lowering effect of exocytosis indubitably has been shown to be crucial for plasma membrane repair of a variety of wounds (reviewed in [35, 119]), several lines of evidence have shown that they are not the last process in the resealing of plasma membranes. Indeed, aside from the notable exceptions of facilitated membrane repair that involves recruitment of additional vesicles originating from the transgolgi network (TGN) [120], there is little to no evidence that large micrometer size wounds are repaired via purely exocytic means. Rather, it seems that exocytosis acts as a preliminary step of other wound-healing process (see Section 4.1.3.2). In fact, there is debate as to whether conclusions made in earlier studies of exocytosis were misinterpretations of endocytic vesicles as an exocytic patch or vesicles, due to the studies being performed in the absence of extracellular endocytic tracers [121]. Similarly, there is also considerable evidence that the synaptotagmin VII/SNARE system may not be the only, or even the main, fusogenic system that mediates Ca^{2+}-dependent exocytosis following injury, at least in cells that are under constant mechanical assault such as muscle fibers and muscle cells (see Section 4.1.3).

4.1.3. Muscle cells

4.1.3.1. Dysferlin-mediated exocytosis

Muscle fibers are highly mechanically active and endure constant mechanical stresses from movement and exercise, and therefore are prone to stress-related injury. Indeed, their tubular morphology further facilitates the generation of shear stress along the long axis upon eccentric contraction, in which the muscle fiber lengthens while its constituent sarcomeres contract [122]. T-tubules are invaginations of the sarcolemma that run perpendicular to the overall muscle fiber's long axis. These invaginations penetrate deep into the muscle fiber and mediate depolarization of membrane potential required for proper muscle contraction via excitation-contraction coupling. High levels of normal stress exerted on T-tubules upon eccentric contraction may rupture them, thereby severely disrupting the local sarcolemma [123, 124]. As such, muscle cells, especially muscle fibers, evolved potent single-cell repair mechanisms to cope with the constant duress under which they find themselves. For this reason, muscle cells and muscle fibers were instrumental in the study of mechanisms responsible for mammalian somatic single-cell repair.

Dysferlin was initially identified as genetic causes of limb-girdle muscular dystrophy 2B (LGMD2B) [125] and Miyoshi myopathy [126], and dysferlin has since been shown to be ubiquitously expressed with particularly high levels in skeletal muscle, heart and kidney [127]. Its prominence in muscle membrane repair was experimentally demonstrated when dysferlin-null mice were observed to develop progressive limb-girdle muscular dystrophy 2B due to defects in Ca^{2+}-dependent sarcolemma resealing [128]. Dysferlin is a member of the C2-domain-containing ferlin family, which are known regulators of Ca^{2+}-dependent vesicle fusion for auditory neurotransmission [34, 129, 130] and are believe to be functionally similar to synaptotagmin I [131]. Dysferlin's localization at the sarcolemma [132] has led to its research in the context of sarcolemma repair. Indeed, it appears that in muscle cells, dysferlin is at the center of Ca^{2+}-dependent exocytosis following injury, after which intracellular membranes are delivered to the plasma membrane, and ASM released to the outer leaflet [133].

Molecular events involved in dysferlin-mediated exocytosis are a lot more complex than the one involved in synaptotagmin VII/SNAREs-mediated fusions. Indeed, dysferlin has been shown to bind to or be associated with a relatively high number of proteins including MG53 [134, 135], caveolin-3 [134], annexin I [136] and many others (reviewed in [137]). However, a study of human myoblasts by Lek et al. [50] led to the discovery that a calpain-cleaved product of dysferlin played a direct role in the sarcolemma's exocytic repair mechanism. Briefly, calpains activated by injury-induced Ca^{2+} influx cleave dysferlin, which releases its C-term fragment mini-dysferlinC72 [50, 138, 139]. Following vesicle packaging, mini-dysferlinC72-containing cytoplasmic vesicles are then transported to the wound site. Once localized, mini-dysferlinC72 interacts with MG53 compartments to form an array, which has been proposed to promote repair by way of wound stabilization (see Section 3.2), as well as promote heterotypic fusion between intracellular vesicles [140] and the sarcolemma [50, 138, 139].

Interestingly, dysferlin has also been shown to associate with AHNAK and may be related to enlargeosome exocytosis. Enlargeosomes are small, AHNAK-positive vesicles resistant to nonionic detergents that undergo endocytosis via a nonacidic route and are supposedly distinct form other conventional vesicular compartments [141]. AHNAK [142] is a very large (≈700 KDa) protein involved in a variety of distinct functions and pathologies (reviewed in [143]). The exact nature and contribution of enlargeosomes to dysferlin-mediated repair is still somewhat ill defined and may vary according to wound severity and cell type. Indeed, their regulated exocytoses have been suggested to add significant amount of membrane compo-nents to the injured plasmalemma in neuronal cells [144] and may therefore be involved in either endocytic (see Section 4.1.3.2) or shedding-mediated repair (see Section 4.2.3) [145]. Dysferlin may also modulate plasma membrane repair via its interaction with the AHNAK/S10010A10/Annexin II complex, which is a known organizer of the actin cytoskeleton and plasma membrane architecture [146].

Hence, contrary to oocytes, dysferlin-mediated exocytosis does not exclusively lead to the formation of a "patch," which also results in diminished in-plane membrane tension and ASM release to the outer leaflet.

4.1.3.2. Caveolae-mediated endocytic repair of mechanical wounds

Exocytosis is insufficient to fully explain the repair of membrane disruptions as lesions from pore-forming proteins are readily removed from the plasma membrane (see Section 4.2.1), which is not explainable by exocytosis alone. Also, the repair of SLO and mechanical lesions has been shown not to depend on exocytosis *per se*, but on the injury-induced release of ASM. Indeed, ASM deficiency, as seen in Niemann-Pick disease (NPD) types A and B [147], is capable of Ca^{2+}-dependent exocytosis but have severely limited Ca^{2+}-dependent endocytosis and shows signs of defective plasma membrane repair, both of which can be rescued by exogenously provided ASM [101, 148]. Similarly, inhibition of ASM by desipramine inhibited both endo-cytosis and normal plasma membrane repair [101]. This injury-induced endocytosis had previously been described and suggested to be involved in the endocytic degradation of SLO pores and of mechanical disruptions [149]. The same study identified the endosomes involved to be Ca^{2+}- and cholesterol dependent [149], but did not offer any mechanistic insight into their formation. As previously stated, caveolae are lipid-raft-rich whose formation is dependent on cholesterol, PIP_2 and PS (see Section 3.1), and are known to be facilitated by the transient formation of ceramide on lipid rafts [150, 151]. Once released to extracellular fluid, ASM cleaves the phosphorylcholine heads of sphingomyelin leaflets on the membrane surface to generate ceramide sphingolipids [152]. The resulting ceramide-enriched domains of the phospholipid bilayer are more prone to membrane invaginations due to them encompassing a smaller molecular area relative to other membrane lipids [152], promoting caveolae's endocytic function [153–155]. Similarly, caveolin-3 deficiency causes muscle degeneration in mice [134], which mirrors the limb-girdle muscular dystrophy 1C (LGMD1C) phenotype in humans [156]. As such, exocytosis of lysosomes and dysferlin vesicles after plasma membrane injury may not heal the membrane directly, but rather facilitate membrane resealing by encouraging caveolae formation. Indeed, upon heterotypic fusion with the membrane, ASM is released to the outer surface of the membrane, which potentiates the formation of ceramide-rich platforms that have been shown to trigger invagination of the plasmalemma [157] and formation of caveolae-derived endosomes (reviewed [158]). Indeed, transmission electron microscopy (TEM) has shown that caveolae were found to be concentrated next to mechanical disruptions of muscle cells [153] and assemble into a single, large merged caveolae-like structure around the large wounds generated in primary muscle fibers [153]. As Corrotte et al. correctly pointed out, these very large endocytic vesicles and invaginations may have initially been identified as related to the exocytic "patch" that was initially proposed to cover and eventually heal wounds in muscle cells (see Section 4.1.3.1). Alternatively, Corrotte et al. [153] proposed an endocytic-mediated model of plasma membrane repair. Briefly, large caveolae-like invaginations are formed as a consequence of a combination of the lower in-plane tension provided by the exocytosis of lysosomes, dysferlin-positive vesicles, changes in plasma membrane shape that follows release of ASM, and the presence of proteins such as dysferlin and caveolins. The growth and eventual fusion of those caveolae-like invaginations provides a "constriction force" that promotes plasmalemma resealing [153].

Endocytosis leads to a decrease in total plasma membrane surface area, increasing in-plane membrane tension and providing the force necessary for the mechanical wound removal. It is, however, important to consider that exocytosis of ASM lysosomes always precedes caveolae-mediated endocytosis. The corresponding in-plane membrane tension increases likely readjusts overall apparent membrane tension back to the cell's pre-injury levels, as type-I alveolar epithelial cells are known to remediate to hypertonic shock by increased caveolae-mediated endocytosis [159]. In fact, endocytic repair seems not to be as muscle specific as it was once thought since alveolar cell repair has been suggested to be linked to MG53 and caveolin-1 [160, 161].

4.2. Small wounds: ectocytic repair, blebbing and membrane shedding

4.2.1. Ectocytic repair of pore-forming toxins and blebbing of small mechanical wounds

As previously stated, caveolae-mediated endocytosis was shown to mediate the repair of membrane disruptions created by pore-forming toxins [45]. Indeed, SLO was directly visualized entering cells within caveolar vesicles [153]. Post-internalization, the pore has been shown to be ubiquitinated and eventually degraded by lysosomal hydrolysis [45].

While endocytic repair of SLO pores is now a widely accepted mechanism, it still raises some questions as SLO pores were shown to be successfully removed from the neurites of SH-SY5Y neuroblastoma cells [162]. SH-SY5Y cells are devoid of lysosomes and hence cannot undergo caveolae-mediated endocytosis.

As discussed in Section 3.3.1, Ca^{2+} entry can lead to local actin depolymerization, which in turn leads to a diminution of apparent membrane tension, and the formation of membrane blebs [163]. Indeed, bleb formation seems to principally depend on osmotic pressure and MCAs, the contribution of in-plane tension being minimal [164, 165]. Formation of membrane blebs can be initiated by laser ablation of the cortex cytoskeletal structures [163]. This also explains why formation of membrane blebs is inhibited by drugs that leads to depolymerization [166] or stabilization [167] of the actin cytoskeleton.

SLO pores cause localized Ca^{2+} entry and actin depolymerization without creating large plasma membrane tears-related increases in membrane tension (see Section 3.3.1). As such, it is not surprising that small blebs may be involved in the removal of SLO pores [168]. It should be noted that the same observations strongly suggest that SLO pore insertion, pore assembly, pore clustering and even bleb formation may be Ca^{2+}-independent [168]. This is controversial, however, as it would imply that SLO pore insertion could possibly displace proteins responsible of the interaction of the plasmalemma with the cytoskeleton. This also poses a problem, as other teams have shown a Ca^{2+} [169] and actin disruption [162] dependence for the survival of SLO-treated cells [169], and for the shedding of SLO-laden microvesicles [162]. In this alternate model [162], pore disruption of the membrane elevates local Ca^{2+} concentration which in turn activates annexins and calpains. Calpains then disrupt the underlying actin cytoskeleton, thereby facilitating bleb formation [170] and shedding of SLO vesicles.

4.2.2. ESCRT-mediated shedding of small disruptions

The endosomal sorting complex required for transport (ESCRT) complexes are factors of the lysosomal pathway during protein processing and are involved in various membrane remodeling events such as lysosomal targeting of ubiquitinated proteins and multivesicular body biogenesis, as well as cytokinetic abscission ([171]; reviewed by Olmos and Carlton [172]). There are five currently known ESCRT complexes: ESCRT-0, ESCRT-I, ESCRT-II, ESCRT-III and ESCRT-IV. Of these, ESCRT-III has since been found to modulate much of the membrane remodeling processes, while ESCRT-0, ESCRT-I and ESCRT-II facilitate its targeting to specific cellular compartments, ESCRT-IV orchestrating the disassembly of the ESCRT-III complex for subunit recycling (reviewed in [173]). An additional function of ESCRT-III in plasma membrane repair was proposed in a recent study, which suggested that ESCRT-III is involved in the pinching out or shedding of wounded membranes in HeLa cells [74]. Indeed, injury-induced Ca^{2+} increase results in Ca^{2+} binding of apoptosis-linked gene-2 (ALG-2) around the site of disruption. Active ALG-2 initiates ESCRT machinery assembly by facilitating the accumulation of ALG-2-interacting protein X (ALIX) near the wound site, after which ALG-2 and ALIX recruit ESCRT-III and vacuolar protein sorting-associated protein 4 (Vps4) to the injured plasma membrane [74, 174]. These subunits form a complex, which cleave and shed the wound from the plasma membrane to extracellular space [174]. ESCRT-mediated shedding leads to a decrease in total plasma membrane surface area, increasing in-plane membrane tension.

5. Conclusion

Injury-induced disruptions to the plasma membrane's shape and composition directly affect the cell's tensegrity. The different active membrane repair mechanisms that have been discussed in this chapter are perhaps best seen as a single interconnected pathway, in which the type and size of the wound determine the extent and severity of factors such as tension change and Ca^{2+} entry. These factors in turn dictate the healing mechanisms being used (**Table 1** and

Figure 2). Mechanical lesions lead to high, localized levels of membrane integrity loss, tension change and Ca^{2+} influx. These physical tears of the plasma membrane are often repaired by targeted exocytosis and endocytosis. Contrastingly, smaller injuries such as those generated by electroporation and osmotic shock induce low levels of membrane disruption, tension change and Ca^{2+} influx across large membrane areas. These in turn facilitate processes such as cytoskeletal remodeling or caveolae flattening. Conversely, membranes disrupted by toxic pores do not lead to substantial increase in plane tension. As such, they can either be rapidly shed or degraded following caveolae-mediated endocytosis. Furthermore, it appears that the wound-healing mechanisms prevalent in a given cell-type fall not only in accordance with the prevalence of specific injury types (i.e., PFTs vs. tears vs. ablations), but also according to cell type-specific differences in cell tensegrity and polarity (e.g., muscle cells vs. epithelial cells).

Similar to the plasma membrane and cytoskeletal elements interact to create tensegrity in the single-cell scale, adhesive forces of single cells and the extracellular matrix (ECM) provide structural stiffness to tissues [1]. Considering the above, it should be no surprise that successful single-cell repair influences the success of tissue repair. Indeed, contrary to tissue repair, single-cell repair is largely a binary event: it either takes place allowing the cell's survival, or not, leading to lysis or apoptotic removal. While relevant to wound healing at the tissue-level, these events have little to no relevance for single-cell wound healing outside of the modification of the environment of other injured cells in the surrounding area (asymmetric binding, change in ROS, Ca^{2+} concentration, etc.). Conversely, it seems that successful repair in one cell may lead to an increased repair potential in surrounding cells [175, 176]. This "potentiated" repair has been shown to involve purinergic and nitric oxide (NO)/PKG-signaling pathways [175, 176]. Similarly, repeated insults to a cell's structural and membrane integrity presumably affect a cell's ability to undergo subsequent membrane resealing and cytoskeletal repair, which would be reflected in its long-term viability in a given tissue. Indeed, the prominent view of the origin of the phenotypes associated with muscular dystrophies point toward a heighted susceptibly to repeated mechanical wounding, leading in turn in a higher rate of single-cell repair failure (reviewed in [177, 178]).

Another parallel between single-cell and tissue wound-healing mechanisms is their reliance on contractile arrays. This similarity has been confirmed in multicellular models such as *Xenopus* embryos [179], Caco-2 intestinal epithelial monolayers [180] and Madin-Darby canine kidney (MDCK) epithelial monolayers [181].

Wound closure in epithelial sheets has been demonstrated to be driven by the coupling of actomyosin contraction and collective cell migration [182–185]. The relative contribution of each mechanism in overall re-epithelialization depends on numerous biomechanical factors, including wound geometry [182–184], wound size [182, 186], tissue stiffness [186] and ECM composition [182]. In particular, wounds of cultured bovine corneal endothelial cell monolayers in ECM-deprived conditions were observed to reseal predominantly through actomyosin activity [182]. This is intriguing since cytoskeletal dynamics greatly influence single-cell wound-healing processes (see Section 3.3) and exhibits the ECM and cytoskeleton's analogous relationship across biological scales in the context of wound healing. These observations suggest that the importance of tensegrity components in wound repair are conserved across single-cell and multicellular models.

Considering the single cell's tensegral context in future wound-healing study will help further characterize an increasingly complex unified pathway theory of plasma membrane repair.

Author details

Eric Boucher, Tatsuya Kato and Craig A. Mandato[*]

*Address all correspondence to: craig.mandato@mcgill.ca

Department of Anatomy and Cell Biology, Faculty of Medicine, McGill University, Montreal, Quebec, Canada

References

[1]   Ingber, D.E., N. Wang, and D. Stamenovic, *Tensegrity, cellular biophysics, and the mechanics of living systems*. Rep Prog Phys, 2014. 77(4): p. 046603.

[2]   Fuller, R.B., *Tensegrity*. Portfolio Art News Annu, 1961. 4: pp. 112–27, 144, 148.

[3]   Wang, N., et al., *Mechanical behavior in living cells consistent with the tensegrity model*. Proc Natl Acad Sci U S A, 2001. 98(14): pp. 7765–70.

[4]   Mendez, M.G., D. Restle, and P.A. Janmey, *Vimentin enhances cell elastic behavior and protects against compressive stress*. Biophys J, 2014. 107(2): pp. 314–23.

[5]   Chen, C., et al., *Effects of vimentin disruption on the mechanoresponses of articular chondrocyte*. Biochem Biophys Res Commun, 2016. 469(1): pp. 132–7.

[6]   Diz-Munoz, A., D.A. Fletcher, and O.D. Weiner, *Use the force: membrane tension as an organizer of cell shape and motility*. Trends Cell Biol, 2013. 23(2): pp. 47–53.

[7]   Xue, F., et al., *Effect of membrane stiffness and cytoskeletal element density on mechanical stimuli within cells: an analysis of the consequences of ageing in cells*. Comput Methods Biomech Biomed Engin, 2015. 18(5): pp. 468–76.

[8]   Knoll, R., *A role for membrane shape and information processing in cardiac physiology*. Pflugers Arch, 2015. 467(1): pp. 167–73.

[9]   Chatterjee, S., et al., *Shear stress-related mechanosignaling with lung ischemia: lessons from basic research can inform lung transplantation*. Am J Physiol Lung Cell Mol Physiol, 2014. 307(9): pp. L668–80.

[10] Vuckovic, A., et al., *Alveolarization genes modulated by fetal tracheal occlusion in the rabbit model for congenital diaphragmatic hernia: a randomized study.* PLoS One, 2013. 8(7): p. e69210.

[11] Myers, K.A., et al., *Hydrostatic pressure sensation in cells: integration into the tensegrity model.* Biochem Cell Biol, 2007. 85(5): pp. 543–51.

[12] Parsegian, V.A., R.P. Rand, and D. Gingell, *Lessons for the study of membrane fusion from membrane interactions in phospholipid systems.* Ciba Found Symp, 1984. 103: pp. 9–27.

[13] Zhelev, D.V. and D. Needham, *Tension-stabilized pores in giant vesicles: determination of pore size and pore line tension.* Biochim Biophys Acta, 1993. 1147(1): pp. 89–104.

[14] Hoffman, J.F., *On red blood cells, hemolysis and resealed ghosts.* Adv Exp Med Biol, 1992. 326: pp. 1–15.

[15] Kay, J.G. and S. Grinstein, *Sensing phosphatidylserine in cellular membranes.* Sensors (Basel), 2011. 11(2): pp. 1744–55.

[16] Riske, K.A. and R. Dimova, *Electro-deformation and poration of giant vesicles viewed with high temporal resolution.* Biophys J, 2005. 88(2): pp. 1143–55.

[17] Gozen, I. and P. Dommersnes, *Pore dynamics in lipid membranes.* European Physical Journal-Special Topics, 2014. 223(9): pp. 1813–1829.

[18] Thompson, N.L. and D. Axelrod, *Reduced lateral mobility of a fluorescent lipid probe in cholesterol-depleted erythrocyte membrane.* Biochim Biophys Acta, 1980. 597(1): pp. 155–65.

[19] Golan, D.E., et al., *Lateral mobility of phospholipid and cholesterol in the human erythrocyte membrane: effects of protein-lipid interactions.* Biochemistry, 1984. 23(2): pp. 332–9.

[20] Rand, R.P. and V.A. Parsegian, *Physical force considerations in model and biological membranes.* Can J Biochem Cell Biol, 1984. 62(8): pp. 752–9.

[21] Johnson, R.M. and D.H. Kirkwood, *Loss of resealing ability in erythrocyte membranes. Effect of divalent cations and spectrin release.* Biochim Biophys Acta, 1978. 509(1): pp. 58–66.

[22] McNeil, P.L., K. Miyake, and S.S. Vogel, *The endomembrane requirement for cell surface repair.* Proc Natl Acad Sci U S A, 2003. 100(8): pp. 4592–7.

[23] Tsai, P.S., et al., *Syntaxin and VAMP association with lipid rafts depends on cholesterol depletion in capacitating sperm cells.* Mol Membr Biol, 2007. 24(4): pp. 313–24.

[24] Zitranski, N., et al., *The "acrosomal synapse": Subcellular organization by lipid rafts and scaffolding proteins exhibits high similarities in neurons and mammalian spermatozoa.* Commun Integr Biol, 2010. 3(6): pp. 513–21.

[25] Correia, J., F. Michelangeli, and S. Publicover, *Regulation and roles of Ca2+ stores in human sperm.* Reproduction, 2015. 150(2): pp. R65–76.

[26] Chander, A., et al., *Annexin A7 trafficking to alveolar type II cell surface: possible roles for protein insertion into membranes and lamellar body secretion.* Biochim Biophys Acta, 2013. 1833(5): pp. 1244–55.

[27] Ichimura, H., et al., *Lung surfactant secretion by interalveolar Ca2+ signaling.* Am J Physiol Lung Cell Mol Physiol, 2006. 291(4): pp. L596–601.

[28] Miklavc, P., et al., *Ca2+-dependent actin coating of lamellar bodies after exocytotic fusion: a prerequisite for content release or kiss-and-run.* Ann N Y Acad Sci, 2009. 1152: pp. 43–52.

[29] Cardenas, A.M. and F. Marengo, *How the stimulus defines the dynamics of vesicle pool recruitment, fusion mode and vesicle recycling in neuroendocrine cells.* J Neurochem, 2016. DOI: 10.1111/jnc.13565.

[30] Chung, C. and J. Raingo, *Vesicle dynamics: how synaptic proteins regulate different modes of neurotransmission.* J Neurochem, 2013. 126(2): pp. 146–54.

[31] de Jong, A.P. and D. Fioravante, *Translating neuronal activity at the synapse: presynaptic calcium sensors in short-term plasticity.* Front Cell Neurosci, 2014. 8: p. 356.

[32] Shin, O.H., *Exocytosis and synaptic vesicle function.* Compr Physiol, 2014. 4(1): pp. 149–75.

[33] Pangrsic, T., E. Reisinger, and T. Moser, *Otoferlin: a multi-C2 domain protein essential for hearing.* Trends Neurosci, 2012. 35(11): pp. 671–80.

[34] Beurg, M., et al., *Control of exocytosis by synaptotagmins and otoferlin in auditory hair cells.* J Neurosci, 2010. 30(40): pp. 13281–90.

[35] Boucher, E. and C.A. Mandato, *Plasma membrane and cytoskeleton dynamics during single-cell wound healing.* Biochim Biophys Acta, 2015. 1853(10 Pt A): pp. 2649–61.

[36] Yamada, E., *The fine structure of the gall bladder epithelium of the mouse.* J Biophys Biochem Cytol, 1955. 1(5): pp. 445–58.

[37] Dulhunty, A.F. and C. Franzini-Armstrong, *The relative contributions of the folds and caveolae to the surface membrane of frog skeletal muscle fibres at different sarcomere lengths.* J Physiol, 1975. 250(3): pp. 513–39.

[38] Kozera, L., E. White, and S. Calaghan, *Caveolae act as membrane reserves which limit mechanosensitive I(Cl,swell) channel activation during swelling in the rat ventricular myocyte.* PLoS One, 2009. 4(12): p. e8312.

[39] Calaghan, S., L. Kozera, and E. White, *Compartmentalisation of cAMP-dependent signalling by caveolae in the adult cardiac myocyte.* J Mol Cell Cardiol, 2008. 45(1): pp. 88–92.

[40] Sinha, B., et al., *Cells respond to mechanical stress by rapid disassembly of caveolae.* Cell, 2011. 144(3): pp. 402–13.

[41] Kovtun, O., et al., *Cavin family proteins and the assembly of caveolae.* J Cell Sci, 2015. 128(7): pp. 1269–78.

[42] Shvets, E., A. Ludwig, and B.J. Nichols, *News from the caves: update on the structure and function of caveolae*. Curr Opin Cell Biol, 2014. 29: pp. 99–106.

[43] Hagiwara, Y., et al., *Caveolin-3 deficiency causes muscle degeneration in mice*. Hum Mol Genet, 2000. 9(20): pp. 3047–54.

[44] Wolfmeier, H., et al., *Ca-dependent repair of pneumolysin pores: A new paradigm for host cellular defense against bacterial pore-forming toxins*. Biochim Biophys Acta, 2015. 1853 (9): p. 2045-54.

[45] Corrotte, M., et al., *Toxin pores endocytosed during plasma membrane repair traffic into the lumen of MVBs for degradation*. Traffic, 2012. 13(3): pp. 483–94.

[46] Gerke, V. and S.E. Moss, *Annexins: from structure to function*. Physiol Rev, 2002. 82(2): pp. 331–71.

[47] Voges, D., et al., *Three-dimensional structure of membrane-bound annexin V. A correlative electron microscopy-X-ray crystallography study*. J Mol Biol, 1994. 238(2): pp. 199–213.

[48] Cezanne, L., et al., *Organization and dynamics of the proteolipid complexes formed by annexin V and lipids in planar supported lipid bilayers*. Biochemistry, 1999. 38(9): pp. 2779–86.

[49] Bouter, A., et al., *Annexin-A5 assembled into two-dimensional arrays promotes cell membrane repair*. Nat Commun, 2011. 2: p. 270.

[50] Lek, A., et al., *Calpains, cleaved mini-dysferlinC72, and L-type channels underpin calcium-dependent muscle membrane repair*. J Neurosci, 2013. 33(12): pp. 5085–94.

[51] Togo, T., et al., *The mechanism of facilitated cell membrane resealing*. J Cell Sci, 1999. 112 (Pt 5): pp. 719–31.

[52] Xie, X.Y. and J.N. Barrett, *Membrane resealing in cultured rat septal neurons after neurite transection: evidence for enhancement by Ca(2+)-triggered protease activity and cytoskeletal disassembly*. J Neurosci, 1991. 11(10): pp. 3257–67.

[53] Miyake, K., et al., *An actin barrier to resealing*. J Cell Sci, 2001. 114(Pt 19): pp. 3487–94.

[54] Chen, X., et al., *Single-site sonoporation disrupts actin cytoskeleton organization*. J R Soc Interface, 2014. 11(95): p. 20140071.

[55] Deguchi, S. and M. Sato, *Biomechanical properties of actin stress fibers of non-motile cells*. Biorheology, 2009. 46(2): pp. 93–105.

[56] Sato, K., et al., *Quantitative evaluation of threshold fiber strain that induces reorganization of cytoskeletal actin fiber structure in osteoblastic cells*. J Biomech, 2005. 38(9): pp. 1895–901.

[57] Costa, K.D., W.J. Hucker, and F.C. Yin, *Buckling of actin stress fibers: a new wrinkle in the cytoskeletal tapestry*. Cell Motil Cytoskeleton, 2002. 52(4): pp. 266–74.

[58] Matsui, T.S., et al., *Non-muscle myosin II induces disassembly of actin stress fibres independently of myosin light chain dephosphorylation*. Interface Focus, 2011. 1(5): pp. 754–66.

[59] Wu, T. and J.J. Feng, *A biomechanical model for fluidization of cells under dynamic strain.* Biophys J, 2015. 108(1): pp. 43–52.

[60] De La Cruz, E.M., J.L. Martiel, and L. Blanchoin, *Mechanical heterogeneity favors fragmentation of strained actin filaments.* Biophys J, 2015. 108(9): pp. 2270–81.

[61] Hayakawa, K., H. Tatsumi, and M. Sokabe, *Mechano-sensing by actin filaments and focal adhesion proteins.* Commun Integr Biol, 2012. 5(6): pp. 572–7.

[62] Hirata, H., et al., *Non-channel mechanosensors working at focal adhesion-stress fiber complex.* Pflugers Arch, 2015. 467(1): pp. 141–55.

[63] Hayakawa, K., H. Tatsumi, and M. Sokabe, *Actin filaments function as a tension sensor by tension-dependent binding of cofilin to the filament.* J Cell Biol, 2011. 195(5): pp. 721–7.

[64] Bernstein, B.W. and J.R. Bamburg, *ADF/cofilin: a functional node in cell biology.* Trends Cell Biol, 2010. 20(4): pp. 187–95.

[65] Orlova, A., et al., *Actin-destabilizing factors disrupt filaments by means of a time reversal of polymerization.* Proc Natl Acad Sci U S A, 2004. 101(51): pp. 17664–8.

[66] Martinac, B., *Mechanosensitive ion channels: molecules of mechanotransduction.* J Cell Sci, 2004. 117(Pt 12): pp. 2449–60.

[67] Muallem, S., et al., *Actin filament disassembly is a sufficient final trigger for exocytosis in nonexcitable cells.* J Cell Biol, 1995. 128(4): pp. 589–98.

[68] Biro, E.N. and S.Y. Venyaminov, *Depolymerization of actin in concentrated solutions of divalent metal chlorides.* Acta Biochim Biophys Acad Sci Hung, 1979. 14(1–2): pp. 31–42.

[69] Zechel, K., *Stability differences of muscle F-actin in formamide in the presence of Mg2+ and Ca2+.* Biochim Biophys Acta, 1983. 742(1): pp. 135–41.

[70] Ono, Y. and H. Sorimachi, *Calpains: an elaborate proteolytic system.* Biochim Biophys Acta, 2012. 1824(1): pp. 224–36.

[71] Nayal, A., D.J. Webb, and A.F. Horwitz, *Talin: an emerging focal point of adhesion dynamics.* Curr Opin Cell Biol, 2004. 16(1): pp. 94–8.

[72] Gasman, S., et al., *Regulated exocytosis in neuroendocrine cells: a role for subplasmalemmal Cdc42/N-WASP-induced actin filaments.* Mol Biol Cell, 2004. 15(2): pp. 520–31.

[73] Goodson, H.V., C. Valetti, and T.E. Kreis, *Motors and membrane traffic.* Curr Opin Cell Biol, 1997. 9(1): pp. 18–28.

[74] Jimenez, A.J., et al., *ESCRT machinery is required for plasma membrane repair.* Science, 2014. 343(6174): p. 1247136.

[75] Terasaki, M., K. Miyake, and P.L. McNeil, *Large plasma membrane disruptions are rapidly resealed by Ca2+-dependent vesicle-vesicle fusion events.* J Cell Biol, 1997. 139(1): pp. 63–74.

[76] McNeil, P.L., et al., *Patching plasma membrane disruptions with cytoplasmic membrane*. J Cell Sci, 2000. 113 (Pt 11): pp. 1891–902.

[77] Abreu-Blanco, M.T., J.M. Verboon, and S.M. Parkhurst, *Cell wound repair in Drosophila occurs through three distinct phases of membrane and cytoskeletal remodeling*. J Cell Biol, 2011. 193(3): pp. 455–64.

[78] Karasaki, S., *Studies on amphibian yolk 1. The ultrastructure of the yolk platelet*. J Cell Biol, 1963. 18: pp. 135–51.

[79] Glover, L. and R.H. Brown, Jr., *Dysferlin in membrane trafficking and patch repair*. Traffic, 2007. 8(7): pp. 785–94.

[80] Han, R. and K.P. Campbell, *Dysferlin and muscle membrane repair*. Curr Opin Cell Biol, 2007. 19(4): pp. 409–16.

[81] Andrews, N.W., P.E. Almeida, and M. Corrotte, *Damage control: cellular mechanisms of plasma membrane repair*. Trends Cell Biol, 2014. 24(12): pp. 734–742.

[82] Mandato, C.A. and W.M. Bement, *Contraction and polymerization cooperate to assemble and close actomyosin rings around Xenopus oocyte wounds*. J Cell Biol, 2001. 154(4): pp. 785–97.

[83] Wang, L., et al., *Vacuole fusion at a ring of vertex docking sites leaves membrane fragments within the organelle*. Cell, 2002. 108(3): pp. 357–69.

[84] McNeil, P.L. and T. Kirchhausen, *An emergency response team for membrane repair*. Nat Rev Mol Cell Biol, 2005. 6(6): pp. 499–505.

[85] Darenfed, H. and C.A. Mandato, *Wound-induced contractile ring: a model for cytokinesis*. Biochem Cell Biol, 2005. 83(6): pp. 711–20.

[86] Benink, H.A. and W.M. Bement, *Concentric zones of active RhoA and Cdc42 around single cell wounds*. J Cell Biol, 2005. 168(3): pp. 429–39.

[87] Bement, W.M., H.A. Benink, and G. von Dassow, *A microtubule-dependent zone of active RhoA during cleavage plane specification*. J Cell Biol, 2005. 170(1): pp. 91–101.

[88] Kawano, Y., et al., *Phosphorylation of myosin-binding subunit (MBS) of myosin phosphatase by Rho-kinase in vivo*. J Cell Biol, 1999. 147(5): pp. 1023–38.

[89] Bishop, A.L. and A. Hall, *Rho GTPases and their effector proteins*. Biochem J, 2000. 348 Pt 2: pp. 241–55.

[90] Egile, C., et al., *Activation of the CDC42 effector N-WASP by the Shigella flexneri IcsA protein promotes actin nucleation by Arp2/3 complex and bacterial actin-based motility*. J Cell Biol, 1999. 146(6): pp. 1319–32.

[91] Rohatgi, R., et al., *The interaction between N-WASP and the Arp2/3 complex links Cdc42-dependent signals to actin assembly*. Cell, 1999. 97(2): pp. 221–231.

[92] Taunton, J., et al., *Actin-dependent propulsion of endosomes and lysosomes by recruitment of N-WASP*. J Cell Biol, 2000. 148(3): pp. 519–30.

[93] Burkel, B.M., et al., *A Rho GTPase signal treadmill backs a contractile array*. Dev Cell, 2012. 23(2): pp. 384–96.

[94] Vaughan, E.M., et al., *Lipid domain-dependent regulation of single-cell wound repair*. Mol Biol Cell, 2014. 25(12): pp. 1867–76.

[95] Yu, H.Y. and W.M. Bement, *Control of local actin assembly by membrane fusion-dependent compartment mixing*. Nat Cell Biol, 2007. 9(2): pp. 149–59.

[96] Arun, S.N., et al., *Cell wounding activates phospholipase D in primary mouse keratinocytes*. J Lipid Res, 2013. 54(3): pp. 581–91.

[97] Abreu-Blanco, M.T., J.M. Verboon, and S.M. Parkhurst, *Coordination of Rho family GTPase activities to orchestrate cytoskeleton responses during cell wound repair*. Curr Biol, 2014. 24(2): pp. 144–55.

[98] Steinhardt, R.A., G. Bi, and J.M. Alderton, *Cell membrane resealing by a vesicular mechanism similar to neurotransmitter release*. Science, 1994. 263(5145): pp. 390–3.

[99] Jaiswal, J.K., N.W. Andrews, and S.M. Simon, *Membrane proximal lysosomes are the major vesicles responsible for calcium-dependent exocytosis in nonsecretory cells*. J Cell Biol, 2002. 159(4): pp. 625–35.

[100] Reddy, A., E.V. Caler, and N.W. Andrews, *Plasma membrane repair is mediated by Ca(2+)-regulated exocytosis of lysosomes*. Cell, 2001. 106(2): pp. 157–69.

[101] Tam, C., et al., *Exocytosis of acid sphingomyelinase by wounded cells promotes endocytosis and plasma membrane repair*. J Cell Biol, 2010. 189(6): pp. 1027–38.

[102] Leitz, J. and E.T. Kavalali, *Ca2+ Dependence of synaptic vesicle endocytosis*. Neuroscientist, 2015. DOI: 10.1177/1073858415588265.

[103] Bi, G.Q., J.M. Alderton, and R.A. Steinhardt, *Calcium-regulated exocytosis is required for cell membrane resealing*. J Cell Biol, 1995. 131(6 Pt 2): pp. 1747–58.

[104] Rust, M.B., *ADF/cofilin: a crucial regulator of synapse physiology and behavior*. Cell Mol Life Sci, 2015. 72(18): pp. 3521–9.

[105] Bi, G.Q., et al., *Kinesin- and myosin-driven steps of vesicle recruitment for Ca2+-regulated exocytosis*. J Cell Biol, 1997. 138(5): pp. 999–1008.

[106] McNeil, P.L., *Repairing a torn cell surface: make way, lysosomes to the rescue*. J Cell Sci, 2002. 115(Pt 5): pp. 873–9.

[107] Rizo, J. and J. Xu, *The synaptic vesicle release machinery*. Annu Rev Biophys, 2015. 44: pp. 339–67.

[108] Detrait, E., et al., *Axolemmal repair requires proteins that mediate synaptic vesicle fusion.* J Neurobiol, 2000. 44(4): pp. 382–91.

[109] Detrait, E.R., et al., *Plasmalemmal repair of severed neurites of PC12 cells requires Ca(2+) and synaptotagmin.* J Neurosci Res, 2000. 62(4): pp. 566–73.

[110] Fox, M.A. and J.R. Sanes, *Synaptotagmin I and II are present in distinct subsets of central synapses.* J Comp Neurol, 2007. 503(2): pp. 280–96.

[111] Shen, S.S., et al., *Molecular regulation of membrane resealing in 3T3 fibroblasts.* J Biol Chem, 2005. 280(2): pp. 1652–60.

[112] Chakrabarti, S., et al., *Impaired membrane resealing and autoimmune myositis in synaptotagmin VII-deficient mice.* J Cell Biol, 2003. 162(4): pp. 543–9.

[113] Toops, K.A. and A. Lakkaraju, *Let's play a game of chutes and ladders: lysosome fusion with the epithelial plasma membrane.* Commun Integr Biol, 2013. 6(4): p. e24474.

[114] Shen, S.S. and R.A. Steinhardt, *The mechanisms of cell membrane resealing in rabbit corneal epithelial cells.* Curr Eye Res, 2005. 30(7): pp. 543–54.

[115] Rao, S.K., et al., *Identification of SNAREs involved in synaptotagmin VII-regulated lysosomal exocytosis.* J Biol Chem, 2004. 279(19): pp. 20471–9.

[116] Tardieux, I., et al., *Lysosome recruitment and fusion are early events required for trypanosome invasion of mammalian cells.* Cell, 1992. 71(7): pp. 1117–30.

[117] Miyake, K. and P.L. McNeil, *Vesicle accumulation and exocytosis at sites of plasma membrane disruption.* J Cell Biol, 1995. 131(6 Pt 2): pp. 1737–45.

[118] Togo, T., T.B. Krasieva, and R.A. Steinhardt, *A decrease in membrane tension precedes successful cell-membrane repair.* Mol Biol Cell, 2000. 11(12): pp. 4339–46.

[119] Cooper, S.T. and P.L. McNeil, *Membrane repair: mechanisms and pathophysiology.* Physiol Rev, 2015. 95(4): pp. 1205–40.

[120] Togo, T. and R.A. Steinhardt, *Nonmuscle myosin IIA and IIB have distinct functions in the exocytosis-dependent process of cell membrane repair.* Mol Biol Cell, 2004. 15(2): pp. 688–95.

[121] Andrews, N.W., M. Corrotte, and T. Castro-Gomes, *Above the fray: surface remodeling by secreted lysosomal enzymes leads to endocytosis-mediated plasma membrane repair.* Semin Cell Dev Biol, 2015. 45: pp. 10–7.

[122] Stauber, W.T., *Eccentric action of muscles: physiology, injury, and adaptation.* Exerc Sport Sci Rev, 1989. 17: pp. 157–85.

[123] Proske, U. and D.L. Morgan, *Muscle damage from eccentric exercise: mechanism, mechanical signs, adaptation and clinical applications.* J Physiol, 2001. 537(Pt 2): pp. 333–45.

[124] Takekura, H., et al., *Eccentric exercise-induced morphological changes in the membrane systems involved in excitation-contraction coupling in rat skeletal muscle.* J Physiol, 2001. 533(Pt 2): pp. 571–83.

[125] Bashir, R., et al., *A gene related to Caenorhabditis elegans spermatogenesis factor fer-1 is mutated in limb-girdle muscular dystrophy type 2B.* Nat Genet, 1998. 20(1): pp. 37–42.

[126] Liu, J., et al., *Dysferlin, a novel skeletal muscle gene, is mutated in Miyoshi myopathy and limb girdle muscular dystrophy.* Nat Genet, 1998. 20(1): pp. 31–6.

[127] Anderson, L.V., et al., *Dysferlin is a plasma membrane protein and is expressed early in human development.* Hum Mol Genet, 1999. 8(5): pp. 855–61.

[128] Bansal, D., et al., *Defective membrane repair in dysferlin-deficient muscular dystrophy.* Nature, 2003. 423(6936): pp. 168–72.

[129] Pangrsic, T., et al., *Hearing requires otoferlin-dependent efficient replenishment of synaptic vesicles in hair cells.* Nat Neurosci, 2010. 13(7): pp. 869–76.

[130] Johnson, C.P. and E.R. Chapman, *Otoferlin is a calcium sensor that directly regulates SNARE-mediated membrane fusion.* J Cell Biol, 2010. 191(1): pp. 187–97.

[131] Reisinger, E., et al., *Probing the functional equivalence of otoferlin and synaptotagmin 1 in exocytosis.* J Neurosci, 2011. 31(13): pp. 4886–95.

[132] Piccolo, F., et al., *Intracellular accumulation and reduced sarcolemmal expression of dysferlin in limb – girdle muscular dystrophies.* Ann Neurol, 2000. 48(6): pp. 902–12.

[133] McDade, J.R., A. Archambeau, and D.E. Michele, *Rapid actin-cytoskeleton-dependent recruitment of plasma membrane-derived dysferlin at wounds is critical for muscle membrane repair.* FASEB J, 2014. 28(8): pp. 3660–70.

[134] Cai, C., et al., *Membrane repair defects in muscular dystrophy are linked to altered interaction between MG53, caveolin-3, and dysferlin.* J Biol Chem, 2009. 284(23): pp. 15894–902.

[135] Matsuda, C., et al., *The C2A domain in dysferlin is important for association with MG53 (TRIM72).* PLoS Curr, 2012. 4: p. e5035add8caff4.

[136] Waddell, L.B., et al., *Dysferlin, annexin A1, and mitsugumin 53 are upregulated in muscular dystrophy and localize to longitudinal tubules of the T-system with stretch.* J Neuropathol Exp Neurol, 2011. 70(4): pp. 302–13.

[137] Cacciottolo, M., et al., *Reverse engineering gene network identifies new dysferlin-interacting proteins.* J Biol Chem, 2011. 286(7): pp. 5404–13.

[138] Redpath, G.M., et al., *Calpain cleavage within dysferlin exon 40a releases a synaptotagmin-like module for membrane repair.* Mol Biol Cell, 2014. 25(19): pp. 3037–48.

[139] Fuson, K., et al., *Alternate splicing of dysferlin C2A confers Ca(2)(+)-dependent and Ca(2)(+)-independent binding for membrane repair.* Structure, 2014. 22(1): pp. 104–15.

[140] McDade, J.R. and D.E. Michele, *Membrane damage-induced vesicle-vesicle fusion of dysferlin-containing vesicles in muscle cells requires microtubules and kinesin*. Hum Mol Genet, 2014. 23(7): pp. 1677–86.

[141] Cocucci, E., et al., *Enlargeosome, an exocytic vesicle resistant to nonionic detergents, undergoes endocytosis via a nonacidic route*. Mol Biol Cell, 2004. 15(12): pp. 5356–68.

[142] Shtivelman, E., F.E. Cohen, and J.M. Bishop, *A human gene (AHNAK) encoding an unusually large protein with a 1.2-microns polyionic rod structure*. Proc Natl Acad Sci U S A, 1992. 89(12): pp. 5472–6.

[143] Davis, T.A., B. Loos, and A.M. Engelbrecht, *AHNAK: the giant jack of all trades*. Cell Signal, 2014. 26(12): pp. 2683–2693.

[144] Borgonovo, B., et al., *Regulated exocytosis: a novel, widely expressed system*. Nat Cell Biol, 2002. 4(12): pp. 955–62.

[145] Cocucci, E., et al., *Enlargeosome traffic: exocytosis triggered by various signals is followed by endocytosis, membrane shedding or both*. Traffic, 2007. 8(6): pp. 742–57.

[146] Benaud, C., et al., *AHNAK interaction with the annexin 2/S100A10 complex regulates cell membrane cytoarchitecture*. J Cell Biol, 2004. 164(1): pp. 133–44.

[147] Schuchman, E.H., *Acid sphingomyelinase, cell membranes and human disease: lessons from Niemann-Pick disease*. FEBS Lett, 2010. 584(9): pp. 1895–900.

[148] Zha, X., et al., *Sphingomyelinase treatment induces ATP-independent endocytosis*. J Cell Biol, 1998. 140(1): pp. 39–47.

[149] Idone, V., et al., *Repair of injured plasma membrane by rapid Ca2+-dependent endocytosis*. J Cell Biol, 2008. 180(5): pp. 905–14.

[150] Gulbins, E. and R. Kolesnick, *Raft ceramide in molecular medicine*. Oncogene, 2003. 22(45): pp. 7070–7.

[151] van Blitterswijk, W.J., et al., *Ceramide: second messenger or modulator of membrane structure and dynamics?* Biochem J, 2003. 369(Pt 2): pp. 199–211.

[152] Holopainen, J.M., M.I. Angelova, and P.K. Kinnunen, *Vectorial budding of vesicles by asymmetrical enzymatic formation of ceramide in giant liposomes*. Biophys J, 2000. 78(2): pp. 830–8.

[153] Corrotte, M., et al., *Caveolae internalization repairs wounded cells and muscle fibers*. Elife, 2013. 2: p. e00926.

[154] Nabi, I.R. and P.U. Le, *Caveolae/raft-dependent endocytosis*. J Cell Biol, 2003. 161(4): pp. 673–7.

[155] Nichols, B., *Caveosomes and endocytosis of lipid rafts*. J Cell Sci, 2003. 116(Pt 23): pp. 4707–14.

[156] Nigro, V. and M. Savarese, *Genetic basis of limb-girdle muscular dystrophies: the 2014 update*. Acta Myol, 2014. 33(3): pp. 1–12.

[157] Trajkovic, K., et al., *Ceramide triggers budding of exosome vesicles into multivesicular endosomes*. Science, 2008. 319(5867): pp. 1244–7.

[158] Draeger, A. and E.B. Babiychuk, *Ceramide in plasma membrane repair*. Handb Exp Pharmacol, 2013(216): pp. 341–53.

[159] Wang, S., et al., *Endocytic response of type I alveolar epithelial cells to hypertonic stress*. Am J Physiol Lung Cell Mol Physiol, 2011. 300(4): pp. L560–8.

[160] Kim, S.C., et al., *TRIM72 is required for effective repair of alveolar epithelial cell wounding*. Am J Physiol Lung Cell Mol Physiol, 2014. 307(6): pp. L449–59.

[161] Jia, Y., et al., *Treatment of acute lung injury by targeting MG53-mediated cell membrane repair*. Nat Commun, 2014. 5: p. 4387.

[162] Atanassoff, A.P., et al., *Microvesicle shedding and lysosomal repair fulfill divergent cellular needs during the repair of streptolysin O-induced plasmalemmal damage*. PLoS One, 2014. 9(2): p. e89743.

[163] Tinevez, J.Y., et al., *Role of cortical tension in bleb growth*. Proc Natl Acad Sci U S A, 2009. 106(44): pp. 18581–6.

[164] Charras, G.T., et al., *Life and times of a cellular bleb*. Biophys J, 2008. 94(5): pp. 1836–53.

[165] Dai, J. and M.P. Sheetz, *Membrane tether formation from blebbing cells*. Biophys J, 1999. 77(6): pp. 3363–70.

[166] Charras, G.T., et al., *Non-equilibration of hydrostatic pressure in blebbing cells*. Nature, 2005. 435(7040): pp. 365–9.

[167] Cunningham, C.C., *Actin polymerization and intracellular solvent flow in cell surface blebbing*. J Cell Biol, 1995. 129(6): pp. 1589–99.

[168] Keyel, P.A., et al., *Streptolysin O clearance through sequestration into blebs that bud passively from the plasma membrane*. J Cell Sci, 2011. 124(Pt 14): pp. 2414–23.

[169] Babiychuk, E.B., et al., *Blebbing confers resistance against cell lysis*. Cell Death Differ, 2011. 18(1): pp. 80–9.

[170] Gauthier, N.C., et al., *Temporary increase in plasma membrane tension coordinates the activation of exocytosis and contraction during cell spreading*. Proc Natl Acad Sci U S A, 2011. 108(35): pp. 14467–72.

[171] Morita, E., et al., *Human ESCRT and ALIX proteins interact with proteins of the midbody and function in cytokinesis*. EMBO J, 2007. 26(19): pp. 4215–27.

[172] Olmos, Y. and J.G. Carlton, *The ESCRT machinery: new roles at new holes*. Curr Opin Cell Biol, 2016. 38: pp. 1–11.

[173] Schuh, A.L. and A. Audhya, *The ESCRT machinery: from the plasma membrane to endosomes and back again.* Crit Rev Biochem Mol Biol, 2014. 49(3): pp. 242–61.

[174] Scheffer, L.L., et al., *Mechanism of Ca(2)(+)-triggered ESCRT assembly and regulation of cell membrane repair.* Nat Commun, 2014. 5: p. 5646.

[175] Togo, T., *Cell membrane disruption stimulates NO/PKG signaling and potentiates cell membrane repair in neighboring cells.* PLoS One, 2012. 7(8): p. e42885.

[176] Togo, T., *Short-term potentiation of membrane resealing in neighboring cells is mediated by purinergic signaling.* Purinergic Signal, 2014. 10(2): pp. 283–90.

[177] Cooper, S.T. and S.I. Head, *Membrane injury and repair in the muscular dystrophies.* Neuroscientist, 2014. 21(6): p. 653–68.

[178] Allen, D.G., N.P. Whitehead, and S.C. Froehner, *Absence of dystrophin disrupts skeletal muscle signaling: Roles of Ca2+, reactive oxygen species, and nitric oxide in the development of muscular dystrophy.* Physiol Rev, 2016. 96(1): pp. 253–305.

[179] Clark, A.G., et al., *Integration of single and multicellular wound responses.* Curr Biol, 2009. 19(16): pp. 1389–95.

[180] Russo, J.M., et al., *Distinct temporal-spatial roles for rho kinase and myosin light chain kinase in epithelial purse-string wound closure.* Gastroenterology, 2005. 128(4): pp. 987–1001.

[181] Tamada, M., et al., *Two distinct modes of myosin assembly and dynamics during epithelial wound closure.* J Cell Biol, 2007. 176(1): pp. 27–33.

[182] Grasso, S., J.A. Hernandez, and S. Chifflet, *Roles of wound geometry, wound size, and extracellular matrix in the healing response of bovine corneal endothelial cells in culture.* Am J Physiol Cell Physiol, 2007. 293(4): pp. C1327–37.

[183] Klarlund, J.K., *Dual modes of motility at the leading edge of migrating epithelial cell sheets.* Proc Natl Acad Sci U S A, 2012. 109(39): pp. 15799–804.

[184] Ravasio, A., et al., *Gap geometry dictates epithelial closure efficiency.* Nat Commun, 2015. 6: p. 7683.

[185] Brugués, A., et al., *Forces driving epithelial wound healing.* Nat Phys, 2014. 10(9): pp. 683–90.

[186] Wu, M. and M. Ben Amar, *Growth and remodelling for profound circular wounds in skin.* Biomech Model Mechanobiol, 2015. 14(2): pp. 357–70.

7

The Use of Amniotic Membrane in the Management of Complex Chronic Wounds

Gregorio Castellanos, Ángel Bernabé-García,
Carmen García Insausti, Antonio Piñero,
José M. Moraleda and Francisco J. Nicolás

Abstract

Chronic wounds do not follow the usual wound healing process; instead, they are stuck in the inflammatory or proliferative phase. This is particularly evident in large, massive wounds with considerable tissue loss, which become senescent and do not epithelialize. In these wounds, we need to remove all the factors that prevent or delay normal wound healing. After that, soft tissue granulation is stimulated by local negative pressure therapy. Lastly, after the granulation is completed, the epithelialization process must be activated. Although a plethora of wound dressings and devices are available, chronic wounds persist as a unresolved medical concern. We have been using frozen amniotic membrane (AM) to treat this type of wounds with good results. Our studies have shown that AM is able to induce epithelialization in large wounds that were unable to epithelialize. AM induces several signaling pathways involved in cell migration and/or proliferation. Among those, we can highlight the mitogen-activated protein kinase (MAPK) and Jun N-terminal kinase (JNK) signaling pathways. Additionally, AM is able to selectively antagonise the anti-proliferative effect of TGFß by modifying its genetic program on keratinocytes. The combined effect of AM on keratinocytes, promoting cell proliferation/migration and antagonising TGFß-effect, is the perfect combination allowing chronic wounds to progress into epithelialization.

Keywords: soft-tissue chronic wounds, amniotic membrane, TGF-β, epithelialization

1. Introduction

The evolution of knowledge about the biology of wound healing makes it possible to predict the sequence and prognosis of the events that occur in this complex process. However, there are wounds in which healing can be either prolonged over time or not fully achieved [1, 2].

Therefore, The keys to providing adequate and efficient treatment involve identifying, as soon as possible, the combination of either internal or external factors that contribute to the complexity of the wound and affect the healing process, and to detect at an early stage when it is likely that a wound would be slow or difficult to heal.

The actions undertaken should be aimed at reducing the aspects that lead to complexity, including factors related to the patient, the wound, relationships with healthcare personnel, and available resources. Only by assessing and understanding the interaction between these factors and their effect on healing will it be possible to develop efficient and appropriate strategies for improving results. Similarly, certain characteristics of the wound, such as its anatomical location, time duration, size, depth, and the state of the wound bed, are correlated with adequate healing [3–5].

The presence of necrotic tissue, crusts, slough, or foreign bodies in the wound bed, which are all obstacles for wound assessment, can lead to a delay in healing, and they can also be a focus of infection. Therefore, it is important to provide frequent, extensive, and efficient debridement until healthy tissue is found [6]. There are other situations that can have an influence and cause healing to fail, such as ischemia. Poor perfusion deprives tissue of an efficient oxygen and metabolic exchange, and causes an increase in vascular permeability, leukocyte retention, synthesis and the liberation of oxygen free radicals and proteolytic enzymes [7]. Inflammation in chronic wounds brings about a prolongation in healing time, resulting in an exacerbated inflammatory reaction, which in turn causes the hyperproduction of pro-inflammatory cytokines and proteolytic enzymes. This activity is combined with a decrease in the secretion of metalloproteinase tissue inhibitors, and it intensifies as the wound bed pH alters. As a consequence, we find that in the wound bed there is a sustained inflammation with matrix degradation, a limited bioavailability of growth factors and intense fibroblast aging, all of which reduce tissue repair, cell proliferation, and angiogenesis [8, 9].

In the same way, chronic wounds are characterized by the presence of one or more bacterial strains, with antibiotic-resistant microorganisms, and the presence of biofilms within which the bacteria are protected against the action of the silver-based antimicrobials [10–13].

The initial response to treatment is indicative of the viability of the tissue and its capacity to heal. When a patient's wound does not heal in the planned period of time using conventional treatment, it is essential to reassess the patient and modify the therapeutic guidelines [14, 15].

Thus, tissue wound healing usually follows a predictable sequence, although in some cases, it is prolonged over time or it is never achieved. The wound healing process is the result of a complex interaction between the patient and wound factors, the treatment adopted, and the skills and knowledge of healthcare professionals. Only by carrying out a detailed initial assessment and repeated treatment assessment will it be possible to identify the factors that contribute to the complexity of the wound and to assess its potential state. The challenge for professionals is to utilize the most efficient therapeutic strategies at the right time and in the most cost-effective way, in order to reduce the complex nature of wounds, to treat the symptoms, and whenever possible, to achieve wound healing.

2. How should chronic and complex soft-tissue wounds be managed?

2.1. Management and treatment strategies

Chronic and complex soft-tissue wounds usually involve difficult healing, which means that they require an appropriate management-treatment strategy using a comprehensive and dynamic approach, applying new therapies to confront this old problem: wound healing [16]. In order to carry out this comprehensive approach, we should take into account the complex nature of the wound and its healing, its relationship with psychosocial factors and delays in wound healing, together with the economic cost for the patient, family, community, and the healthcare system. The steps to follow in order to achieve this approach should take into account the complete assessment of the patient, the control of causal factors, general healthcare, and the preparation of the wound bed.

2.2. Preparation of the wound bed

The preparation of the wound bed is an essential and dynamic process that provides an appropriate framework for a structured approach to wound management. This notion stresses a comprehensive and systematic approach with the aim of assessing and eliminating barriers to the normal wound healing process. It develops the appropriate treatment strategies to be directed at the patient in general and for treating the underlying condition causing the wound. Its objective is to create an optimum healing setting, a well-vascularized wound, with a stable and balanced bed in terms of exudate production, aimed at reducing scar healing time and facilitating the efficiency of other therapeutic measures. The wound bed should be prepared in each phase of the wound healing process following an agreed-upon procedure.

The "Tissue, Inflammation-infection, Moisture, Edge" (T.I.M.E.) scheme, proposed by the European Wound Management Association (EWMA), is based on the research of the International Wound Bed Preparation Advisory Board (IWBPAB), which established an algorithm through the development of the acronym T.I.M.E., whose objective is to describe the characteristics of chronic wounds during wound bed preparation. Following on from this, the concept was updated by placing emphasis on the treatment of the cause of the wound and general patient factors during treatment, before dealing with local wound factors. This algorithm consists of four components that cover the different physiopathological alterations present in chronic wounds: the management and conditioning of non-viable tissue, the monitoring of inflammation and infection, the disequilibrium of moisture due to excess exudate, and the stimulation and progression of the wound edges. So we can see that the T.I.M.E. framework involves the overall strategies that can be applied to the management of different kinds of wound with the aim of maximizing the ability to heal wounds [16–18] (**Figure 1**).

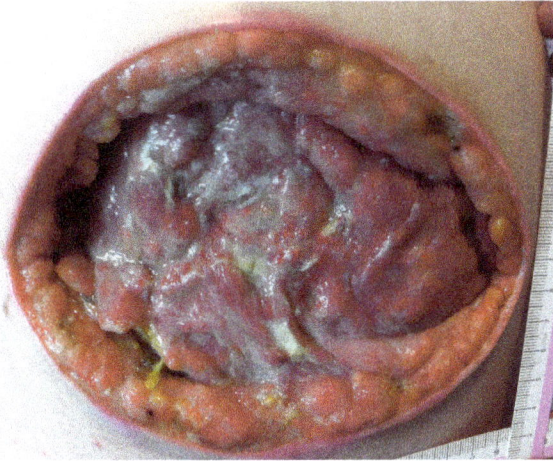

Figure 1. Complex and traumatic soft-tissue wound. Management and treatment of wound bed.

Wound treatment is initiated with a hydrodynamic washing using 0.9% saline solution at room temperature, with a 1–4 kg/cm effective washing pressure, without any damage being caused (a 20-ml syringe, with a 0.9-mm-diameter catheter), and the surrounding area is washed with a soapy antiseptic solution consisting of chlorhexidine digluconate.

For the monitoring of the non-viable tissues (necrotic tissue, crust, slough, and foreign bodies), episodic or continuous debridement is carried out until healthy tissue is found. It can be surgical, using tangential hydrodissection (Versajet™Plus, Smith & Nephew, London, United Kingdom); enzymatic, applying exogenous enzymes locally (collagenase, fibrolysine, trypsin, or chymotrypsin); chemical (cadexomer iodine); autolytic (due to the conjunction of three factors: hydration of the bed, fibrinolysis and the action of the endogenous enzymes on the devitalized tissue); or osmotic (hyperosmotic solutions). On occasions, an instillation therapy can also be used (VeraFlo™, KCI, Acelity LPI, San Antonio, TX) either in deep wounds with a viscous exudate or in uncontrolled infections on prosthetic materials, in order to eliminate the biofilm, reduce the pain, and reactivate healing. A noninvasive treatment option, for the debridement of chronic wounds, is low-frequency guided ultrasound [3].

In the management of the bacterial load (a contaminated or colonized lesion, with critical or infected colonization), foci of local and/or systemic infection have to be removed, which is why it is necessary to clean and debride the wound; take a wound culture; monitor the wound proteases; and use topical antimicrobials (silver, cadexomer iodine), systemic antibiotics according to the antibiogram data, anti-inflammatory drugs, and protease inhibitors if required.

It is important to monitor the exudate and achieve the equilibrium in the moisture, given that a dry wound makes it difficult for cell migration and exudate encourages infection and macerates the perilesional skin area. We should be aware that scarring is faster with wounds in an optimally moist environment in which the physiological and atmospheric conditions of the wound bed are maintained, thus fostering basal keratinocyte migration. A moist environment also prevents cell desiccation, encourages cell migration, promotes angiogenesis, stimulates collagen synthesis, and facilitates intercellular communication. A moist wound environment preserves a slightly acid pH and a low oxygen tension on the surface of the wound [18–20].

Thus, the edges of the wound do not advance because there are keratinocytes that do not migrate, senescent cells, and alterations in the extracellular matrix secondary to the disequilibrium in protease activity.

2.3. Clinical protocols

The preparation of the wound bed requires specific management protocols, which can be grouped into three sections following the T.I.M.E. procedure:

- Nonsurgical debridement with moisture monitoring and dressing every 48 h (**Table 1**).

- Local infection with moisture monitoring and dressing every 72 h (**Table 2**).

- A granulation phase with moisture monitoring and dressing every 72 h (**Table 3**).

Protocol 1: (T/M= Tissue and moisture) **-Non-viable tissue and moisture monitoring** **-Non-surgical debridement** **-Dressing every 48 h**			
-Type of wound	-Necrotic tissue -Low exudate	-Sloughy tissue -Moderate exudate	-Infected sloughy tissue -High exudate
-Debridement	-Collagenase + hydrogel	-Collagenase	-Cadexomer iodine + alginate
-Moist dressing	-Hydrocellular with acrylic adhesive or silicone adhesive	-Hydrocellular with acrylic adhesive or silicone adhesive	-Hydrocellular with acrylic adhesive or silicone adhesive

Table 1. Preparing the wound bed: management protocol (T/M).

Protocol 2: (I/M = Infection and moisture) **-Infection and moisture monitoring** **-Wounds with local infection** **-Dressing every 72 h**			
-Type of wound	-Infection -Low exudate	-Infection -Moderate exudate	-Infection -High exudate
-Decrease in bacterial load	-Nanocrystalline silver or -Silver-impregnated activated carbon+ hydrogel	-Nanocrystalline silver or -Silver-impregnated activated carbon	-Nanocrystalline silver or -Silver-impregnated activated carbon + alginate
-Moist dressing	-Hydrocellular with acrylic adhesive or silicone adhesive	-Hydrocellular with acrylic adhesive or silicone adhesive	-Hydrocellular with acrylic adhesive or silicone adhesive

Table 2. Preparing the wound bed: management protocol (I/M).

Protocol 3: (E/M = Edges and moisture)

-Epithelialization of edges and moisture monitoring

-Wounds in the granulation phase

-Dressing every 72 h

-Type of wound	-Granulation tissue	-Granulation tissue
	-Low or moderate exudate	-High exudate
-Granulation	-Collagen with silver protease modulator matrix or -Powder collagen	-Collagen with silver protease modulator matrix or -Powder collagen + alginate
-Moist dressing	-Hydrocellular with acrylic adhesive or silicone adhesive	-Hydrocellular with acrylic adhesive or silicone adhesive

Table 3. Preparing the wound bed: management protocol (E/M).

After finalizing the preparation of the wound bed, the wound remains open ready for its closure by secondary intention with granulation tissue and the re-establishment of the epidermis. At this point, the surgeon comes across two new problems: how to granulate the wound, and afterwards, how to epithelialize it.

2.4. Wound granulation using negative topical pressure therapy

For the granulation, we use a noninvasive topical negative pressure wound therapy (NPWT) (**Figure 2**), using aspirated drainage to eliminate the secretions, facilitate the closure and prevent complications. Its scientific fundamentals and physiopathology are based on the application of mechanical stress on the tissues, by creating a negative pressure on the surface of the wound [21]. The effect of the macrotension on the tissues is carried out using a sponge dressing (polyurethane-polyvinyl alcohol), with open pores, that contract under the negative pressure, bringing the edges closer together [22], eliminating the exudate, the non-viable tissue, and the soluble wound healing inhibitors (cytokines and matrix metalloproteinases) [23]. Other effects are a reduction in the edema, an increase in neutrophils and monocytes on the bacterial load and an improvement in local perfusion [24]. The effect of microtension, at the cell level, triggers cell stretching, which increases fibroblasts, the formation and division of new cells and the rapid growth of granulation tissue [25], the migration of fibroblasts to the area of the wound (displacing new cells to its surface), the formation of new blood vessels [26], and the formation of granulation tissue through mitosis stimulation. In this way, moist healing of the wound helps wound debridement (**Figure 3**).

The NPWT is contraindicated when either the wound has not been well explored, it has necrotic tissue with eschar or it has weakened blood vessels due to irradiation or suture. Also, NPWT is contraindicated in case of intestinal anastomosis, exposed nerves, the presence of tumors or untreated osteomyelitis. Equally, it is not advisable for either enterocutaneous or enteroatmospheric fistulas. Finally, active bleeding wounds and/or patients treated with anticoagulants are not suitable for NPWT treatment.

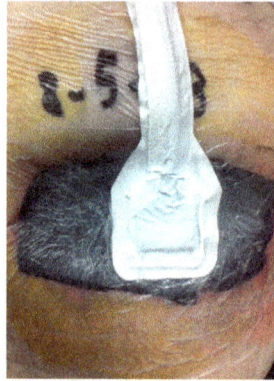

Figure 2. Complex and traumatic soft-tissue wound. Treatment with TNP therapy.

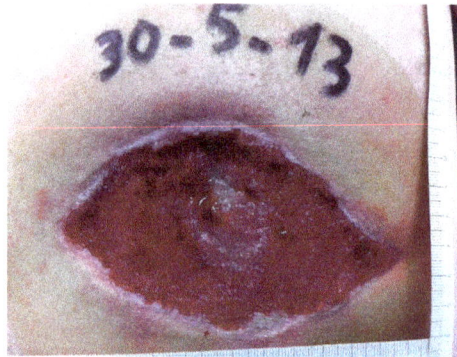

Figure 3. Complex and traumatic soft-tissue wound. Completed granulation after TNP therapy.

2.5. Epithelialization of the chronic and complex soft-tissue wounds

A large variety of wound coverings and procedures have become available over the past two decades, including several types of synthetic dressings and allo-skin or auto-skin substitutes, although their cost is too high for routine clinical practice [27, 28]. New technologies involving growth factors and bioengineered tissues are relatively new and have produced relatively good results; however, they are quite expensive.

2.6. Amniotic membrane and wound healing

Amniotic membrane (AM), the innermost layer of the placenta, has a fetal origin and can easily be separated from the placenta by blunt dissection. AM, due to its special structure, biological properties and immunological characteristics, is a tissue of particular interest as a biological dressing. AM exhibits low immunogenicity and well-documented reepithelialization effects. Moreover, AM shows anti-inflammatory, antifibrotic, antimicrobial, analgesic and nontumori-genic properties. This diversity of its effects is related to its capacity to synthesize and release biologically active molecules including cytokines and signaling factors such as tumor necrosis factor (TNF)-α, transforming growth factor (TGF)-α, TGF-β, basic fibroblast growth factor (b-FGF), epidermal growth factor (EGF), keratinocyte growth factor (KGF), hepatic growth factor (HGF), interleukin-4 (IL-4), IL-6, IL-8, natural inhibitors of metalloproteases, β-defensins, and prostaglandins among others [29–31]. Moreover, AM is a biomaterial that can be easily obtained, processed, and transported. On the other hand, AM may function as a substrate where cells can easily proliferate and differentiate [32]. When compared to skin transplantation, AM treatment offers considerable advantages. Its application does not produce rejection because it has low immunogenicity and does not induce uncontrolled proliferation [33]. All these effects are related to its capacity for the production and release of biologically active substances (see above).

AM has been applied in medicine for more than 100 years. In 1910, Davis [34] reported a comprehensive review of 550 cases of skin transplantation to various types of burns and wounds using natural AM obtained from labor and delivery at the Johns Hopkins University. In 1913, Sabella [35] and Stern [36] separately reported on the use of preserved AM in skin grafting for burns and ulcers. Since then, there have been several reports of the uses of AM in the treatment of wounds of different etiologies and other applications: first, in the reconstructive surgery of different tissues and organs including the mouth, tongue, nasal mucosa, larynx, eardrum, vestibule, bladder, urethra, vagina, and tendons [37–43]; second, as a peritoneum substitute in reconstruction procedures of pelvic exenteration surgery; third, in adherence prevention in the abdomen and pelvic surgery; and finally, as a covering of onphaloceles and the like [34–37, 44].

In ophthalmology, the use of AM was reported for the first time in 1940 by De Rötth, who used fresh fetal membranes, namely amnion and chorion, at the ocular surface as a biological dressing in the management of conjunctival alterations [45]. Later, Sorsby et al. [46] used preserved AM as a temporary coating in the treatment of acute caustic ocular lesions. Even though the results were favorable, its use was abandoned for almost four decades. In 1995, with the reconstitution assays of rabbit corneas with limbic disorder using human preserved AM, by Kim and Tseng [47], there was a renewed widespread interest in the use of AM in ophthalmology. Several publications appeared related to the efficacy of the AM in various ocular surface conditions and in diseases like epidermolysis bullosa [44, 48, 49]. Nowadays, AM is a resource widely used in ophthalmology [49–51] and to a lesser degree in the treatment of wounds, burns lesions, and chronic ulcers of the legs [48, 52–54] and in other surgical and nonsurgical procedures [38–43, 55–59].

3. Using AM in chronic wound healing

Once granulation of the wound is finalized, the process of epithelialization by using AM can be initiated. The source of AM for wound healing is donated placenta. AM has been used for wound healing either as intact AM without epithelium removal or as denuded AM, without the epithelium, [60, 61]. In some cases, AM was used fresh, and in others AM was preserved. Nowadays, it is known that the use of fresh AM is not practical for clinical use [62]. Methods

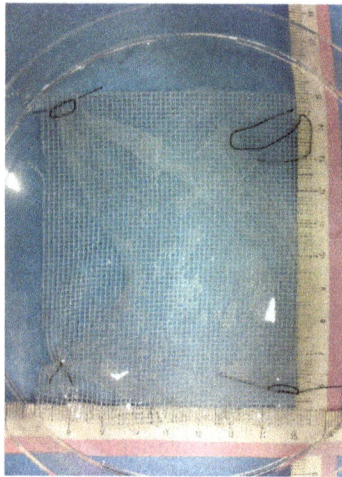

Figure 4. Amniotic membrane fixed to sterile petrolatum gauze (Tulgrasum®) ready for its application.

to remove the epithelium or preserve AM are very diverse and exceed the scope of this chapter. In our case, the placenta is obtained from an uncomplicated elective cesarean of a healthy mother, excluding patients with positive human immunodeficiency virus (HIV), hepatitis B virus (HBV), and hepatitis C virus (HCV) serology. Using an aseptic technique, AM is separated from the subjacent chorion by blunt dissection and stored in saline solution or phosphate buffered saline with antibiotics (cotrimoxazol, tobramycin, vancomycin, and amphotericin B). In this solution, AM is taken to the clean room [55]. Then, its processing, under sterile conditions, is carried out in a type II vertical laminar flow cabinet (HEPA filter). Then it is cut up into fragments measuring 10 × 10cm, which are then placed on a sterile scaffold of sterile petrolatum gauze (Tulgrasum®) and fixed with silk points at their ends (**Figure 4**). Finally, individual fragments are introduced into a bag with cryopreservative solution to freeze them in liquid nitrogen. These fragments cannot be used in the clinical practice until 3 months have passed, when there is a certainty that their donor has not been seroconverted to HIV, HBV, or HCV. After its defrosting in a 37°C bath, they are taken back to the surgical area and are applied on the wounds of the selected patient [55] (**Figures 5** and **6**).

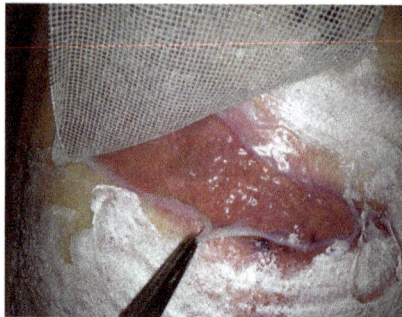

Figure 5. Complex and traumatic soft-tissue wound. Application of the amniotic membrane.

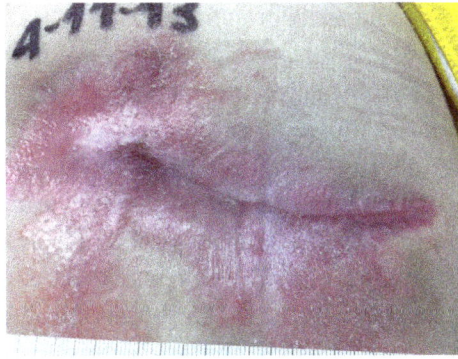

Figure 6. Complex and traumatic soft-tissue wound. Complete epithelialization after amniotic membrane treatment.

3.1. Molecular mechanisms underlying AM-induced skin reepithelialization

The molecular mechanisms underlying AM-induced skin reepithelialization are largely unknown. AM might have a wound healing effect by improving keratinocyte migration from the wound edge and stimulating its differentiation, thereby generating an intact epithelium [63]. Niknejad et al. [64] reflected that the stimulatory effect on epithelialization from the wound bed and/or the wound edge is facilitated by growth factors and progenitor cells released by AM. In addition, it has been described that the preservation of the integrity of the basement membrane and stromal matrix increases the healing potency of AM and is crucial in promoting a fast reepithelialization [65].

Insausti et al. [55] had previously worked on HaCaT cells, a spontaneously immortalized human keratinocyte cell line, as a model to comprehend the molecular consequences of AM application on human wounds [66]. This research showed that HaCaT cells exhibited different molecular reactions upon stimulation with AM that were attributed to the effects of soluble AM-released factors on HaCaT cells [55]. The application of AM to keratinocytes induced the activation of the phosphorylation of ERK1/2, JNK1/2, and p38 [55]. Also, AM-conditioned medium induced similar responses, suggesting a trans-effect of AM on the triggering of these events. Additionally, the authors reported that HaCaT cells stimulated with AM showed an increased expression of *c-JUN*. Members of the AP1 family had been involved in keratinocyte migration and the wound healing process [67–70]. AM induced the phosphorylation of Jun N-terminal kinase (JNK)1 and two kinases in HaCaT cells [55]; JNK1 is a positive regulator of c-JUN, contributing to its phosphorylation and stabilization [71, 72]. Finally, the expression of c-Jun in the wounds treated with AM was very strong, and particularly evident at the basal epithelium near the leading edge and at the dermal leading edge or keratinocyte tongue, indicating that c-Jun expression might be an important event for epithelialization occurring at the AM-stimulated wound borders [55].

3.2. Chronic wound healing, AM, and TGF-β

Wound fluid derived from chronic venous leg ulcers is rich in pro-inflammatory cytokines such as TNF-α, interleukin-1β (IL-1β), and TGF-β1 [73]. In addition, the quantities of these cytokines drop as the chronic wound commences to heal, denoting a strong correlation between non-healing wounds and an increased level of pro-inflammatory cytokines [74]. TGF-β has a critical role in regulating multiple cellular responses that occur in all phases of wound healing [75]. Of the many cytokines shown to influence the wound healing process, TGF-β has the broadest spectrum of action because it affects the behavior of a wide variety of cell types and mediates a diverse range of cellular functions [76]. Platelets are thought to be the primary source of TGF-β at the wound site; also, activation of latent TGF-β occurs immediately after wounding [75]. The TGF-β signaling pathway is considered as a promising target for the treatment of many pathological skin conditions including chronic non-healing wounds [75]. Keratinocytes, fibroblasts, and monocytes are among the targeted cells in the TGF-β management of the wound [76]. Monocytes/macrophages and fibroblasts then contribute to autocrine-perpetuated high concentrations of TGF-β at the wound site [76].

TGF-β exerts its effect on cells by increasing the phosphorylation of members of the receptor activated (R-)Smad family (Smad2 and 3). Additionally, non-Smad pathways are also activated, including the extracellular-signal-regulated kinase (ERK), JNK, and p38 mitogen-activated protein (MAP) kinase pathways, the tyrosine kinase Src, and phosphatidylinositol 3-kinase (PI3K) [77, 78]. Once receptor-induced phosphorylation has taken place, R-Smads form complexes with the common-mediator (Co-) Smad4, which are translocated to the nucleus [79] where they, in cooperation with other transcription factors, co-activators, and corepressors, regulate the transcription of specific genes [80].

The effects of TGF-β on full-thickness wound reepithelialization have been studied in a transgenic mouse. The study in the ear mouse model suggests that TGF-β has an inhibitory effect on epithelialization when the wound involves all the layers of the skin [81]. Also, the overexpression of TGF-β, at the epidermis level, causes a decrease in reepithelialization [82, 83]. Abolishing part of the TGF-β signaling pathway has been suggested as a way to improve wound healing, so abolishing part of the TGF-β-stimulated Smad pathways may enhance wound healing and benefit the effect of TGF-β signaling over matrix synthesis by fibroblasts, for instance [76]. TGF-β causes the growth arrest of epithelial cells. The mechanisms, which differ somewhat between different cell types, involve the inhibition of the expression of the transcription factor Myc and members of the Id family, and the transcriptional induction of the cell cycle inhibitors CDKN2B (p15) and CDKN1A (p21) [84].

In order to further unravel the molecular mechanism by which AM may contribute to the epithelialization and wound border proliferation in chronic post-traumatic wounds, Alcaraz et al. [85] analyzed the association between TGF-β signaling and AM regulation in wound healing using keratinocytes. Strikingly, AM was capable of attenuating the TGF-β-induced phosphorylation of Smad2 and Smad3 in HaCaT cells. Both the strength and duration of TGF-β signaling, expressed as sustained phosphorylation of Smads, are essential to achieve proper cell responses to TGF-β; the impossibility to do so produces a loss of the cell cycle arrest in response to TGF-β [86]. AM attenuates TGF-β-induced Smad2 and Smad3 phosphorylation and hence attenuates CDKN2B (p15) and CDKN1A (p21) expression [85], which has been connected to cell cycle regulation [86]. Therefore, the presence of AM counteracts the cell cycle arrest induced by TGF-β on keratinocytes, releasing them from the restrain imposed by TGFß [85]. The effect of AM on TGF-β-regulated genes is not indiscriminate, and not all genes are affected by the presence of AM. Interestingly, genes that positively participate in wound healing such as *SNAI-2* and *PAI-1* were synergistically up-regulated by the presence of AM and TGF-β [85]. Finally, the expression of c-Jun was maximal when both TGF-β and AM were present in either HaCaT or primary keratinocyte cells [85].

It has been suggested that AM might exert its wound healing effect by increasing keratinocyte migration speed from the wound edge [63]. Growth factors and progenitor cells released by AM [64] are supposed to mediate the epithelialization stimulatory effect. AM induces cell migration in a wound healing assay in keratinocytes and mesenchymal cells [85]. Furthermore, in keratinocytes, inhibition of cell proliferation with mitomycin C, affected the migrating properties of AM. In the same study, the use of JNK1 inhibitors prevented AM-induced cell migration in both cell types. Moreover, a closer inspection of the margins of the scratch wound healing assays showed a high expression of c-JUN in the AM-stimulated cells engaged in the migratory wave. The AM-induced high expression of c-JUN at the wound border was prevented by inhibitors SP600125 and PD98059, which is consistent with the fact that AM induces the activation of a signaling cascade that produces the phosphorylation of ERK1/2 and JNK1/2. A local increase of c-JUN was observed in the patient wound border when the wound had been treated with AM. This is coherent with the AM effect on cell migration. In fact, in the examination of patient wound borders a few days after AM application, a clear proliferation/ migration was observed [85]. This correlates well with the robust expression of c-Jun at the wound border, which is particularly robust at the *stratum basale* of the epidermis that overlaps the keratinocyte tongue, the area where the migration of keratinocytes happens to epithelialize the wound [85]. Additionally, in that investigation, the authors revealed that the application of AM promotes healing in chronic wounds by refashioning the TGF-β-induced genetic program, stimulating keratinocyte migration and proliferation [85]. Additionally, there might be a synergy of AM and TGF-β signaling for the resolution of chronic wounds [85, 87]. Thus, stimulation of keratinocytes with both AM and TGF-β was synergistic when compared to both stimulus being added separately [85]. Moreover, the treatment of cells with TGF-β signaling inhibitors hampered the effect of AM, indicating that both AM and TGF-β signaling positively contribute to cell migration [87]. The down-regulation of Smad3 has been suggested as a possible way of improving wound healing [76]. In this sense, the effect of R-Smads, Smad2 or 3, seems to be different given that the overexpression of Smad2 increased AM-induced cell migration while the overexpression of Smad3 prevented it [87]. Notably, the ability of keratinocytes to sense TGF-β through Smad3 prevents the cell proliferation of keratinocytes and consequently prevents wound healing resolution when the levels of TGF-β are high [88].

Presently, in order to evaluate the effect of AM on chronic post-traumatic wounds, a clinical trial is being conducted in our hospital, with exceptional results. The TGF-β-stimulated Smad pathway has also been involved in the production of fibrosis and inflammation in response to TGF-β. Thus, interfering with TGF-β signaling may be a good way of interfering with fibrosis and improving the evolution of wound healing [76]. In different experimental models, the application of AM is able to ameliorate fibrosis [89–92]. Currently, we are exploring whether the application of AM is able to reduce fibrosis and inflammation in chronic wounds.

4. Summary

To summarize, AM is a biological dressing that stimulates proper epithelialization in chronic wounds. It has several advantages; among them, it is economical, easy to obtain, and in endless supply. Additionally, AM can be cryopreserved at a low temperature while preserving all its biological functions. Finally, it can be used as a treatment in the outpatient clinic, which reduces costs even more. Thus, AM must be taken into account as a consolidated treatment option for chronic wounds.

Acknowledgements

We would like to thank other members of the different laboratories who contribute in our daily task of increasing our knowledge of AM and chronic wound healing. Ana M García, María D. López and Mónica Rodríguez working in the clean room and providing AM. Paola Romencín, José E. Millán, David García and Noemi Marín, working on AM and animal models, and Miguel Blanquer, working in the cell therapy group. Antonia Alcaraz, Catalina Ruiz-Cañada, Ania Mrowiec, Eva M. García, and Sergio Liarte working on molecular aspects of AM and wound healing using cell models. This work was supported by a grant from the Fundación Séneca de la Región de Murcia and a grant from the Instituto de Salud Carlos III, Fondo de Investigaciones Sanitarias. Plan Estatal I+D+i and the Instituto de Salud Carlos III-Subdirección General de Evaluación y Fomento de la Investigación (Grant no.: PI13/00794) http://www.isciii.es/Fondos FEDER (ERDF funds) http://ec.europa.eu/regional_policy/es/funding/erdf/. We are indebted to the Hospital Clínico Universitario Virgen de la Arrixaca for strongly supporting this research.

Author details

Gregorio Castellanos[1], Ángel Bernabé-García[2], Carmen García Insausti[3], Antonio Piñero[1], José M. Moraleda[3] and Francisco J. Nicolás[2]*

*Address all correspondence to: Franciscoj.nicolas2@carm.es

1 Surgery Service, Virgen de la Arrixaca University Clinical Hospital, El Palmar, Murcia, Spain

2 Molecular Oncology and TGFβ, Research Unit, Virgen de la Arrixaca University Hospital, El Palmar, Murcia, Spain

3 Cell Therapy Unit, Virgen de la Arrixaca University Clinical Hospital, El Palmar, Murcia, Spain

References

[1] Troxler M, Vowden K, Vowden P. Integrating adjunctive therapy into practice: the importance of recognising 'hard-to-heal' wounds. World Wide Wounds (online) 2006; available from URL: http://www.worldwidewounds.com/2006/december/Troxler/Integrating-Adjunctive-Therapy-Into-Practice.html.

[2] Falanga V, Saap LJ, Ozonoff A. Wound bed score and its correlation with healing of chronic wounds. Dermatol Ther. 2006;19(6):383–90.

[3] Doerler M, Reich-Schupke S, Altmeyer P, Stucker M. Impact on wound healing and efficacy of various leg ulcer debridement techniques. J Dtsch Dermatol Ges. 2012;10(9): 624–32.

[4] Margolis DJ, Berlin JA, Strom BL. Risk factors associated with the failure of a venous leg ulcer to heal. Arch Dermatol. 1999;135(8):920–6.

[5] Henderson EA. The potential effect of fibroblast senescence on wound healing and the chronic wound environment. J Wound Care. 2006;15(7):315–8.

[6] Steed DL. Clinical evaluation of recombinant human platelet-derived growth factor for the treatment of lower extremity diabetic ulcers. Diabetic Ulcer Study Group. J Vasc Surg. 1995;21(1):71–8; discussion 9–81.

[7] Mogford J., Mustoe T. Experimental models of wound healing.In: Falanga V., editor. Cutaneous Wound Healing. London: Martin Dunitz Ltd.; 2001. p. 109–22.

[8] Medina A, Scott PG, Ghahary A, Tredget EE. Pathophysiology of chronic nonhealing wounds. J Burn Care Rehabil. 2005;26(4):306–19.

[9] Shukla VK, Shukla D, Tiwary SK, Agrawal S, Rastogi A. Evaluation of pH measurement as a method of wound assessment. J Wound Care. 2007;16(7):291–4.

[10] Bowler PG, Duerden BI, Armstrong DG. Wound microbiology and associated approaches to wound management. Clin Microbiol Rev. 2001;14(2):244–69.

[11] Ngo Q, Vickery K, Deva AK. PR21 Role of Bacterial Biofilms in Chronic Wounds. ANZ Journal of Surgery. 2007;77:A66.

[12] Percival SL, Bowler PG, Dolman J. Antimicrobial activity of silver-containing dressings on wound microorganisms using an in vitro biofilm model. Int Wound J. 2007;4(2):186–91.

[13] Bjarnsholt T, Kirketerp-Moller K, Kristiansen S, Phipps R, Nielsen AK, Jensen PO, et al. Silver against Pseudomonas aeruginosa biofilms. APMIS. 2007;115(8):921–8.

[14] Attinger CE, Janis JE, Steinberg J, Schwartz J, Al-Attar A, Couch K. Clinical approach to wounds: débridement and wound bed preparation including the use of dressings and wound-healing adjuvants. Plast Reconstr Surg. 2006;117(7 Suppl):72S–109S.

[15]　Baharestani M, de Leon J, Mendez-Eastman S, et al. Consensus statement: a practical guide for managing pressure ulcers with negative pressure wound therapy utilizing vacuum-assisted closure-understanding the treatment algorithm. Adv Skin Wound Care. 2008(21(Suppl 1)):1–20.

[16]　EWMA, editor. Position Document: Wound Bed Preparation in Practice. (EWMA). London: MEP Ltd.; 2004.

[17]　Falanga V. Classifications for wound bed preparation and stimulation of chronic wounds. Wound Repair Regen. 2000;8(5):347–52.

[18]　Sibbald RG, Williamson D, Orsted HL, Campbell K, Keast D, Krasner D, et al. Preparing the wound bed--debridement, bacterial balance, and moisture balance. Ostomy Wound Manage. 2000;46(11):14–22, 4–8, 30–5; quiz 6–7.

[19]　Falanga V. Wound bed preparation: science applied to practice. In: (EWMA). EWMA, editor. Position Document: Wound Bed Preparation in Practice. London: MEP Ltd.; 2004. p. 2–5.

[20]　Halim AS, Khoo TL, Saad AZ. Wound bed preparation from a clinical perspective. Indian J Plast Surg. 2012;45(2):193–202.

[21]　Morykwas MJ, Argenta LC, Shelton-Brown EI, McGuirt W. Vacuum-assisted closure: a new method for wound control and treatment: animal studies and basic foundation. Ann Plast Surg. 1997;38(6):553–62.

[22]　Banwell PE, Musgrave M. Topical negative pressure therapy: mechanisms and indications. Int Wound J. 2004;1(2):95–106.

[23]　Stechmiller JK, Kilpadi DV, Childress B, Schultz GS. Effect of vacuum-assisted closure therapy on the expression of cytokines and proteases in wound fluid of adults with pressure ulcers. Wound Repair Regen. 2006;14(3):371–4.

[24]　Timmers MS, Le Cessie S, Banwell P, Jukema GN. The effects of varying degrees of pressure delivered by negative-pressure wound therapy on skin perfusion. Ann Plast Surg. 2005;55(6):665–71.

[25]　Saxena V, Hwang CW, Huang S, Eichbaum Q, Ingber D, Orgill DP. Vacuum-assisted closure: microdeformations of wounds and cell proliferation. Plast Reconstr Surg. 2004;114(5):1086–96; discussion 97–8.

[26]　Greene AK, Puder M, Roy R, Arsenault D, Kwei S, Moses MA, et al. Microdeformational wound therapy: effects on angiogenesis and matrix metalloproteinases in chronic wounds of 3 debilitated patients. Ann Plast Surg. 2006;56(4):418–22.

[27]　Greaves NS, Iqbal SA, Baguneid M, Bayat A. The role of skin substitutes in the management of chronic cutaneous wounds. Wound Repair Regen. 2013;21(2):194–210.

[28]　Lorenz HP, Longaker M. Wounds: biology, pathology, and management. Essential practice of surgery. New York: Springer; 2003. p. 77–88.

[29] Yang L, Shirakata Y, Shudou M, Dai X, Tokumaru S, Hirakawa S, et al. New skin-equivalent model from de-epithelialized amnion membrane. Cell Tissue Res. 2006;326(1):69–77.

[30] Parolini O, Soncini M. Human placenta: a source of progenitor/stem cells? J Reproduktionsmed Endokrinol. 2006;3(2):117–126.

[31] Parolini O, Alviano F, Bagnara GP, Bilic G, Buhring HJ, Evangelista M, et al. Concise review: isolation and characterization of cells from human term placenta: outcome of the first International Workshop on Placenta Derived Stem Cells. Stem Cells. 2008;26(2): 300–11.

[32] Miki T, Strom SC. Amnion-derived pluripotent/multipotent stem cells. Stem Cell Rev. 2006;2(2):133–42.

[33] Insausti CL, Blanquer M, Bleda P, Iniesta P, Majado MJ, Castellanos G, et al. The amniotic membrane as a source of stem cells. Histol Histopathol. 2010;25(1):91–8.

[34] Davis JS. A method of splinting skin grafts. Skin transplantation. 1910; 21:44.

[35] Sabella N. Use of fetal membranes in skin grafting. Med Records NY. 1913;83:478–80.

[36] Stern M. The grafting of preserved amniotic membrane to burned and ulcerated surfaces, substituing skin grafts: a preliminary report. J Am Med Assoc. 1913;60(13): 973–4.

[37] Ganatra MA. Amniotic membrane in surgery. J Pak Med Assoc. 2003;53(1):29–32.

[38] Tolhurst DE, van der Helm TW. The treatment of vaginal atresia. Surg Gynecol Obstet. 1991;172(5):407–14.

[39] Georgy M, Aziz N. Vaginoplasty using amnion graft: new surgical technique using the laparoscopic transillumination light. J Obstet Gynecol. 1996;16(4):262–4.

[40] Morton KE, Dewhurst CJ. Human amnion in the treatment of vaginal malformations. Br J Obstet Gynaecol. 1986;93(1):50–4.

[41] Fishman IJ, Flores FN, Scott FB, Spjut HJ, Morrow B. Use of fresh placental membranes for bladder reconstruction. J Urol. 1987;138(5):1291–4.

[42] Brandt FT, Albuquerque CD, Lorenzato FR. Female urethral reconstruction with amnion grafts. Int J Surg Investig. 2000;1(5):409–14.

[43] Zohar Y, Talmi YP, Finkelstein Y, Shvili Y, Sadov R, Laurian N. Use of human amniotic membrane in otolaryngologic practice. Laryngoscope. 1987;97(8 Pt 1):978–80.

[44] Trelford JD, Trelford-Sauder M. The amnion in surgery, past and present. Am J Obstet Gynecol. 1979;134(7):833–45.

[45] de Rötth A. Plastic repair of conjunctival defects with fetal membranes. Arch Ophthalmol. 1940;23(3):522–5.

[46] Sorsby A, Symons HM. Amniotic membrane grafts in caustic burns of the eye: (burns of the second degree). Br J Ophthalmol. 1946;30(6):337–45.

[47] Kim JC, Tseng SC. Transplantation of preserved human amniotic membrane for surface reconstruction in severely damaged rabbit corneas. Cornea. 1995;14(5):473-84.

[48] Mermet I, Pottier N, Sainthillier JM, Malugani C, Cairey-Remonnay S, Maddens S, et al. Use of amniotic membrane transplantation in the treatment of venous leg ulcers. Wound Repair Regen. 2007;15(4):459–64.

[49] Gomes JA, Romano A, Santos MS, Dua HS. Amniotic membrane use in ophthalmology. Curr Opin Ophthalmol. 2005;16(4):233–40.

[50] Dua HS, Gomes JAP, King AJ, Maharajan VS. The amniotic membrane in ophthalmology. Surv Ophthalmol. 2004;49(1):51–77.

[51] Baradaran-Rafii A, Aghayan HR, Arjmand B, Javadi MA. Amniotic membrane transplantation. Iranian J Ophthalmic Res. 2007;2(1):58–75.

[52] Colocho G, Graham WP, Iii, Greene AE, Matheson DW, Lynch D. Human amniotic membrane as a physiologic wound dressing. Arch Surg. 1974;109(3):370–3.

[53] Singh R, Chouhan US, Purohit S, Gupta P, Kumar P, Kumar A, et al. Radiation processed amniotic membranes in the treatment of non-healing ulcers of different etiologies. Cell Tissue Bank. 2004;5(2):129–34.

[54] Hasegawa T, Mizoguchi M, Haruna K, Mizuno Y, Muramatsu S, Suga Y, et al. Amnia for intractable skin ulcers with recessive dystrophic epidermolysis bullosa: report of three cases. J Dermatol. 2007;34(5):328–32.

[55] Insausti CL, Alcaraz A, Garcia-Vizcaino EM, Mrowiec A, Lopez-Martinez MC, Blanquer M, et al. Amniotic membrane induces epithelialization in massive posttraumatic wounds. Wound Repair Regen. 2010;18(4):368–77.

[56] Sangwan VS, Matalia HP, Vemuganti GK, Fatima A, Ifthekar G, Singh S, et al. Clinical outcome of autologous cultivated limbal epithelium transplantation. Indian J Ophthalmol. 2006;54(1):29–34.

[57] Díaz-Prado S, Rendal-Vázquez ME, Muiños-López E, Hermida-Gómez T, Rodríguez-Cabarcos M, Fuentes-Boquete I, et al. Potential use of the human amniotic membrane as a scaffold in human articular cartilage repair. Cell Tissue Bank. 2010;11(2):183–95.

[58] Yeager AM, Singer HS, Buck JR, Matalon R, Brennan S, O'Toole SO, et al. A therapeutic trial of amniotic epithelial cell implantation in patients with lysosomal storage diseases. Am J Med Genet. 1985;22(2):347–55.

[59] Redondo P, Giménez de Azcarate A, Marqués L, García-Guzman M, Andreu E, Prósper F. Amniotic membrane as a scaffold for melanocyte transplantation in patients with stable vitiligo. Dermatol Res Pract. 2011;2011:6.

[60] Akle C, McColl I, Dean M, Adinolfi M, Brown S, Fensom AH, et al. Transplantation of amniotic epithelial membranes in patients with mucopolysaccharidoses. Exp Clin Immunogenet. 1985;2(1):43–8.

[61] Wilshaw SP, Kearney JN, Fisher J, Ingham E. Production of an acellular amniotic membrane matrix for use in tissue engineering. Tissue Eng. 2006;12(8):2117–29.

[62] Zelen CM, Snyder RJ, Serena TE, Li WW. The use of human amnion/chorion membrane in the clinical setting for lower extremity repair: a review. Clin Podiatr Med Surg. 2015;32(1):135–46.

[63] Lee SH, Tseng SC. Amniotic membrane transplantation for persistent epithelial defects with ulceration. Am J Ophthalmol. 1997;123(3):303–12.

[64] Niknejad H, Peirovi H, Jorjani M, Ahmadiani A, Ghanavi J, Seifalian AM. Properties of the amniotic membrane for potential use in tissue engineering. Eur Cell Mater. 2008;15:88–99.

[65] Kubo M, Sonoda Y, Muramatsu R, Usui M. Immunogenicity of human amniotic membrane in experimental xenotransplantation. Invest Ophthalmol Vis Sci. 2001;42(7):1539–46.

[66] Boukamp P, Petrussevska RT, Breitkreutz D, Hornung J, Markham A, Fusenig NE. Normal keratinization in a spontaneously immortalized aneuploid human keratinocyte cell line. J Cell Biol. 1988;106(3):761–71.

[67] Angel P, Szabowski A, Schorpp-Kistner M. Function and regulation of AP-1 subunits in skin physiology and pathology. Oncogene. 2001;20(19):2413–23.

[68] Yates S, Rayner TE. Transcription factor activation in response to cutaneous injury: role of AP-1 in reepithelialization. Wound Repair Regen. 2002;10(1):5–15.

[69] Gangnuss S, Cowin AJ, Daehn IS, Hatzirodos N, Rothnagel JA, Varelias A, et al. Regulation of MAPK activation, AP-1 transcription factor expression and keratinocyte differentiation in wounded fetal skin. J Invest Dermatol. 2004;122(3):791–804.

[70] Li G, Gustafson-Brown C, Hanks SK, Nason K, Arbeit JM, Pogliano K, et al. c-Jun is essential for organization of the epidermal leading edge. Dev Cell. 2003;4(6):865–77.

[71] Ronai Z. JNKing Revealed. Mol Cell. 2004;15(6):843–4.

[72] Sabapathy K, Hochedlinger K, Nam SY, Bauer A, Karin M, Wagner EF. Distinct roles for JNK1 and JNK2 in regulating JNK activity and c-Jun-dependent cell proliferation. Mol Cell. 2004;15(5):713–25.

[73] Harris IR, Yee KC, Walters CE, Cunliffe WJ, Kearney JN, Wood EJ, et al. Cytokine and protease levels in healing and non-healing chronic venous leg ulcers. Exp Dermatol. 1995;4(6):342–9.

[74] Trengove NJ, Bielefeldt-Ohmann H, Stacey MC. Mitogenic activity and cytokine levels in non-healing and healing chronic leg ulcers. Wound Repair Regen. 2000;8(1):13–25.

[75] Finnson KW, McLean S, Di Guglielmo GM, Philip A. Dynamics of transforming growth factor beta signaling in wound healing and scarring. Advances Wound Care. 2013;2(5): 195–214.

[76] Ashcroft GS, Roberts AB. Loss of Smad3 modulates wound healing. Cytokine Growth Factor Rev. 2000;11(1–2):125–31.

[77] Moustakas A, Heldin CH. Non-Smad TGF-beta signals. J Cell Sci. 2005;118(Pt 16):3573–84.

[78] Mu Y, Gudey SK, Landstrom M. Non-Smad signaling pathways. Cell Tissue Res. 2012;347(1):11–20.

[79] Pierreux CE, Nicolas FJ, Hill CS. Transforming growth factor beta-independent shuttling of Smad4 between the cytoplasm and nucleus. Mol Cell Biol. 2000;20(23): 9041–54.

[80] Heldin CH, Moustakas A. Role of Smads in TGFbeta signaling. Cell Tissue Res. 2012;347(1):21–36.

[81] Tredget EB, Demare J, Chandran G, Tredget EE, Yang L, Ghahary A. Transforming growth factor-beta and its effect on reepithelialization of partial-thickness ear wounds in transgenic mice. Wound Repair Regen. 2005;13(1):61–7.

[82] Chan T, Ghahary A, Demare J, Yang L, Iwashina T, Scott PG, et al. Development, characterization, and wound healing of the keratin 14 promoted transforming growth factor-beta1 transgenic mouse. Wound Repair Regen. 2002;10(3):177–87.

[83] Yang L, Chan T, Demare J, Iwashina T, Ghahary A, Scott PG, et al. Healing of burn wounds in transgenic mice overexpressing transforming growth factor-beta 1 in the epidermis. Am J Pathol. 2001;159(6):2147–57.

[84] Heldin CH, Landstrom M, Moustakas A. Mechanism of TGF-beta signaling to growth arrest, apoptosis, and epithelial-mesenchymal transition. Curr Opin Cell Biol. 2009;21(2):166–76.

[85] Alcaraz A, Mrowiec A, Insausti CL, Bernabe-Garcia A, Garcia-Vizcaino EM, Lopez-Martinez MC, et al. Amniotic membrane modifies the genetic program induced by TGFss, stimulating keratinocyte proliferation and migration in chronic wounds. PLoS One. 2015;10(8):e0135324.

[86] Nicolas FJ, Hill CS. Attenuation of the TGF-beta-Smad signaling pathway in pancreatic tumor cells confers resistance to TGF-beta-induced growth arrest. Oncogene. 2003;22(24):3698–711.

[87] Ruiz-Canada C, Bernabé-García A, Angosto D, Castellanos G, Insausti CL, Moraleda JM, et al. Amniotic membrane stimulates migration by modulating TFG-β signaling. (In press).

[88] Ashcroft GS, Yang X, Glick AB, Weinstein M, Letterio JL, Mizel DE, et al. Mice lacking Smad3 show accelerated wound healing and an impaired local inflammatory response. Nat Cell Biol. 1999;1(5):260–6.

[89] Hodge A, Lourensz D, Vaghjiani V, Nguyen H, Tchongue J, Wang B, et al. Soluble factors derived from human amniotic epithelial cells suppress collagen production in human hepatic stellate cells. Cytotherapy. 2014;16(8):1132–44.

[90] Cargnoni A, Gibelli L, Tosini A, Signoroni PB, Nassuato C, Arienti D, et al. Transplantation of allogeneic and xenogeneic placenta-derived cells reduces bleomycin-induced lung fibrosis. Cell Transplant. 2009;18(4):405–22.

[91] Cargnoni A, Piccinelli EC, Ressel L, Rossi D, Magatti M, Toschi I, et al. Conditioned medium from amniotic membrane-derived cells prevents lung fibrosis and preserves blood gas exchanges in bleomycin-injured mice-specificity of the effects and insights into possible mechanisms. Cytotherapy. 2014;16(1):17–32.

[92] Cargnoni A, Ressel L, Rossi D, Poli A, Arienti D, Lombardi G, et al. Conditioned medium from amniotic mesenchymal tissue cells reduces progression of bleomycin-induced lung fibrosis. Cytotherapy. 2012;14(2):153–61.

8

Surgical Management of Wounds

Peter Mekhail, Shuchi Chaturvedi and

Shailesh Chaturvedi

Abstract

In surgical speciality, understanding of the wound healing is absolutely necessary. There are different kinds of wounds that require treatment which is most appropriate to them. In this chapter, we have discussed treatment for different types of wounds in four main types according to WHO Classification. Pros and cons of different types of materials used for cleaning and dressing are discussed. Dressing materials are discussed in detail. We have described the process of wound healing. There are various factors that influence wound healing and we have specifically described how they differ in primary and secondary wound healing. Usage of various kinds of dressing materials and their mechanism of action is described in detail. We have specifically highlighted the role of community nurses and tissue viability nurses. Since the availability and the recognition of tissue viability nurses, the cost of wound treatment has come down considerably and it is also very popular with the patients. Vacuum-assisted closure (VAC) therapy is very helpful in large wounds that are producing a lot of exudates. The VAC pulls the skin edges together and removes the exudate. Other adjunctive therapies are also mentioned but they are not available in most hospitals and therefore detailed descriptions are not provided.

Keywords: wound, closer, techniques, infection, surgical

1. Introduction

Wound management is considered one of the main pillars of patients' care at all levels of health service. The financial burden on the health service and the community in relation to wound management are due to prolonged stay, the cost of different materials required for wound care, delayed discharge, loss of earnings, continuous input and follow up at primary care level. No reliable data are available for the cost of treating the wound which do not close with primary intention. A report by Lewis et al. [1] has carried out a comprehensive review of the literature and has found that the cost of dressings and other material alone could be as high as £37 million per year in England. Data for primary care are easily available as they purchase on Form 10 but the data for secondary care are difficult to find as most hospitals buy directly from manufacturers at specially negotiated price, therefore factoring this in is quite difficult and no reliable study has been found on literature search. If patient stays in hospital the cost of stay in hospital could be as high as £400–500 per day depending upon the geographic location of hospital. Additionally, the cost of staffing, local or general anaesthetic, has to be factored in as well.

Significant developments have taken place with regards to wound management over the course of the years. Thanks to the evolving technology, better understanding of the healing process and relevant contributing factors we are now able to address the problem in a timely, cost-effective and efficient manner. It is a developing area and therefore the means of management will only improve with time.

2. Understanding tissue healing

Understanding tissue healing is fundamental in wound management. Such a complex physiological process is proven to be dependent on multiple inter-related factors [2].

Wound healing can be defined as the process by which the body restores and replaces function to damaged tissues [3]. Following tissue trauma, healing can be initiated through one of the two mechanisms:

1. Regeneration, which means replacement of damaged tissue by an identical type of tissue. This process is only confined to a few types of cells, for example epithelial, liver and nerve cells [2].

2. Repair, where damaged tissues are replaced by connective tissue to form a scar. This mechanism occurs in vast majority of cases [2].

3. Stages of wound healing

In general terms, the wound healing process can be divided into four stages with some potential overlap between the stages. Identification and recognition of the wound stage enables appropriate treatment objectives for that particular stage. When treating, practitioner at times may fail to establish correct treatment objectives due to failure to correctly recognise the healing stage of that particular wound.

3.1. Stage 1 (vascular response)

Tissue trauma leads to activation of coagulation cascade resulting in formation of a fibrin mesh to fill the gap within the tissue. It usually lasts up to 3 days [3].

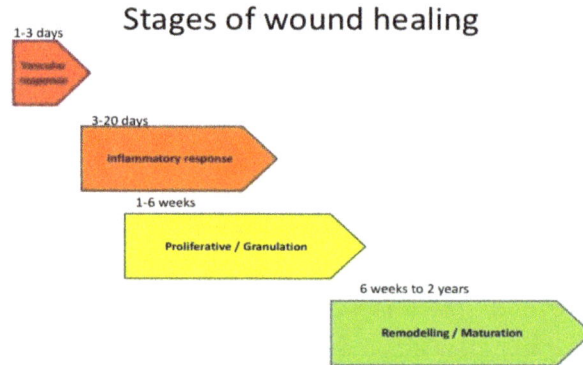

Scheme 1. Stages of Wound healing.

3.2. Stage 2 (inflammatory response)

At this stage, vasodilatation and increased permeability of the adjacent blood vessels are noted. This is the result of inflammatory mediators like histamine and prostaglandins released by mast cells. Clinically, this is characterised by redness, swelling, localised heat, pain and functional limitation. Clinical presentation at this stage might be confused with wound infection, as hyperaemia occurs in the first 3 weeks of healing.

Increased capillary permeability at this phase leads to exudates production containing essential growth factors, nutrients and enzymes mandatory for wound healing in addition to their anti-microbial characteristics [4].

Immuno-compromised patients might not be able to produce appropriate inflammatory response resulting in failure of activation of normal healing process [5].

3.3. Stage 3 (proliferative/granulation phase)

New connective tissue starts to fill the wound and a decrease of the wound size is noted. This occurs as a result of epithelialisation, wound contraction and granulation [2]. Collagen and other extra-cellular materials form scaffolding on which the new capillaries grow (angiogenesis) to form connective tissue. The process is referred to as granulation formation [2]. Angiogenesis is promoted by material produced by macrophages including transforming growth factor (TGF) and tumour necrosis factor (TNF) [6].

Fibroblast contraction that takes place during this stage is responsible for wound contraction and hence reducing wound size. This is considered to be a crucial part of a large and open wound healing [7].

Growth factor	Abbreviation	Main origins	Effects
Epidermal growth factor	EGF	Activated macrophages	Keratinocyte and fibroblast mitogen Keratinocyte migration Granulation tissue formation
Transforming growth factor-α	TGF-α	Activated macrophages T-lymphocytes Keratinocytes	Hepatocyte and epithelial cell proliferation Expression of anti-microbial peptides Expression of chemotactic cytokines
Hepatocyte growth factor	HGF	Mesenchymal cells	Epithelial and endothelial cell proliferation Hepatocyte motility
Vascular endothelial growth factor	VEGF	Mesenchymal cells	Vascular permeability Endothelial cell proliferation
Platelet-derived growth factor	PDGF	Platelets Macrophages Endothelial cells Smooth muscle cells Keratinocytes	Granulocyte, macrophage, fibroblast and smooth muscle cell chemotaxis Granulocyte, macrophage and fibroblast activation Fibroblast, endothelial cell and smooth muscle cell proliferation Matrix metalloproteinase, fibronectin and hyaluronan production Angiogenesis Wound remodelling Integrin expression regulation
Fibroblast growth factors 1 and 2	FGF-1, -2	Macrophages Mast cells T-lymphocytes Endothelial cells Fibroblasts	Fibroblast chemotaxis Fibroblast and keratinocyte proliferation Keratinocyte migration Angiogenesis Wound contraction Matrix (collagen fibres) deposition
Transforming growth factor-β	TGF-β	Platelets T-lymphocytes Macrophages Endothelial cells Keratinocytes Smooth muscle cells Fibroblasts	Granulocyte, macrophage, lymphocyte, fibroblast and smooth muscle cell chemotaxis TIMP synthesis Angiogenesis Fibroplasia Matrix metalloproteinase production inhibition Keratinocyte proliferation
Keratinocyte growth factor	KGF	Keratinocytes	Keratinocyte migron and differentiation

Table 1. Various growth factors involved in wound healing [10].

During the final phase of proliferation, re-epithelialisation takes place across the wound surface. This process will be delayed until the wound bed is filled with granulation tissue in cases of wound healing with secondary intention [2].

3.4. Stage 4 (remodelling/maturation phase)

This is the fourth and final stage of wound healing and it might extend up to 2 years from the time of tissue trauma. During this stage, the raised and reddish scar becomes more flat, smooth and lighter in colour. This relates to a reduction in the blood supply. Mature scars are hairless, avascular and do not contain sweat or sebaceous glands.

Collagen fibres are reorganised to maximise tensile strength, a process called remodelling and it is stimulated by macrophages [8].

Hypertrophic scar and keloid formation are two known abnormalities associated with this stage. While the former takes place after initial repair, the latter occurs sometime after healing is completed and continues to grow afterwards [9]. Keloid formation occurs 10 times more commonly in the Black Afro-Caribbean population in comparison to Caucasian population [9] **Table 1**.

4. Wound classification

Surgical wounds are commonly classified according to the degree of contamination and breaching of the aerodigestive tract epithelium into four categories:

A. Clean

Uncontaminated wounds without breaching of the respiratory, gastrointestinal (GI) or genitourinary (GU) tract. Examples include mastectomy, neck dissection, thyroid surgery and hernia surgery. These wounds are commonly managed with primary closure.

B. Clean-contaminated

Gastrointestinal, respiratory or Genitourinary tracts are entered in a controlled fashion. Usually no gross contamination or spillage should happen if proper precautions, i.e. minimising spillage, protecting the wound edges, etc., are taken. Examples of these types of wounds include cholecystectomy, Whipple operation, elective colonic or gastric surgery.

C. Contaminated

Any gross spillage of GI tract contents or major breach in the sterile technique either as causative agent or accidental can lead to contamination of wound. Perforated appendicitis, bile spillage, diverticular perforation or penetrating wounds come within this category. Although primary closure is still feasible in these wounds, thorough washout with copious amount of saline to remove as much contaminating agent, i.e. faeces or pus, as possible and prophylactic intra-operative antibiotics are advisable. Most randomised controlled trials (RCTs) prove the reduction in major sepsis though minor wound infection may still occur. In cases of gross contamination of abdominal cavity with faecal matter and when one is not sure of complete removal of contaminating agent it is better to leave the abdomen open and covered with wet packs for 48 hours and then re-checking the abdomen under general anaesthetic by removing the pack. If the abdominal cavity looks clean and there is no dead tissue or bowel then the closure can be attempted. These wounds are best closed in one layer with whole thickness sutures with either nylon or prolene as tension sutures.

D. Dirty wounds

This refers to old traumatic wounds with necrotic tissue, ongoing infection or perforation and presence of known organisms in the wound prior to intervention. Primary closure is not advisable and debridement is essential. Examples include abscesses, perforated bowel and faecal peritonitis. In cases of gross contamination of abdominal cavity with faecal matter and when one is not sure of complete removal of contaminating agent it is better to leave the abdomen open and covered with wet packs for 48 hours and then re-checking the abdomen under general anaesthetic by removing the pack. If the abdominal cavity looks clean and there is no dead tissue or bowel then the closure can be attempted. These wounds are best closed in one layer with whole thickness suture with either nylon or prolene as tension sutures.

Techniques of wound closure:

A. Closure by primary intention

In this technique, approximation of wound edges and deeper tissue layers is meticulously carried out with appropriate sutures in layers. Skin is approximated by sub-cuticular sutures or staples. Sterstrips™ are used to relieve tension on suture line and to give more aesthetically pleasing and functional scar. Elimination of dead space minimises new tissue formation, and careful epidermal alignment minimises scar formation [11, 12].

B. Closure by secondary intention

This is considered an adequate alternative to primary intention closure, particularly in cases where major tissue loss or gross contamination is expected. It might include closure of deeper facial planes while leaving the skin open [13].

5. Factors affecting wound healing [14]

The World Health Organisation (WHO) considers wound healing a multi-factorial process and each factor contributes to the healing process either directly or indirectly.

A. Patient-related factors

a. Age

b. Nutritional status

c. Underlining co-morbidity including diabetes, anaemia and compromised immunity

d. Patients' physiological status, for instance, multi-organ dysfunction, inotropic/vasopressor support

B. Wound-related factors

a. Type of organ or tissue

b. Extent/severity of injury

c. Nature of injury, e.g. clean laceration versus crushing injury

d. Wound contamination

e. Time lapse between the injury and initiation of treatment

C. Local factors related to the surgical technique itself

a. Appropriate haemostasis to ensure viable and well vascularised wound edges is a necessity but at the same time there should be no continuous oozing

b. Decision to perform (or not to perform) wound debridement as part of the surgical wound management does affect the final outcome

c. Timing of closure can be as important as any of the above factors in determining the fate of the wound

6. Surgical approaches to wound management [14]

There are certain golden surgical principles that must be followed in order to achieve adequate wound management.

6.1. For primary repair

A. Primary closure requires clean, well approximated and tension free suturing technique.

B. Infection and delayed healing are almost inevitable when primary closure of contaminated wound takes place without proper debridement or washout.

C. Various suturing techniques mean each technique is ideal for certain types of wounds. For example, while a subcuticular skin suture is considered to be an excellent option of good alignment for the wound edges, it is not the best haemostatic technique and in wounds with oozing edges or expected oozing a continuous mattress suture might be a better option in those cases where oozing is expected.

D. Choosing the correct suture material is vital in ensuring a desirable outcome. In general, a monofilament stitch carries less risk of infection in comparison to braided (multifilament) stitches [15]. Correct tensile strength of the material used is essential in maintaining the integrity of the wound until the healing is complete [15].

E. Size of sutures and interval between stitches should be proportional to the thickness of approximated tissues.

F. Deep wounds should be closed in layers whenever possible.

G. Timing of suture removal is determined by site and vascularity. For example, while skin stitches on the face can be removed as early as in 3 days, abdominal closure, usually, necessitate keeping suture material for up to 7–10 days.

H. Some operations that leave quite a large raw area may require drains as the chances of haematoma formation are high. The most common example is mastectomy. In these cases use of human fibrin glue spray reduces the drainage and also Seroma formation is reduced to a significant degree [16]. The product ARTISS is produced by Baxter Ltd. It contains 5% fibrin and 95% prothrombin and comes loaded in syringe. The product must be connected to a pressurised air source and before using the temperature of fluid must be at 25°C. This solution is good where one may need adjusting the flaps as it takes roughly 3 minutes for it to work [16]. If immediate fixation of the surfaces is required, Tessil (Baxter) is a good product [17]. This contains 95% fibrin and 5% prothrombin and adheres immediately. This is very useful in thoracotomy where it is sprayed straight to the chest wall and pleura [17].

For delayed primary closure:

A. Delayed primary closure is a good alternative in clean contaminated wounds and whenever washout is required. Wounds can be left open with saline-soaked sterile gauze and then patient should be taken back to the theatre, the gauze is removed and if wound looks clean and free of contaminant, sutures can be applied after 48 hours.

6.2. For healing with secondary intention

A. Promote healing with secondary intention after performing surgical debridement.

B. Surgical debridement includes washout of wound edges with antiseptic solutions, thorough washout with copious amounts of saline, excising dead and necrotic tissue down to healthy bleeding edges and gentle tissue handling to minimise iatrogenic tissue trauma.

7. Post-operative wound care

Regardless of the nature of the wound, healing mechanism or the type of closure, the aims of post-operative wound care remain the same. The main goal is to promote fast, complication-free healing with the best possible functional and aesthetic outcome [18]. Special consideration is given to wound healing with primary intention. As there is minimal tensile strength at the wound edges due to lack of remodelling collagen fibres, additional support in the form of sutures, tapes or staples is usually required until epithelisation takes place [19].

8. Guidance for reducing post-operative surgical site infection (SSI) [20]

A. Dressings and wound cleaning

a. Aim not to disturb the wound in the first 48 hours as this can damage the new delicate layer of epithelium. If necessary, use sterile saline for cleaning wound during this period and not to rub the surface.

b. Aseptic non-touch technique is mandatory for changing/removing dressings.

c. Advise patients that they can have a shower 48 hours post-operatively as by this time the top layer of epithelium has formed and the wound becomes water tight.

d. Early referral to tissue viability services is preferable in cases of wounds healing by secondary intention.

B. Anti-microbial treatment

a. Consider giving antibiotics whenever SSI (cellulites) is suspected.

b. Antibiotic choice should be broad spectrum initially then spectrum should be narrowed to target specific organisms once the culture and sensitivity report is available [21].

C. Further debridement

a. If debridement becomes necessary, surgical debridement in the theatre is always preferred in grossly contaminated wounds.

b. Avoid gauze dressings as when gauze is removed it damages granulation tissue which sticks to it. Though in certain superficial pussy wounds this method is still used and statistically no difference has been found in the healing time in comparison to more costly dressings.

c. Some non-healing wound with lot of dead tissue can be treated with sterile Green Bottle Larvae (*Lucilia sericata*) which destroy the necrotic tissue with enzyme and then ingest it. Larvae are applied directly to the wound and then held in place with an occlusive dressing. These can be applied to wound infected with MRSA (Methecillin Resistant Staphylococcus Aureus) as the larvae digest the bacteria as well and reduce the chance of continued infection. It is stipulated that the enzyme also produces growth of granulation tissue, however, some patients may find having larvae on their body unacceptable and if left too long the enzyme produced may destroy the keratinised epithelium [2].

d. Different types of special dressings can be applied to absorb the exudates and let the wound heal quicker and with less pain when changing the dressing. There are numerous dressings available for this kind of wounds and are described in the next section.

e. Cleaning the wound with hydrojets and by putting the patient in whirlpool has also been tried and found helpful in cleaning grossly contaminated wounds or quite large wounds. If wound is small and irrigation is required to remove exudates and debris that might interfere with wound healing, gentle irrigation with a syringe filled with saline or sterile water is preferred [3, 22].

f. Irrigation of wounds with antiseptic solution has been tried with hypochloride (*Eusol*) solution, Aserbane™ and hydrogen peroxide as caustic agents have been tried but there are no reliable data available to prove their efficacy [3].

D. Structured wound care approach

a. Using flowcharts and a structured approach with clear guidance is essential to ensure continuity within the team.

b. Continuous education about recent updates in wound care.

E. Methods to avoid

a. Topical antibiotics in wounds healing by primary intention.

b. Moist cotton gauze or mercury-based antiseptic solutions.

F. Post-operative wound complications: The most common and significant post-operative wound complications are wound infection and wound dehiscence. Once suspected, active management should start and this includes swabs for culture and sensitivities, followed by empirical antibiotics administration in the first instance [21]. Debridement in some cases might be necessary to promote wound healing.

9. Dressings

a. The ideal dressing should carry certain characteristics to assist wound healing. It must maintain some moisture at the wound site, act as a barrier against fluid or bacterial contamination, potentially remove excess exudates that might lead to wound maceration and finally it should be adherent to skin but removed with no/minimal trauma [24]. Tegaderm™ and Opsite™ dressings are two such dressings. These are water resistant and allow patient to have a wash next day if the patients wish so.

b. Wound which are producing lot of debris and discharge need cleaning with aseptic technique. There are a number of different materials available, some of the commonly used ones are described below.

- Hydrocolloid dressings. These contain sodium carboxymethylcellulose which is combined to elastomers and applied to a carrier, usually polyurethane foam. The hydrocolloid absorbs the exudates and becomes gel and when dressing is removed the whole lot lifts off without disturbing the granulation tissue. Common ones are Granuflex™, Comfeel Plus™, Aqua-cel™ and DuoDerm Extra Thin™.

- Polysaccharide beads. This comes in powder form and swells when it comes in contact with fluid or exudates. This can be left in place for a few days and then removed with gentle wash with saline. It is available as Debrisan (Pharmacia Ltd) and Iodosorb (Perstrop).

- Alginates. These are made from the sodium salts of algenic acid. Alginic acid is produced from seaweed. When exposed to fluid it is activated and forms a gel and absorbs the exudates. It comes in different size and shape as flat squares and ribbons. It is very commonly used in UK. Flat square and ribbons are manufactured by many pharmaceuticals. Kaltostat (Convatec) is the most widely used in our institute.

- Foam dressing. These are made from polyurethane or silicon which absorbs liquid by capillary action. They can be applied to wound as a filler for the cavities. Dressings can be removed every couple of days and the foam can be washed and cut to size for re-application. Lyofoam (Seton) and Silastic (Dow Corning Ltd) are common examples.

- Silver impregnated dressings. These dressings also come as squares or ribbon. They are made of alginate, carboxymethylcellulose and silver impregnated nylon fibres. Silver is used for its anti-microbial action and at the same time the alginate absorbs the exudate to form gel. It is quite effective for the superficial wounds infected with gram positive bacteria and as ribbon for the cavities after surgery for pilonidal sinuses. Most common one is Silver-cel (Systagenix). Aquacel™ is also available with silver.

- Iodine containing dressings. These are gauze dressings impregnated with iodine which is usually good for quite superficial wounds. Iodine acts as antiseptic. Inadine (Systagenix) is readily available. The only problem with this dressing is that it sticks to the granulation tissue, so have to soak the wound in saline for 5 minutes before removing the dressing.

- Allograft and Xenograft for challenging skin loss situations [22, 23]

Skin is considered the largest organ of the human body representing about 16% of the total body weight. Skin loss is commonly encountered in problems such as burns or de-gloving injuries. The skin plays a vital role in terms of immunity, protection and thermoregulation of the human body. Consequently, skin loss can be associated with significant morbidities and even mortalities. Over decades, Research has been carried out to provide biologic skin substitutes that can take the skin function and can be readily available. Cadaveric and porcine grafts have been used for decades as a biologic skin substitutes. When cadaveric grafts are used, they are called allograft as they are originated from the same species. On the contrary, porcine grafts are called xenografts because they are taken from one species and transplanted on to another one.

10. Role of district nurses for wound management

While the journey of wound management starts at the acute hospital, a major part of it takes place in the community. District nurses and practice nurses in the community play a role in wound care. District nurse care is usually provided to patients who cannot physically attend their general practice for various reasons. Once the patients' condition enables them to move freely outside their homes, they are strongly advised to consult the practice nurses in the general practice and this allows appropriate resource allocation and provides a good service for the people who really need it. Moreover, it promotes recovery of the relatively fitter patient population.

11. Tissue viability services [25]

The concept of tissue viability nurses is relatively new though the idea originated in the 1980s. It covers all aspects of skin and soft tissue wounds. Although surgical wound management is a major part of their role, it is not their sole field of expertise. They also cover various soft tissue-related areas such as pressure sores and chronic leg ulceration. In addition to their bedside role, they provide education to the entire healthcare team. Across the UK, they are also working on preventing common hospital-related skin problems like pressure sores, thereby saving costs in the long term. Their role extends into the community where they provide support to district and practice nurses and help them to choose the correct dressing material and other essential tools for wound healing. The Tissue Viability Society has been established since 2014 and it is considered an excellent forum to discuss all new techniques and materials used for wound healing [26].

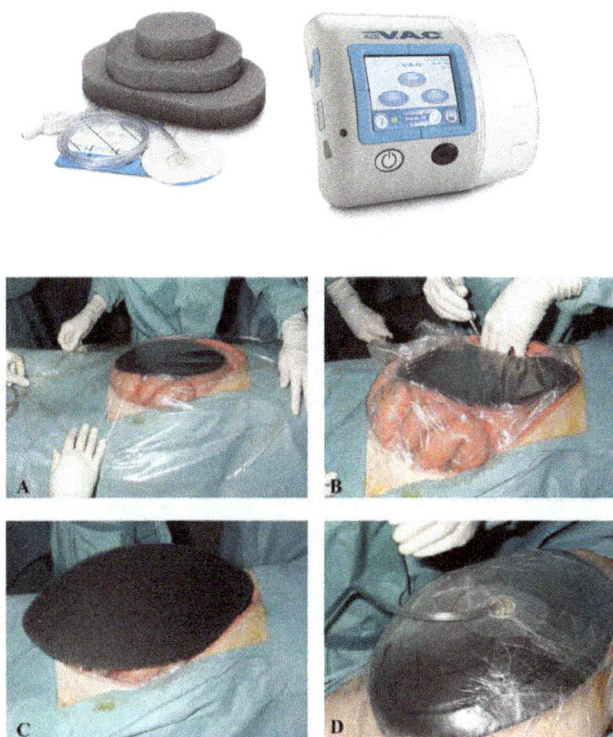

Figure 1. Prospective evaluation of vacuum-assisted closure in abdominal compartment syndrome and severe abdominal sepsis, *J Am Coll Surg.* 2007; **205**: 586–592 (Courtesy of KCI medical).

11.1. Vacuum-assisted closure (VAC) therapy and its role in wound healing

VAC therapy is a simple but effective method of promoting rapid healing. It is currently considered to be an effective means of managing large complex acute and chronic wounds (**Figures 1** and **2**) [27].

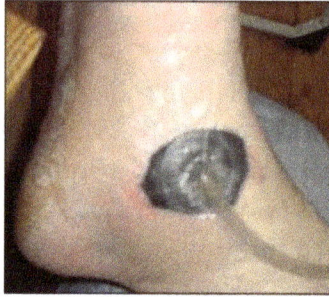

Figure 2. Vacuum dressing or small oozing wound (Courtesy of WWW.REHABPUB.COM).

VAC is an active wound therapy that was first described in 1997 by Morykwas and Argenta [28]. The system applies negative pressure to the wound bed via an open-cell polyurethane foam dressing [28]. The foam will be in direct contact with the wound and connects to a canister via a suction tube. An effective airtight seal is mandatory for the system to function.

Treatment objectives

A. Removal of excessive exudate and promoting a moist rather than wet environment for wound healing [27].

B. Increase angiogenesis which promotes granulation formation [28].

C. Ability to promote healing in complex wounds and wounds that fail to heal with the conventional methods [27, 28].

Wounds that can be treated with VAC therapy [29]

A. Pressure ulcers

B. Diabetic foot ulcers

C. Trauma wounds with tissue loss

D. Burns

E. Leg ulcers

F. Skin grafts

G. Surgical wound dehiscence

Contraindications and precautions [29]

A. Known or suspected malignant wounds

B. Gastrointestinal fistulation

C. Untreated osteomyelitis

D. Direct exposure of large blood vessels due to risk of bleeding

E. Thick/necrotic eschar.

11.2. Adjunctive measurements contributing to wound management

1. Ultrasound waves, electrotherapy or laser therapy. These adjuncts have always been thought to contribute towards better wound management. In a recent RCT, Cullum et al. concluded that there is lack of sufficient reliable evidence to draw conclusions about the contribution of laser therapy, therapeutic ultrasound, electrotherapy and electromagnetic therapy to chronic wound healing [30].

2. Hyperbaric oxygen therapy. Tissue hypoxia is one of the characteristics of chronic wounds. Therefore, means of increasing O_2 supply to tissues could potentially improve chronic wound healing. In a recent Cochrane review of 12 randomised trials, it was concluded that hyperbaric O_2 therapy can improve the chance of healing of diabetic foot ulcers only on short term but not on long term bases [31]. It can also reduce the size of wounds caused by chronic venous insufficiency but it was found to have no effect in wounds/ulcers caused by arterial insufficiency [31].

12. Conclusion

After reading this chapter the reader would have full understanding of types of wounds (WHO Classification) and how to treat them. We have described in details how to deal with different types of wound from clean surgical wound to heavily contaminated wounds. Closure of wounds by primary intention when the wound is clean and debridement and then leaving the wound to heal by secondary intention with or without secondary closure with sutures as deemed necessary. Different types of dressings are described in details with pros and cons of each one of them. Role of all personnel involved in treating the wound is defined. More specific types of method, i.e. laser therapy, ultrasound, hyperbaric oxygen and compression used for treating the wound are enumerated but not described in details as there is not enough evidence available.

Acknowledgements

We would like to express our sincere thanks to Dr Jaina Chauhan and Miss Janaki Solanki for poof reading the article and making linguistic changes where necessary. We would also like to acknowledge the help provided by Miss Shona Stewart in co-ordinating the project.

Author details

Peter Mekhail[1], Shuchi Chaturvedi[2] and Shailesh Chaturvedi[3*]

*Address all correspondence to: s.chaturvedi@nhs.net

1 Aberdeen Royal Infirmary, Aberdeen, UK

2 Kings College London, London, UK

3 Department of General Surgery, Aberdeen Royal Infirmary, Aberdeen, UK

References

[1] Lewis R, Whiting P, ter Riet G, O'Meara S, Glanville J. A rapid and systemic review of the clinical effectiveness and cost effectiveness of debriding agents in treating surgical wounds healing by secondary intention. Health Technol Assess. 2001:5 (14):3–4,26–29,35–39,59–61.

[2] M. Flanagan. The physiology of wound management. Journal of Wound Care. June, Vol 9, No 6, 2000:209–300

[3] Tortora, G.J., Grabowski, S.R. *Principles of Anatomy and Physiology* (8th edn). New York: Harper Collins College Publications, 1996.

[4] Hutchinson, J.J. Prevalence of wound infection under occlusive dressings: a collective survey of reported research. *Wounds* 1989; 1: 123–133.

[5] Baxter, C.R. Immunologic reactions in chronic wounds. *Am J Surgery* 1994; 167: S: 12S–14S.

[6] Nathan, C.F. Secretory products of macrophages. *J Clin Investigation* 1987; 79: 319–326.

[7] Brown, G.L. Acceleration of tensile strength of incisions treated with EGF and TGF. *Annals of Surgery* 1988; 208: 788–794.

[8] Diegelmann, R. et al. The role of macrophages in wound repair: a review. *Plastic Reconstructive Surgery* 1991; 68: 107–113.

[9] Eisenbeiss, W., Peter, P.W., Bakhtiari, C. et al. Hypertrophic scars and keloids. *J Wound Care* 1998; 7: 5, 255–257.

[10] Mitchell, Richard Sheppard; Kumar, Vinay; Abbas, Abdul K;Faust, Nelson (2007). Robins Basic Pathology. Philadelphia: Saunders. ISBN 1-4160-2973-7. 8th Edition.

[11] Kanzler MH, Gorsulowsky DC, Swanson NA. Basic mechanisms in the healing cutaneous wound. *J Dermatol Surg Oncol*. 1986 Nov. 12(11):1156–64.

[12] Singer AJ, Clark RA. Cutaneous wound healing. *N Engl J Med.* 1999 Sep 2. 341(10): 738–46.

[13] Diwan R, Tromovitch TA, Glogau RG, Stegman SJ. Secondary intention healing. The primary approach for management of selected wounds. *Arch Otolaryngol Head Neck Surg.* 1989 Oct. 115(10):1248–9.

[14] Best practice guidelines in disaster situations. WHO/EHT/CPR 2005, formatted 2009.Chapter 9:9–11

[15] Mohan H. Kudur , Sathish B. Pai, H. Sripathi, Smitha Prabhu. Sutures and suturing techniques in skin closure .Indian J Dermatol Venereol Leprol. July-August 2009. Vol 75. Issue 4:425–433.

[16] Benevento R, Santoriello A, Pellino G, Sciaudone G, Candilio G, De Fatico GS, Selvaggi F; EBSQ Colo, Canonico S. The effects of low-thrombin fibrin sealant on wound serous drainage, seroma formation and length of postoperative stay in patients undergoing axillary node dissection for breast cancer. A randomized controlled trial. Int J Surg. 2014 Nov;12(11):1210–5.

[17] Sierra D, Fibrin sealant adhesive systesm: a review of their chemistry, material properties and clinical applications. *J Biomat App* 1993;7:309–352.

[18] Singer AJ, Dagum AB. Current management of acute cutaneous wounds. NEJM 2008;359:1037–46.

[19] Yao K, Bae L, Yew WP. Post-operative wound management. Aust Fam Physician. 2013 Dec;42(12):867–70.

[20] Mark Collier et al. National Institute for Health and Care Excellence. Prevention and treatment of surgical site infections. Available at publications.nice.org.uk/ surgical-site-infection-cg74. Published 2008.

[21] Singhal H, Kaur K, Zammit C. Medscape reference: wound infection treatment and management. Available at emedicine.medscape.com/ article/188988,; Updated Dec. 2015; Section2:2–3.

[22] Benjamin C Wood et al. Skin Grafts and Biologic Skin Substitutes. Available at emedicine.medscape.com/article/1295109-overview; Updated March 2015; Section 3: 3

[23] Ennis WJ, Valdes W, Salzman S, Fishman D, Meneses P. Trauma and wound care. In: Morison MJ, Ovington LG, Wilkie K, editors. Chronic wound care. A problem-based learning approach. London: Mosby Elsevier Limited; 2004. p. 291–307.

[24] Ruszczak Z, Schwartz RA, Joss-Wichman E, Wichman R, Zalewska A. Medscape reference: surgical dressings. Available at emedicine.medscape.com/article/1127868-overview#showall; Section 6–7.

[25] Fanja Pagnamenta. Tissue viability The role of the tissue viability nurse. Wound Essentials 2014, Vol 9 No 2.(65–67).

[26] Tissue Viability Society (2014) Available at: http://tvs.org.uk.

[27] Joseph E, Hamori CA, Bergman S, et al. A prospective randomised trial of vaccum-assisted closure versus standard therapy of chronic nonhealing wounds. Wounds2000; 3:60–7.

[28] Morykwas MJ, Argenta LC, Shelton-Brown EI, et al. Vacuum-assisted closure: a new method for wound control and treatment: animal studies and basic foundation. Ann Plast Surg1997;38:553–62.

[29] Baxter Helena, Ballard Kate. Vacuum Assisted Closure. Nursing Times 2001;Vol 97(35): 51–53.

[30] Cullum N, Nelson EA, Flemming K, Sheldon T. Systematic reviews of wound care management: (5) beds; (6) compression; (7) laser therapy, therapeutic ultrasound, electrotherapy and electromagnetic therapy. Health Technol Assess: 2001:Vol 5(9):161–163.

[31] Kranke P, Bennett MH, Martyn-St James M, Schnabel A, Debus SE, Weibel S. Hyperbaric oxygen therapy for chronic wounds. Cochrane Database of Systematic Reviews 2015, Issue 6. Art. No.: CD004123. DOI: 10.1002/14651858.CD004123.pub4

9

Polarisation of Macrophage and Immunotherapy in the Wound Healing

Yu-Sheng Wu, Fan-Hua Nan, Sherwin Chen and
Shiu-Nan Chen

Abstract

Immune cells are involved in virtually every aspect of the wound repair process, from the initial stages where they participate in haemostasis and work to prevent infection to later stages where they drive scar formation. Immunotherapy is being developed offers some advantageous immunomodulation factors that are known in the field of alternative medicine, such as mushroom beta-glucan, anti-microbial peptides and triterpenoid; these factors represent a novel therapeutic approach for anti-inflammation to promote the wound healing.

Keywords: healing, immunotherapy, inflammation, macrophage, polarisation, wound

1. Inflammation

When an organism is injured by a wound injury or infected by a pathogen, inflammation is a crucial response. Inflammation is a complex interaction with molecular mediators; it includes the function of immune cells in a microenvironment through a response that occurs at all levels of biological organisation [1]. Following previous studies, this paper illustrates that the inflammation response involves cooperation between cells and a wide range of mediators, such as cytokines, chemokines and non-enzyme factors involved in the classical immune response. The macrophage is one of the critical inflammatory immune cells involved in the uptake and degradation of infectious agents and senescent cells and also plays critical roles in tissue growth, tissue remodelling and inflammation by producing oxidants, proteinases and anti-microbial peptides [2–4]. Activated inflammatory cells are sources of reactive oxygen species (ROS) and reactive nitrogen species (RNS) that can initiate changes in cell functions, including cell signalling pathways, transcription factor activation, mediator release and apoptosis. However, whether the ROS and RNS that are produced and released by neutrophils or macrophages are sufficient to diffuse through the extra-cellular matrix, enter epithelial cells and cross the cytoplasm is not clear [5–7]. Even the physiological roles of ROS and RNS in the cellular response are not clear [8–11]. The results obtained from experiments performed on the livers of tilapia showed that extra-cellular hydrogen peroxide (H_2O_2) attracted cell migration. These results suggested that ROS is a crucial factor in initiating the migration of macrophages that trigger cascades of phagocytic activity.

In the microenvironment of inflammation, the platelet-derived growth factor (PDGF), the tumour necrosis factors (TNF)-α and TNF-β, the hepatocyte growth factor, transforming growth factor (TGF)-β2, the epidermal growth factor (EGF) and the fibroblast growth factor all play an important role in physiological immune response. The interleukins (IL)-1, IL-6, IL-8, IL-10, and the interferon gamma (INF-γ) also detain key functions in the natural inflammatory response [12–16]. These factors hold a primordial function in fibroblast activation and regulation, also concerning reactive fibrosis that follows their continuing activation. Although these growth factors are also related to fibroblast migration and activation, particular research was recently focused on the PDGF family of growth factors and their relative receptors [17, 18]. Research has documented that PDGF exerts autocrine, mitogenic effects on keratinocytes to support epidermal proliferation and stabilisation of the epidermal junction during wound closure. In addition, it stimulates vessel maturation by recruiting and differentiating pericytes to the immature-endothelial channel [19–22]. According to these references, we investigate whether the produced ROS/RNS is related to the released factors and (if so) what type of relationship exists among ROS/RNS and these factors.

2. Reactive oxygen species production and physical response

The production and scavenging of ROS may be initiated by adverse environmental factors. Research has shown that intra-cellular levels of ROS may rapidly rise and ROS may be generated by the activation of various oxidases and peroxidases in response to certain environmental changes [23]. ROS forms through energy transfer or through electron transfer reactions. ROS formation causes the formation of singlet oxygen, which results in sequential reduction to superoxide, H_2O_2 and hydroxyl radicals [24]. Mitochondria are a crucial source of ROS production in most cells. This ROS production contributes to mitochondrial stress and plays a critical role in redox signalling from the organelles [25]. Mitochondria have a 4-layer structure composed of the outer mitochondrial membrane, intermembrane space, inner mitochondrial membrane and matrix [26]. NADPH oxidase is an enzymatic source in the mitochondrial structure that generates ROS and plays a fundamental role in maintaining normal cell functions. Recent research has focussed on the influence of this enzyme to cellular oxidative stress that may contribute to various pathophysiological conditions and diseases [27, 28]. A crucial function of NADPH oxidase is modulating multiple redox-sensitive intra-cellular signalling pathways; NADPH modulates these pathways by generating ROS molecules, inhibiting protein tyrosine phosphatases and activating certain redox-sensitive transcription factors. Moreover, the ROS consist of numerous molecular species, including H_2O_2, oxide ions (O_2) and hydroxide (OH^-) [29]. Molecular oxygen is a biradical, containing two unpaired electrons in the outer structure; because these two electrons have the same spin, oxygen can only react with one electron; therefore it is not very reactive when these two electrons have the same spin. Oxygen's unpaired electrons can become excited and can change the spin of one electron. This transforms oxygen into a powerful oxidant because the two electrons with opposing spins can rapidly react with other pairs of electrons [30]. Electrons can be contributed from NADH and FADH2 enzymes and can pass through the electron transport chain, generating superoxide (O_2^-) at complexes I and III. This generated superoxide can be reduced to H_2O_2 by superoxide dismutase and can be completely reduced into water by glutathione peroxidase, as presented in **Figure 1**.

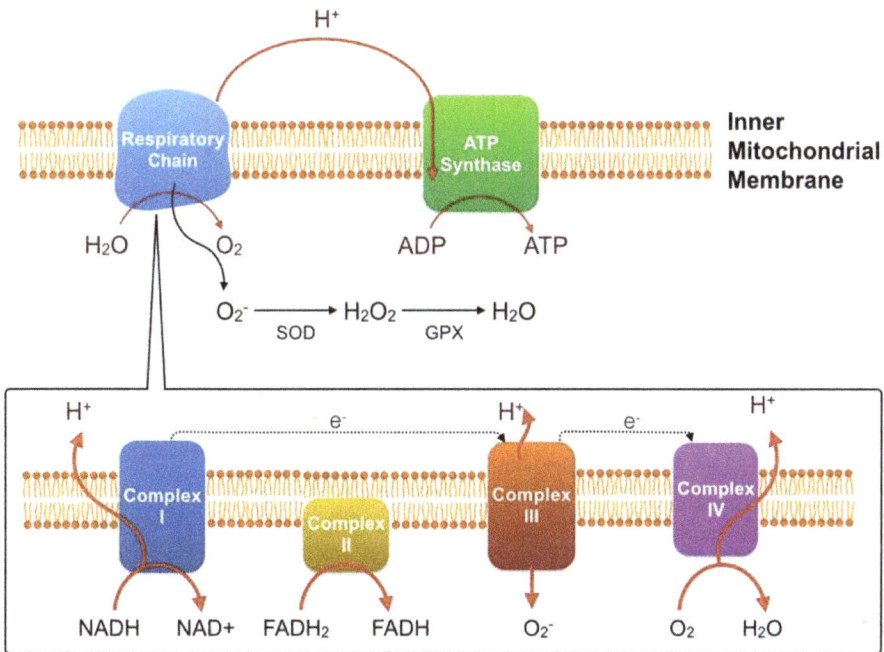

Figure 1. ROS are produced from the electron transport pathway to form superoxide (O_2^-) at complex I and complex III released into the matrix and reduced O_2 to form H_2O at complex IV. Following, the generated O_2^- is transferred to the form of H_2O_2 by superoxide dismutase (SOD) and completely reduced to water (H_2O) by glutathione peroxidase (GPX).

Research has shown that ROS consist of numerous molecular species, including H_2O_2, oxide ions (O_2^-) and OH^{-29}. These molecular species act as signalling molecules in the migration of profibrogenic cells [31] and peripheral blood monocytes [23, 32]. One of the crucial physiological functions of ROS is the modulation of ion channels. Research has illustrated that ROS may act through Ca^{2+} as an intra-cellular second messenger involved in regulating diverse functions, such as fertilisation, electrical signalling, contraction, secretion, memory, gene transcription and cell death [33, 34]. Furthermore, studies have reported that H_2O_2 may affect cell energy stores [35], induce DNA strand breaks [36], enhance cell adhesion [37], increase endothelial tissue permeability [38] and stimulate the release of cytokines.

In the research presented in **Figure 2**, the concentration of ROS seems to be considered the concentration of a crucial signalling molecule. Low concentrations of generated ROS are believed to be critical for metabolic adaptation in the organelle. Moderate concentrations of ROS can be produced and released by stress; pathogen-infected and bacterial endotoxin lipopolysaccharide (LPS) are involved in the inflammatory response. The high concentration of ROS in the induced apoptosis/autophagy process can cause cell death [39] and initiate self-healing [40].

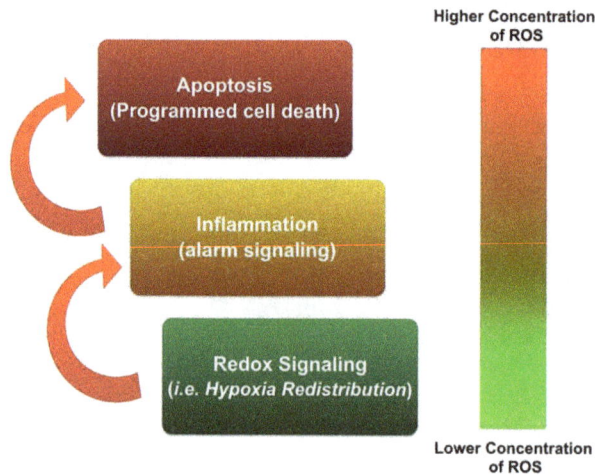

Figure 2. Concentration of generated ROS may involve in the different physiological response. At the low concentration, the ROS regulate in the redox signalling, and at the moderate concentration of induced ROS which participated in the inflammation process. At the high level of ROS concentration increased and was to be involved in the cellular apoptosis.

3. Tissue resident macrophages

Macrophages, which are present in almost all body tissue and display distinct location-specific phenotypes and gene expression profiles, display remarkable functional diversity in innate immune responses, tissue development and tissue homeostasis [41]. In different organs, the resident macrophages are given various appellations: microglia cells have fundamental importance in assessing the pathogenetic significance of perivascular inflammatory phenomena within the brain [42]; Kupffer cells are resident and recruited macrophages that play major roles in the homeostatic function of the liver and in its response to tissue damage [43]; alveolar macrophages are key determinants pulmonary immune responses and in the lung inflammation caused by asthma [44]. Previously, it was hypothesised that tissue macrophages were recruited from circulating blood monocytes. Recent studies have demonstrated that tissue macrophages such as microglia, Kupffer cells and Langerhans cells are established prenatally and arise independently of the hematopoietic transcription factor Myb [45]. Myb is required for developing hematopoietic stem cells (HSCs) and all CD11b[high] monocytes and macrophages but is not required for yolk sac (YS) macrophages and for developing YS-derived F4/80[bright] macrophages. Such macrophages can persist independently of HSCs in several types of tissue in adult mice [46]. Kupffer cells as well as other resident macrophages (e.g., microglia) originate from the YS in a colony-stimulating factor-1/receptor (CSF-1R)-dependent and Myb-independent manner. Researchers have suggested that these macrophages are maintained by local proliferation, which results in extensive mitosis after stress or an exchanged tissue microenvironment [43, 47].

Macrophages are the most crucial and abundant immune cells. They can be categorised into two primary types according to function and differentiation: classically activated macrophages (M1 macrophages) and alternatively activated macrophages (M2 macrophages) [48]. Macrophages are relevant to innate resistance and to the relationship between inflammation and autoimmune disease. In mouse models, macrophages present CD11b, F4/80 and CSF-1R, with F4/80 being the surface proteins for M1 and M2 macrophages [49, 50]. When pathogens enter the organism from the intestinal portal vein, circulating monocytes (surrounding the pathogens and present in the peripheral blood) respond to chemokines (e.g., CCL2) and are exposed to antigens. While interacting with pattern recognition receptors (PRRs), antigens may exert either M1 or M2 polarising activities, depending on the Th1 (IFN-γ) and Th2 (IL-4 and IL-13) cytokines and immune factors [51, 52].

4. Inflammation and macrophages

Inflammation is an important adaptive physiological response of the organism. Inflammation response embodies a complicated interaction among molecular mediators and cells. It globally affects the leukocytes, also the lymphocytes in their micro-environmental function and organisation [48]. Throughout their response, numerous factors are involved in the classical immune response. Macrophages detain a critical role in the uptake and degradation of infectious agents and senescent cells; they also play crucial roles in tissue growth, tissue remodelling and inflammation by producing oxidants, proteinases and anti-microbial peptide [40].

Resident macrophages sense exogenous or endogenous danger signals (e.g., bacterial products or necrotic cell debris) through PRRs. In response to Toll-like receptor (TLR) ligands and interferon-gamma (IFN-γ) or IL-4/IL-13, macrophages undergo M1 (classical) or M2 (alternative) activation. The activation of M1 and M2 macrophages mirrors TH1-TH2 polarisation; M1 and M2 activation span the extremes of a continuum. M1 macrophages, which display a morphology that depends on their tissue location, develop in response to stimulation with IFN-γ and microbial products such as LPS. M1 macrophages can secrete substantial amounts of pro-inflammatory cytokines, such as IL-1β, IL-15, IL-18, TNF-α and IL-12 [53]. M2 macrophages adapt to similarities and differences between IL-4, TLR ligands with IL-10 and glucocorticoids [54].

The phenotypes of M1 and M2 macrophages exhibit observable differences. The M1 phenotype is characterised by the expression of high levels of pro-inflammatory cytokines, high production of reactive nitrogen and oxygen intermediates, promotion of Th1 response and anti-microbial and tumour-inhibiting activity [43]. The M2 macrophage uses immune inhibitory effects to secrete large amounts of IL-10, TGF-β, and C-C motif chemokine ligands 17 (CCL17) and CCL22. Moreover, the M2 macrophage attracts non-cytotoxic T_{reg} and Type 2 T-helper cells (TH2 cells) to aggregate in tumour tissue, inhibit T-cell differentiation and function, lower cytotoxic T-cell function, induce T-cell apoptosis, secrete CCL18 and attract naive T cells [55].

Macrophage	M1	M2
Transcription factor		
Interferon regulatory factor	IRF-3 [61, 62]	IRF-4 [63]
(IRF)		
	IRF-5 [64]	
	IRF-8 [65]	
Nuclear factor	NF-κB [43]	
Signal transducer and activator of transcription	STAT-1 [66]	STAT-3 [43]
(STAT)		
		STAT-5 [67]
		SATA-6 [68]
Suppressor	SOCS-1	
of cytokine signalling	SOCS-2	
(SOCS)	SOCS-3	
	(controversial) [58]	
Phenotype	iNOS [69, 70]	YM-1 [71]
	IL-6 [72]	Arg-1 [73, 74]
	TNF-α [75]	Fizz-1 [76]
		IL-10 [77]

Table 1. Regulators in the M1 and M2 macrophage.

Macrophage polarisation is highly related to expressions of various TLRs on macrophages [56, 57]. The evidence indicates that TLR signalling (e.g., TLR4), which is activated by LPS and other microbial ligands, drives macrophages to prefer the M1 phenotype. In this reaction, MyD88 and TRIF activate a cascade of kinases, including IRAK4, TRAF6 and IKKβ; this results in the activation of nuclear factor kappa B (NF-κB), which drives the macrophage forward to the M1 phenotype. By contrast, IL-4 and IL-13 drive the macrophage's phenotype forward to M2. Activation of STAT6 through the IL-4 receptor alpha (IL-4Rα) and IL-10 induce activation of STAT3 through receptor IL-10R, which activates JAK1 and JAK3 (38), causing STAT6 activation [58, 59]. IL-10, TGF-β, IL-4 and IL-13 enhance inflammation and cellular immune response with NO, which is generated through IFN-γ-induced iNOS and is reduced in macrophages by Arg1 interactions with mast cells, basophils, eosinophils, NKT cells, IgE and selected subclasses of IgG. This promotes allergies and hypersensitivity [60] (**Table 1**).

5. Inflammation and disease

Accumulating evidence indicates that chronic low-grade inflammation contributes to the systemic metabolic dysfunction that is associated with inflammation disorders [78]. Cytokines and pathogen-associated molecular patterns have been shown to co-stimulate cell surface receptors, including TLRs, to initiate intra-cellular signalling that activates NF-κB. NF-κB activation was thought to induce the target gene's expression to promote cellular proliferation and to activate the immune response. However, research has revealed that NF-κB activation can occur in most cell types; recent reports have demonstrated that high level activation of NF-κB signalling pathways in the liver, adipose tissue and central nervous system (CNS) is involved in the development of inflammation-associated metabolic diseases [79]. The mutants of the brain-specific serpin, neuroserpin, also form ordered polymers that accumulate within the ER of neurons; these mutations cause an autosomal-dominant type of dementia known as familial encephalopathy with neuroserpin inclusion bodies, which is believed to be an inflammation disorder [80, 81].

Research has shown that, in specific tissue lesions, extra-cellular lipid droplets are forming a core region surrounded by smooth muscle cells and collagen-rich matrix. Lymphocytes as the T cells, monocyte, macrophages and mast cells are infiltrating in the lesion particularly in regions where the atheroma grows. These immune cells also generate important signals in the defence cascade by producing the inflammatory cytokines, largely involved in the athero-sclerotic process [82]. A case report indicated that Alzheimer's disease (AD) inflammation appears to arise from within the CNS. Little or no involvement of lymphocytes or monocytes in AD was observed beyond their normal brain surveillance. This observation has placed AD outside the realm of conventional neuroimmunologic studies that largely focus on humoral aspects of such CNS inflammatory disorders as multiple sclerosis [83]. Judging from published reports, we believe that metabolic disorders and even neuronal diseases are highly related to abnormal inflammation.

6. Macrophage and T-cell differentiation

In pathogen infection, dendritic cells (DCs) and macrophages primarily act as phagocytotic antigen-presenting cells (APCs) that degrade infected pathogens into fragments, and then move those fragments to the nearby lymphoid organs. The pathogen fragments combine with cell surface histocompatibility complex (major histocompatibility complex) to activate and differentiate T cells. **Figure 3** displays the cooperation of the antigen-presenting cells, co-stimulatory molecules and cytokines.

The metabolic organs, such as the liver, pancreas and adipose tissue, are composed of paren-chymal and stromal cells, which include macrophages to maintain metabolic homeostasis. Bacterial infection innately activates macrophages, causing the secretion of proinflammatory cytokines, such as TNF-α, IL-6 and IL-1β. This promotes peripheral insulin resistance and reduces nutrient storage during the metabolic reaction. Furthermore, some additional physiological mechanism can lead to the activation of macrophages. For these latest, the regulatory T cells (T_{reg}), the Fcγ receptors, the apoptotic cells and the prostaglandins are increasing the number of macrophages involved in the regulation of inflammation and anti-tumour defences [84]. These inflammatory mediators are involved in activating anti-microbial defence mechanisms, including oxidative processes that contribute to killing pathogens and the secreted IL-12 and IL-23. These direct the differentiation and expansion of anti-microbial T_H1 and T_H17 cells that help to drive inflammatory responses [85]. Recent research shows that intestinal antigen-presenting cells can be divided into CD11c$^+$CD11b$^-$, CD11c$^+$CD11b$^+$ and CD11c^{dull}CD11b$^+$ categories. Particularly, the CD11c^{dull}CD11b$^+$ cells are CD103$^-$F4/80$^+$macro-phages, with efficient role in inducing the Foxp3$^+$ regulatory T (T_{reg}) cells [86]. Tumour cells affect the surrounding cellular environment by promoting tumour growth and metastasis by establishing a tumour microenvironment that is conducive to tumour development [87–90]. In the tumour microenvironment, tumour cells secrete inflammatory cytokines, such as TGF-β and IL-10. These cytokines stimulate differentiation of regulatory T and T_{reg} cells [91, 92] as well as differentiation of tumour-associated macrophages (TAMs) into M2 macrophages. This causes the host immune system to locate and attack cancer cells, which generates subsequent tumour cell evasion of this immune surveillance and attack, which enhances tumour growth and metastasis [87, 93–98]. Various cytokines, chemokines and growth factors in the tumour microenvironment are the primary elements that affect the host's anti-tumour ability and evasion of tumour cells [89, 99]. Tumour microenvironments are complicated cellular micro-cosms [89, 97], and numerous immune cells are located throughout tumour microenviron-ments. Macrophages are the most crucial and abundant immune cells in the tumour microenvironment. The two most critical types of macrophages, based on function and differentiation, are M1 and M2 macrophages. M1 macrophages are characterised by tumour

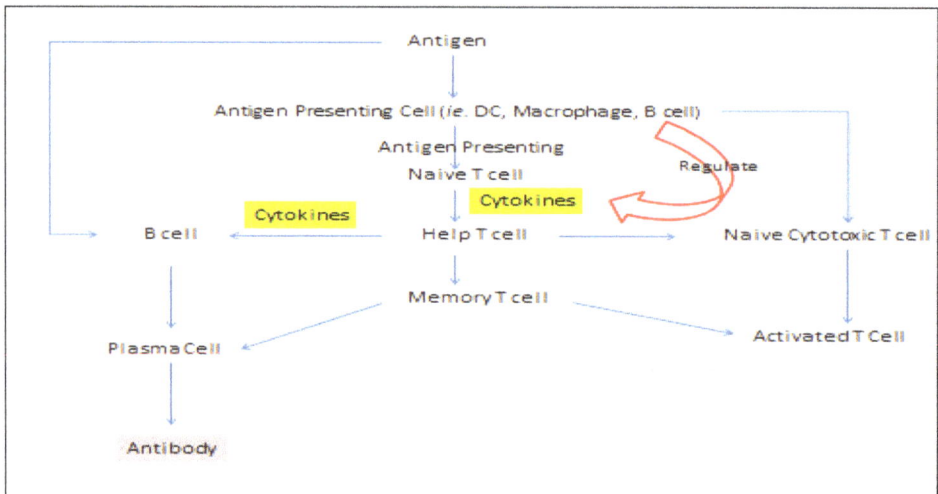

Figure 3. The cooperation of the antigen-presenting cells, costimulatory molecules, and cytokines. Bacterial infection innately activates macrophages, causing the secretion of pro-inflammatory cytokines, such as TNF-α, IL-6, and IL-1β. This promotes peripheral insulin resistance and reduces nutrient storage during the metabolic reaction. Furthermore, several additional mechanisms can also contribute to the activation of macrophages for immune-regulatory activity.

resistance, whereas M2 macrophages are characterised by tumour promotion [98, 100]. In mouse models, macrophages present CD11b, F4/80, CSF-1R and F4/80 as the surface proteins for M1 and M2 macrophages [93, 101]. Recent studies have noted large quantities of TAMs in tumour tissue. TAMs are the most abundant and critical immune cells in the tumour microenvironment [102–104] and are the main factors that enable the tumour microenvironment to exert immune inhibitory effects [101, 102]. In the tumour microenvironment, tumour cells and the surrounding stoma cells secrete cytokines and growth factors that stimulate TAMs and activate the various expression, function, receptor regulation and secretion types of chemokines [103, 105], including anti-tumour M1 macrophages and pro-tumour M2 macrophages [98, 106–108]. In the tumour microenvironment, the proportions of M1 and M2 macrophages are unequal. Tumour microenvironments contain large amounts of transmitters, such as M-CSF, IL-6, IL-10, TGF-β and COX-2, that induce transformation of TAMs into M2 macrophages that secrete immune inhibitory chemokines and have poor antigen-presenting and cytotoxic abilities, which generates tumour growth and metastasis [49, 98, 102–104, 109–114]. M2 macrophages and TAMs have protumour and immune inhibitory effects, secrete large amounts of IL-10, TGF-β, CCL17 and CCL22, attract non-cytotoxic T_{reg} and TH2 cells to aggregate in tumour tissue, inhibit T-cell differentiation and function, lower cytotoxic T-cell function, induce T-cell apoptosis, secrete CCL18 and attract naïve T cells [49, 98, 115]. NADPH oxidase is a major enzymatic source of cellular ROS. NADPH plays a fundamental role in maintaining normal cell functions. Recent research has focussed on this enzyme's role in cellular oxidative stress, which may eventually contribute to various pathophysiological conditions and diseases [27, 28]. Studies have found that NADPH oxidase modulates multiple redox-sensitive intra-cellular signalling pathways by generating ROS molecules. This modulation includes inhibition of protein tyrosine phosphatases and activation of certain redox-sensitive transcription factors [116, 117]. ROS consist of numerous molecular species, including H_2O_2, oxide ions (O_2^-) and OH^{-29}, that act as signalling molecules involved in the migration of hepatic profibrogenic cells [118] and the functioning of peripheral blood monocytes [119]. ROS and RNS, generated endogenously or in response to environmental stress, have long been implicated in tissue injury for a variety of disease states [120, 121]. Stimulation of the mitochondrial apoptotic pathway through ROS and mitochondrial DNA damage promotes outer membrane permeabilisation, which triggers caspase-dependent or caspase-independent cytosolic signalling events [122]. Activated inflammatory cells serve as sources of ROS and RNS that can initiate the alteration of the cell function, gathering specific cellular signalling, transcription factor activation, physiological factors release, the apoptosis process and compensatory cell proliferation. However, it remains unclear whether the ROS or the RNS production and release through neutrophils or macrophages enhance sufficient diffusion into the intra-cellular cytoplasm as to affect the cellular response [123, 124].

7. Wound healing

Immune cells are involved in virtually every aspect of the wound repair process, from the initial stages, where they participate in haemostasis and work to prevent infection, to later stages where they drive scar formation [125, 126]. T lymphocytes exercise crucial in vivo effects on various parameters of healing [127–129]. Neutrophils help control infection during wound healing, but they also release harmful enzymes that damage healthy tissue surrounding the wound site [130–132]. Recent researchers have noted that several specific proteins produced by wound macrophages at the site of injury are involved: (1) in the recruitment and activation of additional macrophages infiltrating in the wound; (2) in the production of growth factors that promote cellular proliferation and tissue recovery synthesis; (3) in stimulating proteases and extra-cellular matrix growth and (4) in the process of tissue remodelling [133]. β-catenin-dependent Wnt pathways, which are classified according to their ability to promote stabilisation of β-catenin in the cytoplasm, act as cellular signals through cytoplasmic stabilisation and accumulation of β-catenin in the nucleus to activate gene transcription [134]. This could enhance wound healing by lymphocytes [135, 136]. Nicotinamide adenine dinucleotide phosphate (NADPH) oxidase modulates multiple redox-sensitive intra-cellular signalling pathways by generating ROS molecules. This includes inhibiting protein tyrosine phosphatases and activating certain redox-sensitive transcription factors [116, 137, 138]. This shows that ROS regulate the expression of key chemical mediators that further modulate the inflammatory response in animal models; it has also been reported that these redox-sensitive processes may include cytokine action, angiogenesis, cell motility and extra-cellular matrix formation [139–141]; this can enable reliable estimates of wound-healing capacity, which is altered by various conditions, such as inflammation. Furthermore, research on one of the ROS has indicated that H_2O_2 plays a critical role in wound repair, inflammation and anti-inflammation mechanisms [142, 143]. Our published research also showed that the production of ROS (i.e., H_2O_2 after an injury has occurred) may cause healing to generate inflammation through the apoptosis of the cell. Over-inhibition of NADPH oxidase activity may reduce the normal progress of apoptosis under the wound and might delay healing [29].

Inflammation enhances vascular permeability, active migration of blood cells and the passage of plasma constituents into the injured tissue [144]. Blood leukocytes actively participate in the defence and inflammation responses, being activated since the earliest phases of atherosclerosis process. Inflammation and atherosclerosis shelter intricate mechanisms relied to leukocytes recruitment [145]. Neuro-inflammation mediators are described to be closely related to brain cells functioning (such as microglia and astrocytes), to the complement system activation and to cytokines, and chemokines production [146]. Regarding cancer development [147], pro-inflammatory cytokines, including IL-1α, IL-1β, IL-6, IL-8, IL-18, chemokines, matrix metallopeptidase-9 and vascular endothelial growth factor, are primarily regulated by the transcription NF-κB, which is active in most tumours and is induced by carcinogens [148]. Cutaneous wound repair is a tightly regulated and dynamic process involving blood clotting, inflammation, formation of new tissue and tissue remodelling [149]. Thrombin is the protease involved in blood coagulation. Its deregulation can cause haemostatic abnormalities, which range from subtle subclinical problems to serious life-threatening coagulopathies (i.e., during septicaemia) [150]. Inflammation and coagulation are both parts of the natural mechanism that protects the organism against infection. The endothelial cells and the platelets are capable to react in the acute, also in the chronic inflammatory environment. They release pro-inflammatory mediators that produce adhesion of molecules, proteases and clotting factors associated to leukocytes recruitment [151]. The elements of the PAR family serve as sensors that detect blood-clotting serine proteinases in the inflamed target cells. Activation of PAR-1 by thrombin and of PAR-2 by other factors on the membrane of endothelial cells generates rapid expression and exposure of adhesive proteins that mediate an acute inflammatory reaction and of the tissue factor that initiates the blood coagulation cascade [152] as presented as **Figure 4**.

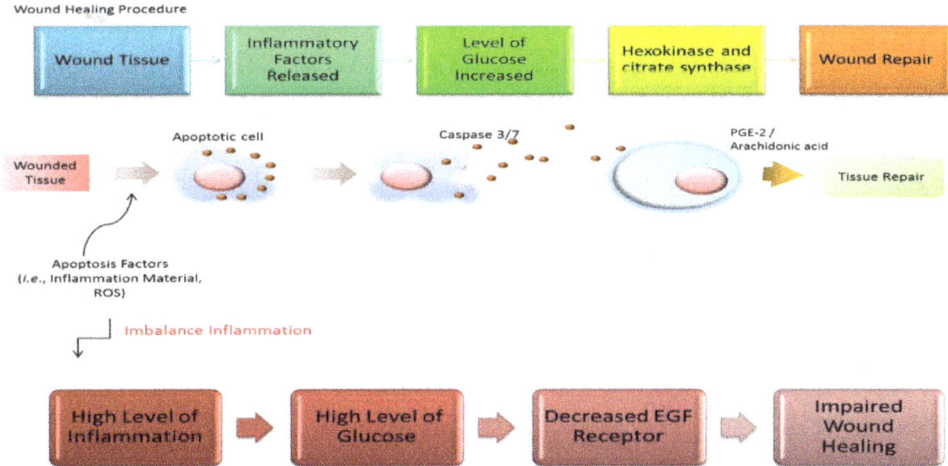

Figure 4. Wound healing was initiated after the injury of the cell, tissue even the organ. In the early stage of the healing, the damaged tissue producing a lot of ROS leading to neighbour cells into the apoptosis, following the apoptotic cells collapsed and released caspases were able to induce the tissue repair. However, the imbalance inflammatory may induce over-production of blood glucose that is leading to decrease the EGF receptor expression further to impair the wound healing.

8. Immunomodulation in anti-inflammation therapy

Nakanishi et al. found that celecoxib can alter the immune inhibitory effects of the tumour microenvironment by promoting transformation of TAMs into M1 macrophages, inhibiting tumour growth [153]. In 1968, Ikekawa et al. found that the fruiting body extracts from *Lentinus edodes*, *Trametes versicolor*, *Ganoderma tsugae*, *Flammulina velutiper* and *Tricholoma matsutake* demonstrated substantial anti-tumour activities towards transplanted tumour cells of Sarcoma 180 [154, 155]. *Autrodia comphorata*-derived beta-glucan inhibited tumour growth for Sarcoma 37, Sarcoma 180, Erlich ascites sarcoma and Yoshida sarcoma as well as inhibited LLC1 transplanted tumour growth [156]. Daily intake of *A. comphorata*-derived beta-glucan for 18 consecutive days was demonstrated to slow tumour growth and reduce the rate of metastasis [157]. Cytotoxic T-cell activity and tumour occurrence rates were observed, and the results illustrated that daily oral intake of *Grifola frondosua*-derived beta-glucan or Lentinan can enhance cytotoxic T-cell activity and reduce tumour occurrence rates [158]. The addition of a conditioned medium along with tumour cells into the progenitor cells of DCs was found to further inhibit maturation of DCs and lower the antigen-presenting capability of the DCs [159]. Tumour cells were found to secrete M-CSF, inhibiting dendritic and T-cell differentiation and anti-tumour ability [87, 159–161]. In the inflammation environment, the amounts of M1 and M2 macrophages are not equal [162]. The tumour environment contains vast quantities of transmitters such as M-CSF, IL-6, IL-10, TGF-β and COX-2 that induce tumour megakaryocytes to differentiate into M2 macrophages, which, in addition to having inferior antigen-presenting and cytotoxic abilities, also secrete factors that inhibit immune cells, resulting in enhanced immune inhibitory effects in the tumour environment [49, 98, 102–104, 109–114]. M2 macrophages in tumour bearing mice enhance tumour growth and immune inhibitory effects. They also secrete cytokines, such as IL-10 and TGF-β, in high quantities, which attract non-cytotoxic T_{reg} cells and TH2 cells to congregate in tumour tissue; those cells inhibit the differentiation and normal function of T cells, including their cytotoxic ability, and further promote T-cell apoptosis [49, 98, 115, 163, 164]. The polarisation of TH1 and TH2 is built on cytokine patterns; polarisation begins when the antigen-presenting cells interact with naive T cells; they polarise into Type 1 (TH1) and TH2 cells in response to the type of antigen encountered [165]. TH1 and TH2 cells secrete different cytokines; TH1 cells rely on IL-2, IFN-γ and TNF, which are involved in cell-mediated immunity against pathogens, but TH2 cells depend mostly on IL-4 and IL-5, which stimulate the production of IgE antibodies and eosinophil responses, resulting in allergic diseases [166, 167]. Although an imbalanced TH1/TH2 immune response is linked to certain hypersensitivity disorders such as allergies, asthma and hay fever [168], studies have suggested that using a biological response modifier to restore the balance between TH1 and TH2 immune response can be a potential treatment option for IgE-dependent hypersensitivity [169]. *Ganoderma lucidum* is a medicinal mushroom that has been widely used as a folk medicine in Asian countries such as China and Japan for hundreds of years for its immuno-modulating and anti-tumour effects. Numerous biologically available substances with immunity enhancement effects, particularly polysaccharides, have been isolated from the extract of *G. lucidum* [170].

Anti-microbial peptides are effective components of innate immunity that exist widely in biological systems. One of the specific anti-microbial peptides, hepcidin, is a 25-amino acid antibiotic peptide synthesised in the liver. Hepcidin is responsible for regulating iron balance and recycling iron in humans and mice. Studies have reported 0–100 μg/ml concentrations of hepcidin incubated with HT1080, Hep-G2 and HeLa for 24 h. The results have indicated higher growth inhibition ratios after 70 μg/ml treatment with hepcidin in HT1080 cells; the treatment has been very effective in inhibiting the growth of fibrosarcoma cells [171, 172]. Tachyplesin is an anti-microbial peptide present in the leukocytes of the horseshoe crab (*Tachypleus tridentatus*); it inhibited the growth of TSU tumour cells on the CAM of chicken embryos as well as the growth of B16 tumour cells in syngenic mice; moreover, it blocked the proliferation of both tumour and endothelial cells in culture in a dose-dependent manner, whereas proliferation was relatively unaffected in non-tumourigenic cell lines Cos-7 and NIH-3T3 [173]. D-K4R2L9 is a peptide comprised of Leu, Lys and Arg residues, totalling 15 amino acid residues that bind to and lyse B16-F10 mouse melanoma cells in culture at concentrations that do not harm normal 3T3 fibroblasts or erythrocytes; this can be conducted to prevent intravenous-injected D122 lung carcinoma cells from forming lung tumours in mice [174, 175]. Bovine lactoferricin (LfcinB), an anti-microbial peptide, is a 25-amino acid long highly basic peptide with a disulfide bridge between two cysteines, thus giving it a cyclic twisted anti-parallel β-sheet solution structure. LfcinB has been tested on neuroblastoma growth *in vivo*; nude rats carrying SH-SY-5Y xenografts were given injections of 1.0 or 2.0 mg LfcinB; these rats' cancer was significantly inhibited after LfcinB treatment, compared with untreated controls [176]. Anti-microbial peptides can activate specific innate immune responses and immunomodulatory effects in the host, even if the host is at risk or has been damaged. Furthermore, researchers have proposed that anti-microbial peptides can modulate the host's immune system through inflammatory responses and can stimulate beneficial inflammation; anti-microbial peptides might be able to inhibit tumour growth.

9. Conclusion

From the injury to the wound recovery, there are a series of physiological responses that occur in relation to immune cells. Polarisation of the macrophage is an important response in wound healing. A series of inflammatory factors are cited having notable function in the differentiation from novel macrophage into the classical macrophage (M1). The cellular mechanism involved in the regulation of classical macrophage (M1) and alternative macrophage (M2) was documented in the wound healing process. At the present time, the M1/M2 differentiation was studied for selected immune responses. However, future studies may allow possible therapeutic targets considering this process in wound healing.

The immunotherapy that is being developed offers some advantageous immunomodulation factors that are known in the field of alternative medicine, such as mushroom beta-glucan, anti-microbial peptides and triterpenoid; these factors represent a novel therapeutic approach for anti-inflammation. These factors may be a viable alternative approach to the problem of drug resistance. Recent insights into wound healing and anti-inflammation are promising; however, exploiting these insights is complex because it involves chemistry, biology, instrumentation science and formulation science. Discovering new methods that are more effective in targets is difficult. Immunotherapy might be an alternative therapy that can be applied in the early phases of clinical therapy. Similarly, immunomodulation might be applicable in the early phases of immune disease.

Author details

Yu-Sheng Wu[1], Fan-Hua Nan[2], Sherwin Chen[1] and Shiu-Nan Chen[1*]

*Address all correspondence to: d97b45004@ntu.edu.tw; snchen@ntu.edu.tw

1 College of Life Science, National Taiwan University, Taipei, Taiwan

2 Department of Aquaculture, National Taiwan Ocean University, Keelung, Taiwan

References

[1] P. Allavena, A. Sica, G. Solinas *et al.*, "The inflammatory micro-environment in tumor progression: the role of tumor-associated macrophages," *Critical Reviews in Oncology/ Hematology*, vol. 66, no. 1, pp. 1–9, 2008.

[2] S. S. Choe, K. C. Shin, S. Ka *et al.*, "Macrophage HIF-2alpha ameliorates adipose tissue inflammation and insulin resistance in obesity," *Diabetes*, vol. 63, no. 10, pp. 3359–71, 2014.

[3] Y. Enoki, T. Sato, S. Tanaka *et al.*, "Netrin-4 derived from murine vascular endothelial cells inhibits osteoclast differentiation in vitro and prevents bone loss in vivo," *FEBS Letters*, vol. 588, no. 14, pp. 2262–9, 2014.

[4] B. Gore, M. Izikki, O. Mercier *et al.*, "Key role of the endothelial TGF-beta/ALK1/ endoglin signaling pathway in humans and rodents pulmonary hypertension," *PLoS One*, vol. 9, no. 6, p. e100310, 2014.

[5] G. Poschmann, M. Grzendowski, A. Stefanski *et al.*, "Redox proteomics reveal stress responsive proteins linking peroxiredoxin-1 status in glioma to chemosensitivity and oxidative stress," *Biochimica et Biophysica Acta*, 2014.

[6] L. Wu, H. Chen, C. Curtis *et al.*, "Go in for the kill," *Virulence*, vol. 5, no. 7, pp. 710–21, 2014.

[7] J. H. Yu, and H. Kim, "Oxidative stress and inflammatory signaling in cerulein pancreatitis," *World Journal of Gastroenterology*, vol. 20, no. 46, pp. 17324–9, 2014.

[8] E. Y. Choi, H. J. Kim, and J. S. Han, "Anti-inflammatory effects of calcium citrate in RAW 264.7cells via suppression of NF-kappaB activation," *Environmental Toxicology and Pharmacology*, vol. 39, no. 1, pp. 27–34, 2014.

[9] C. S. Luo, J. R. Liang, Q. Lin *et al.*, "Cellular responses associated with ROS production and cell fate decision in early stress response to iron limitation in the diatom *Thalassiosira pseudonana*," *Journal of Proteome Research*, vol. 13, no. 12, pp. 5510–23, 2014.

[10] E. McNeill, M. J. Crabtree, N. Sahgal *et al.*, "Regulation of iNOS function and cellular redox state by macrophage Gch1 reveals specific requirements for tetrahydrobiopterin in NRF2 activation," *Free Radical Biology & Medicine*, vol. 79C, pp. 206–16, 2014.

[11] K. A. Redgrove, and E. A. McLaughlin, "The role of the immune response in *Chlamydia trachomatis* infection of the male genital tract: a double-edged sword," *Frontiers in Immunology*, vol. 5, p. 534, 2014.

[12] F. Morescalchi, S. Duse, E. Gambicorti *et al.*, "Proliferative vitreoretinopathy after eye injuries: an overexpression of growth factors and cytokines leading to a retinal keloid," *Mediators Inflammation*, vol. 2013, p. 269787, 2013.

[13] M. J. Kipanyula, P. F. Seke Etet, L. Vecchio *et al.*, "Signaling pathways bridging microbial-triggered inflammation and cancer," *Cellular Signalling*, vol. 25, no. 2, pp. 403–16, 2013.

[14] R. Kisielewski, A. Tolwinska, A. Mazurek *et al.*, "Inflammation and ovarian cancer—current views," *Ginekologia Polska*, vol. 84, no. 4, pp. 293–7, 2013.

[15] E. Przybyt, M. J. van Luyn, and M. C. Harmsen, "Extracellular matrix components of adipose derived stromal cells promote alignment, organization, and maturation of cardiomyocytes in vitro," *Journal of Biomedical Materials Research Part A*, , 2014.

[16] R. Roshani, F. McCarthy, and T. Hagemann, "Inflammatory cytokines in human pancreatic cancer," *Cancer Letters*, vol. 345, no. 2, pp. 157–63, 2014.

[17] R. Nemenoff, "Activation of PPARgamma in myeloid cells promotes lung cancer progression and metastasis," *Oncoimmunology*, vol. 1, no. 3, pp. 403–4, 2012.

[18] R. Nemenoff, "Wound healing: a role for HDACs in inhibition of fibroblast proliferation through repression of PDGF receptor-alpha. Focus on ""Repression of PDGF-R-alpha after cellular injury involves TNF-alpha, formation of a c-Fos-YY1 complex, and negative regulation by HDAC"," *American Journal of Physiology – Cell Physiology*, vol. 302, no. 11, p. C1588–9, 2012.

[19] C. Hellberg, A. Ostman, and C. H. Heldin, "PDGF and vessel maturation," *Recent Results in Cancer Research*, vol. 180, pp. 103–14, 2010.

[20] C. Liu, W. Zhao, W. Meng *et al.*, "Platelet-derived growth factor blockade on cardiac remodeling following infarction," *Molecular and Cellular Biochemistry*, vol. 397, no. 1–2, pp. 295–304, 2014.

[21] S. Shimizu, H. Kouzaki, T. Ogawa *et al.*, "Eosinophil-epithelial cell interactions stimulate the production of MUC5AC mucin and profibrotic cytokines involved in airway tissue remodeling," *American Journal of Rhinology & Allergy*, vol. 28, no. 2, pp. 103–9, –2014.

[22] K. L. Spiller, R. R. Anfang, K. J. Spiller *et al.*, "The role of macrophage phenotype in vascularization of tissue engineering scaffolds," *Biomaterials*, vol. 35, no. 15, pp. 4477–88, 2014.

[23] K. Apel, and H. Hirt, "Reactive oxygen species: metabolism, oxidative stress, and signal transduction," *Annual Review of Plant Biology*, vol. 55, pp. 373–99, 2004.

[24] L. O. Klotz, "Oxidant-induced signaling: effects of peroxynitrite and singlet oxygen," *Biological Chemistry*, vol. 383, no. 3–4, pp. 443–56, 2002.

[25] A. Y. Andreyev, Y. E. Kushnareva, and A. A. Starkov, "Mitochondrial metabolism of reactive oxygen species," *Biochemistry (Moscow)*, vol. 70, no. 2, pp. 200–14, 2005.

[26] X. Li, P. Fang, J. Mai *et al.*, "Targeting mitochondrial reactive oxygen species as novel therapy for inflammatory diseases and cancers," *Journal of Hematology & Oncology*, vol. 6, pp. 19, 2013.

[27] E. C. Chan, F. Jiang, H. M. Peshavariya *et al.*, "Regulation of cell proliferation by NADPH oxidase-mediated signaling: potential roles in tissue repair, regenerative medicine and tissue engineering," *Pharmacology & Therapeutics*, vol. 122, no. 2, pp. 97–108, 2009.

[28] F. Jiang, Y. Zhang, and G. J. Dusting, "NADPH oxidase-mediated redox signaling: roles in cellular stress response, stress tolerance, and tissue repair," *Pharmacolical Reviews*, vol. 63, no. 1, pp. 218–42, 2011.

[29] Y. S. Wu, S. L. Huang, F. H. Nan *et al.*, "Over-inhibition of NADPH oxidase reduce the wound healing in liver of finfish," *Fish and Shellfish Immunology*, vol. 40, no. 1, pp. 174–81, 2014.

[30] J. F. Turrens, "Mitochondrial formation of reactive oxygen species," *Journal of Physiology*, vol. 552, no. Pt 2, pp. 335–44, 2003.

[31] E. Novo, C. Busletta, L. V. Bonzo *et al.*, "Intracellular reactive oxygen species are required for directional migration of resident and bone marrow-derived hepatic pro-fibrogenic cells," *Journal of Hepatology*, vol. 54, no. 5, pp. 964–74, 2011.

[32] A. Van der Goes, D. Wouters, S. M. Van Der Pol *et al.*, "Reactive oxygen species enhance the migration of monocytes across the blood-brain barrier in vitro," *FASEB Journal*, vol. 15, no. 10, pp. 1852–4, 2001.

[33] A. Ghosh, and M. E. Greenberg, "Calcium signaling in neurons: molecular mechanisms and cellular consequences," *Science*, vol. 268, no. 5208, pp. 239–47, 1995.

[34] S. Orrenius, B. Zhivotovsky, and P. Nicotera, "Regulation of cell death: the calcium-apoptosis link," *Nature Reviews Molecular Cell Biology*, vol. 4, no. 7, pp. 552–65, 2003.

[35] R. G. Spragg, D. B. Hinshaw, P. A. Hyslop *et al.*, "Alterations in adenosine triphosphate and energy charge in cultured endothelial and P388D1 cells after oxidant injury," *Journal of Clinical Investigation*, vol. 76, no. 4, pp. 1471–6, 1985.

[36] R. G. Spragg, "DNA strand break formation following exposure of bovine pulmonary artery and aortic endothelial cells to reactive oxygen products," *American Journal of Respiratory Cell and Molecular Biology*, vol. 4, no. 1, pp. 4–10, 1991.

[37] A. C. Gasic, G. McGuire, S. Krater *et al.*, "Hydrogen peroxide pretreatment of perfused canine vessels induces ICAM-1 and CD18-dependent neutrophil adherence," *Circulation*, vol. 84, no. 5, pp. 2154–66, 1991.

[38] A. Siflinger-Birnboim, H. Lum, P. D. Vecchio *et al.*, "Involvement of Ca2+ in the H2O2-induced increase in endothelial permeability," *American Journal of Physiology–Lung Cellular and Molecular Physiology*, vol. 14, no. 6, pp. L973, 1996.

[39] T. Finkel, "Signal transduction by mitochondrial oxidants," *Journal of Biological Chemistry*, vol. 287, no. 7, pp. 4434–40, 2012.

[40] Y.-S. Wu, and S.-N. Chen, "Apoptotic cell: linkage of inflammation and wound healing," *Frontiers in Pharmacology*, vol. 5, 2014.

[41] M. Haldar, and K. M. Murphy, "Origin, development, and homeostasis of tissue-resident macrophages," *Immunological Reviews*, vol. 262, no. 1, pp. 25–35, 2014.

[42] G. J. Guillemin, and B. J. Brew, "Microglia, macrophages, perivascular macrophages, and pericytes: a review of function and identification," *Journal of Leukocyte Biology*, vol. 75, no. 3, pp. 388–97, 2004.

[43] A. Sica, P. Invernizzi, and A. Mantovani, "Macrophage plasticity and polarization in liver homeostasis and pathology," *Hepatology*, vol. 59, no. 5, pp. 2034–42, 2014.

[44] S. Przybranowski, C. Wilke, N. Van Rooijen *et al.*, "Resident alveolar macrophages suppress while recruited macrophages promote allergic lung inflammation in murine models of asthma," *American Journal of Respiratory and Critical Care Medicine*, vol. 189, pp. A3685, 2014.

[45] S. Epelman, K. J. Lavine, A. E. Beaudin *et al.*, "Embryonic and adult-derived resident cardiac macrophages are maintained through distinct mechanisms at steady state and during inflammation," *Immunity*, vol. 40, no. 1, pp. 91–104, 2014.

[46] C. Schulz, E. G. Perdiguero, L. Chorro *et al.*, "A lineage of myeloid cells independent of Myb and hematopoietic stem cells," *Science*, vol. 336, no. 6077, pp. 86–90, 2012.

[47] J.-J. Widmann, and H. Fahimi, "Proliferation of mononuclear phagocytes (Kupffer cells) and endothelial cells in regenerating rat liver. A light and electron microscopic cytochemical study," *The American Journal of Pathology*, vol. 80, no. 3, pp. 349, 1975.

[48] W.-J. Wang, Y.-S. Wu, S. Chen *et al.*, "Mushroom β-glucan may immunomodulate the tumor-associated macrophages in the Lewis lung carcinoma," *BioMed Research International*, 2014.

[49] F. O. Martinez, L. Helming, and S. Gordon, "Alternative activation of macrophages: an immunologic functional perspective," *Annual Review of Immunology*, vol. 27, pp. 451–83, 2009.

[50] R. A. Flavell, S. Sanjabi, S. H. Wrzesinski *et al.*, "The polarization of immune cells in the tumour environment by TGFβ," *Nature Reviews Immunology*, vol. 10, no. 8, pp. 554–67, 2010.

[51] A. Sica, and A. Mantovani, "Macrophage plasticity and polarization: in vivo veritas," *The Journal of Clinical Investigation*, vol. 122, no. 3, pp. 787–95, 2012.

[52] A. Mantovani, S. K. Biswas, M. R. Galdiero *et al.*, "Macrophage plasticity and polarization in tissue repair and remodelling," *The Journal of Pathology*, vol. 229, no. 2, pp. 176–85, 2013.

[53] F. O. Martinez, A. Sica, A. Mantovani *et al.*, "Macrophage activation and polarization," *Frontiers in Bioscience: A Journal and Virtual Library*, vol. 13, pp. 453–61, 2007.

[54] A. Mantovani, S. Sozzani, M. Locati *et al.*, "Macrophage polarization: tumor-associated macrophages as a paradigm for polarized M2 mononuclear phagocytes," *Trends in Immunology*, vol. 23, no. 11, pp. 549–55, 2002.

[55] F. R. Smiderle, G. Alquini, M. Z. Tadra-Sfeir *et al.*, "*Agaricus bisporus* and *Agaricus brasiliensis* (1→6)-β-d-glucans show immunostimulatory activity on human THP-1 derived macrophages," *Carbohydrate Polymers*, vol. 94, no. 1, pp. 91–9, 2013.

[56] R.-S. Sauer, D. Hackel, L. Morschel *et al.*, "Toll like receptor (TLR)-4 as a regulator of peripheral endogenous opioid-mediated analgesia in inflammation," *Molecular Pain*, vol. 10, no. 1, pp. 10, 2014.

[57] J. S. Orr, M. J. Puglisi, K. L. Ellacott *et al.*, "Toll-like receptor 4 deficiency promotes the alternative activation of adipose tissue macrophages," *Diabetes*, vol. 61, no. 11, pp. 2718–27, 2012.

[58] N. Wang, H. Liang, and K. Zen, "Molecular mechanisms that influence the macrophage M1–M2 polarization balance," *Frontiers in Immunology*, vol. 5, 2014.

[59] C. S. Whyte, E. T. Bishop, D. Rückerl *et al.*, "Suppressor of cytokine signaling (SOCS) 1 is a key determinant of differential macrophage activation and function," *Journal of Leukocyte Biology*, vol. 90, no. 5, pp. 845–54, 2011.

[60] S. Gordon, and F. O. Martinez, "Alternative activation of macrophages: mechanism and functions," *Immunity*, vol. 32, no. 5, pp. 593–604, 2010.

[61] H. Zhou, J. Liao, J. Aloor *et al.*, "CD11b/CD18 (Mac-1) is a novel surface receptor for extracellular double-stranded RNA to mediate cellular inflammatory responses," *The Journal of Immunology*, vol. 190, no. 1, pp. 115–25, 2013.

[62] Y. S. Schwartz, and A. Svistelnik, "Functional phenotypes of macrophages and the M1-M2 polarization concept. Part I. Proinflammatory phenotype," *Biochemistry (Moscow)*, vol. 77, no. 3, pp. 246–60, 2012.

[63] U. S. Rangaswamy, and S. H. Speck, "Murine gammaherpesvirus M2 protein induction of IRF4 via the NFAT pathway leads to IL-10 expression in B cells," *PLoS Pathogens*, vol. 10, no. 1, pp. e1003858, 2014.

[64] I. A. Udalova, T. Krausgruber, T. Smallie *et al.*, "IRF5 promotes inflammatory macro-phage polarization and Th1/Th17 response," *Nature Immunology*, 2011.

[65] H. Xu, J. Zhu, S. Smith *et al.*, "Notch-RBP-J signaling regulates the transcription factor IRF8 to promote inflammatory macrophage polarization," *Nature Immunology*, vol. 13, no. 7, pp. 642–50, 2012.

[66] H. J. Lee, Y. K. Oh, M. Rhee *et al.*, "The role of STAT1/IRF-1 on synergistic ROS production and loss of mitochondrial transmembrane potential during hepatic cell death induced by LPS/d-GalN," *Journal of Molecular Biology*, vol. 369, no. 4, pp. 967–84, 2007.

[67] W. Xiao, H. Hong, Y. Kawakami *et al.*, "Regulation of myeloproliferation and M2 macrophage programming in mice by Lyn/Hck, SHIP, and Stat5," *The Journal of Clinical Investigation*, vol. 118, no. 3, pp. 924, 2008.

[68] Y. Ji, S. Sun, A. Xu *et al.*, "Activation of natural killer T cells promotes M2 macrophage polarization in adipose tissue and improves systemic glucose tolerance via interleukin-4 (IL-4)/STAT6 protein signaling axis in obesity," *Journal of Biological Chemistry*, vol. 287, no. 17, pp. 13561–71, 2012.

[69] J. Wan, M. Benkdane, F. Teixeira-Clerc *et al.*, "M2 Kupffer cells promote M1 Kupffer cell apoptosis: a protective mechanism against alcoholic and nonalcoholic fatty liver disease," *Hepatology*, vol. 59, no. 1, pp. 130–42, 2014.

[70] M. Heusinkveld, P. J. d. V. van Steenwijk, R. Goedemans *et al.*, "M2 macrophages induced by prostaglandin E2 and IL-6 from cervical carcinoma are switched to activated M1 macrophages by CD4+ Th1 cells," *The Journal of Immunology*, vol. 187, no. 3, pp. 1157–65, 2011.

[71] D. Zhou, C. Huang, Z. Lin *et al.*, "Macrophage polarization and function with emphasis on the evolving roles of coordinated regulation of cellular signaling pathways," *Cellular Signalling*, vol. 26, no. 2, pp. 192–7, 2014.

[72] A. J. Covarrubias, and T. Horng, "IL-6 strikes a balance in metabolic inflammation," *Cell Metabolism*, vol. 19, no. 6, pp. 898–9, 2014.

[73] P. Kell, T. Ennis, K. Chang *et al.*, "Macrophages mediate the ability of the receptor for advanced glycation end products to prevent formation of abdominal aortic aneurysm in a murine model," *Arteriosclerosis, Thrombosis, and Vascular Biology*, vol. 34, no. Suppl 1, p. A114, 2014.

[74] A. Gal, T. T. Tapmeier, and R. J. Muschel, "Plasticity of tumor associated macrophages in a metastatic melanoma model in the mouse," *Cancer Research*, vol. 72, no. 8 Suppl, pp. 402, 2012.

[75] K. L. Spiller, S. Nassiri, C. E. Witherel *et al.*, "Sequential delivery of immunomodulatory cytokines to facilitate the M1-to-M2 transition of macrophages and enhance vascularization of bone scaffolds," *Biomaterials*, vol. 37, pp. 194–207, 2015.

[76] X. Cai, Y. Yin, N. Li *et al.*, "Re-polarization of tumor-associated macrophages to pro-inflammatory M1 macrophages by microRNA-155," *Journal of Molecular Cell Biology*, vol. 4, no. 5, pp. 341–3, 2012.

[77] J.-H. Lee, G. T. Lee, S. H. Woo *et al.*, "BMP-6 in renal cell carcinoma promotes tumor proliferation through IL-10–dependent M2 polarization of tumor-associated macrophages," *Cancer Research*, vol. 73, no. 12, pp. 3604–14, 2013.

[78] N. Ouchi, J. L. Parker, J. J. Lugus *et al.*, "Adipokines in inflammation and metabolic disease," *Nature Reviews Immunology*, vol. 11, no. 2, pp. 85–97, 2011.

[79] R. G. Baker, M. S. Hayden, and S. Ghosh, "NF-κB, inflammation, and metabolic disease," *Cell Metabolism*, vol. 13, no. 1, pp. 11–22, 2011.

[80] B. Gooptu, and D. A. Lomas, "Polymers and inflammation: disease mechanisms of the serpinopathies," *The Journal of Experimental Medicine*, vol. 205, no. 7, pp. 1529–34, 2008.

[81] R. L. Davis, A. E. Shrimpton, P. D. Holohan *et al.*, "Familial dementia caused by polymerization of mutant neuroserpin," *Nature*, vol. 401, no. 6751, pp. 376–9, 1999.

[82] G. K. Hansson, "Inflammation, atherosclerosis, and coronary artery disease," *New England Journal of Medicine*, vol. 352, no. 16, pp. 1685–95, 2005.

[83] H. Akiyama, S. Barger, S. Barnum *et al.*, "Inflammation and Alzheimer's disease," *Neurobiology of Aging*, vol. 21, no. 3, pp. 383–421, 2000.

[84] T. A. Wynn, A. Chawla, and J. W. Pollard, "Macrophage biology in development, homeostasis and disease," *Nature*, vol. 496, no. 7446, pp. 445–55, 2013.

[85] A. Sica, and A. Mantovani, "Macrophage plasticity and polarization: in vivo veritas," *Journal of Clinical Investigation*, vol. 122, no. 3, pp. 787–95, 2012.

[86] T. L. Denning, B. A. Norris, O. Medina-Contreras *et al.*, "Functional specializations of intestinal dendritic cell and macrophage subsets that control Th17 and regulatory T cell responses are dependent on the T cell/APC ratio, source of mouse strain, and regional localization," *The Journal of Immunology*, vol. 187, no. 2, pp. 733–47, 2011.

[87] J. A. Joyce, and J. W. Pollard, "Microenvironmental regulation of metastasis," *Nature Reviews Cancer*, vol. 9, pp. 239–52, 2009.

[88] L. M. Coussens, and Z. Werb, "Inflammation and cancer," *Nature*, vol. 420, pp. 860–67, 2002.

[89] G. Baronzio, G. Fiorentini, and C. R. Cogle, *Cancer microenvironment and therapeutic implications*. Springer, 2009.

[90] F. Xing, J. Saidou, and K. Watabe, "Cancer associated fibroblasts (CAFs) in tumor microenvironment," *Frontiers in Bioscience (Landmark Ed)*, vol. 15, pp. 166–79, 2010.

[91] G. Castello, S. Scala, G. Palmieri *et al.*, "HCV-related hepatocellular carcinoma: From chronic inflammation to cancer," *Clinical Immunology*, vol. 134, pp. 237–50, 2010.

[92] C. A. Janeway, M. Walport, and P. Travers, *Immunobiology: the immune system in health and disease*. Garland Science, 2005.

[93] D. I. Gabrilovich, and A. A. Hurwitz, *Tumor-induced immune suppression*. Springer, 2008.

[94] W. Zou, "Immunosuppressive networks in the tumour environment and their therapeutic relevance," *Nature Reviews Cancer*, vol. 5, pp. 263–74, 2005.

[95] G. P. Dunn, A. T. Bruce, H. Ikeda *et al.*, "Cancer immunoediting: from immunosurveillance to tumor escape," *Nature Immunology*, vol. 3, pp. 991–8, 2002.

[96] G. P. Dunn, L. J. Old, and R. D. Schreiber, "The immunobiology of cancer immunosurveillance and immunoediting," *Immunity*, vol. 21, pp. 137–48, 2004.

[97] B. Z. Qian, and J. W. Pollard, "Macrophage diversity enhances tumor progression and metastasis," *Cell*, vol. 141, pp. 39–51, 2010.

[98] D. W. Siemann, *"Tumor microenvironment.* Wiley Online Library, 2011.

[99] N. Mach, S. Gillessen, S. B. Wilson *et al.*, "Differences in dendritic cells stimulated *in vivo* by tumors engineered to secrete granulocyte-macrophage colony-stimulating factor of flt3-ligand," *Cancer Research*, vol. 60, pp. 3239–46, 2000.

[100] S. K. Biswas, and A. Mantovani, "Macrophage plasticity and interaction with lymphocyte subsets: cancer as a paradigm," *Nature Immunology*, vol. 11, pp. 889–96, 2010.

[101] B. Ruffell, N. I. Affara, and L. M. Coussens, "Differential macrophage programming in the tumor microenvironment," *Trends in Immunology*, vol. 33, pp. 119–126, 2012.

[102] R. A. Flavell, S. Sanjabi, S. H. Wrzesinski *et al.*, "The polarization of immune cells in the tumour environment by TGFbeta," *Nature Reviews Immunology*, vol. 10, pp. 554–67, 2010.

[103] L. Bingle, N. J. Brown, and C. E. Lewis, "The role of tumour-associated macrophages in tumour progression: implications for new anticancer therapies," *The Journal of Pathology*, vol. 196, pp. 254–65, 2002.

[104] J. W. Pollard, "Tumour-educated macrophages promote tumour progression and metastasis," *Nature Reviews Cancer*, vol. 4, pp. 71–78, 2004.

[105] A. Mantovani, A. Sica, S. Sozzani *et al.*, "The chemokine system in diverse forms of macrophage activation and polarization," *Trends in Immunology*, vol. 25, pp. 677–86, 2004.

[106] A. Mantovani, and A. Sica, "Macrophages, innate immunity and cancer: balance, tolerance, and diversity," *Current Opinion in Immunology*, vol. 22, pp. 231–7, 2010.

[107] A. Mantovani, A. Sica, P. Allavena *et al.*, "Tumor-associated macrophages and the related myeloid-derived suppressor cells as a paradigm of the diversity of macrophage activation," *Human Immunology*, vol. 70, pp. 325–30, 2009.

[108] C. Steidl, T. Lee, S. P. Shah *et al.*, "Tumor-associated macrophages and survival in classic Hodgkin's Lymphoma," *The New England Journal of Medicine*, vol. 362, pp. 875–85, 2010.

[109] K. D. Elgert, D. G. Alleva, and D. W. Mullins, "Tumor-induced immune dysfunction: the macrophage connection," *Journal of Leukocyte Biology*, vol. 64, pp. 275–90, 1998.

[110] C. Sunderkötter, M. Goebeler, K. Schulze-Osthoff *et al.*, "Macrophage-derived angiogenesis factors," *Pharmacology & Therapeutics*, vol. 51, pp. 195–216, 1991.

[111] E. Giraudo, M. Inoue, and D. Hanahan, "An amino-bisphosphonate targets MMP-9-expressing macrophages and angiogenesis to impair cervical carcinogenesis," *The Journal of Clinical Investigation*, vol. 114, pp. 623–33, 2004.

[112] A. Ben-Baruch, "Inflammation-associated immune suppression in cancer: the roles played by cytokines, chemokines and additional mediators," *Seminars in Cancer Biology*, vol. 16, pp. 38–52, 2006.

[113] M. Mitsuhashi, J. Liu, S. Cao *et al.*, "Regulation of interleukin-12 gene expression and its anti-tumor activities by prostaglandin E2 derived from mammary carcinomas," *Journal of Leukocyte Biology*, vol. 76, pp. 322–32, 2004.

[114] A. Mantovani, S. Sozzani, M. Locati *et al.*, "Macrophage polarization: tumor-associated macrophages as a paradigm for polarized M2 mononuclear phagocytes," *Trends in Immunology* vol. 23, pp. 549–55, 2002.

[115] G. Solinas, G. Germano, A. Mantovani *et al.*, "Tumor-associated macrophages (TAM) as major players of the cancer-related inflammation," *Journal of Leukocyte Biology*, vol. 86, pp. 1065–73, 2009.

[116] M. P. Fink, "Role of reactive oxygen and nitrogen species in acute respiratory distress syndrome," *Current Opinion in Critical Care*, vol. 8, no. 1, pp. 6–11, 2002.

[117] F. Dong, X. C. Zhang, S. Y. Li *et al.*, "Possible involvement of NADPH oxidase and JNK in homocysteine-induced oxidative stress and apoptosis in human umbilical vein endothelial cells," *Cardiovascular Toxicology*, vol. 5, no. 1, pp. 9–20, 2005.

[118] E. Novo, C. Busletta, L. V. Bonzo *et al.*, "Intracellular reactive oxygen species are required for directional migration of resident and bone marrow-derived hepatic pro-fibrogenic cells," *Journal of Hepatology*, vol. 54, no. 5, pp. 964–74, 2011.

[119] A. Van der Goes, D. Wouters, S. M. Van Der Pol *et al.*, "Reactive oxygen species enhance the migration of monocytes across the blood-brain barrier in vitro," *FASEB Journal : Official Publication of the Federation of American Societies for Experimental Biology*, vol. 15, no. 10, pp. 1852–4, 2001.

[120] J. W. Park, S. W. Ryter, and A. M. Choi, "Functional significance of apoptosis in chronic obstructive pulmonary disease," *COPD*, vol. 4, no. 4, pp. 347–53, 2007.

[121] S. W. Ryter, H. P. Kim, A. Hoetzel *et al.*, "Mechanisms of cell death in oxidative stress," *Antioxid Redox Signal*, vol. 9, no. 1, pp. 49–89, 2007.

[122] M. L. Circu, and T. Y. Aw, "Reactive oxygen species, cellular redox systems, and apoptosis," *Free Radical Biology and Medicine*, vol. 48, no. 6, pp. 749–62, 2010.

[123] B. T. Mossman, "Introduction to serial reviews on the role of reactive oxygen and nitrogen species (ROS/RNS) in lung injury and diseases," *Free Radical Biology and Medicine*, vol. 34, no. 9, pp. 1115–6, 2003.

[124] S. I. Grivennikov, F. R. Greten, and M. Karin, "Immunity, Inflammation, and Cancer," *Cell*, vol. 140, no. 6, pp. 883–899, 2010.

[125] T. A. Wilgus, "Immune cells in the healing skin wound: influential players at each stage of repair," *Pharmacological Research*, vol. 58, no. 2, pp. 112–6, 2008.

[126] R. Alinovi, M. Goldoni, S. Pinelli *et al.*, "Oxidative and pro-inflammatory effects of cobalt and titanium oxide nanoparticles on aortic and venous endothelial cells," *Toxicology In Vitro*, vol. 29, no. 3, pp. 426–37, 2014.

[127] G. Pellegrini, G. Rasperini, G. Obot *et al.*, "Soft tissue healing in alveolar socket preservation technique: histologic evaluations," *International Journal of Periodontics Restorative Dent*, vol. 34, no. 4, pp. 531–9, –2014.

[128] V. Kumar, "Innate lymphoid cells: new paradigm in immunology of inflammation," *Immunology Letters*, vol. 157, no. 1–2, pp. 23–37, 2014.

[129] A. Barbul, and M. C. Regan, "The regulatory role of T lymphocytes in wound healing," *Journal of Trauma*, vol. 30, no. 12 Suppl, pp. S97–100, 1990.

[130] T. A. Petrie, N. S. Strand, C. Tsung-Yang *et al.*, "Macrophages modulate adult zebrafish tail fin regeneration," *Development*, vol. 141, no. 13, pp. 2581–91, 2014.

[131] M. Sugaya, "Chemokines and skin diseases," *Archivum Immunologiae et Therapia Experimentalis (Warsz)*, 2014.

[132] S. Zhang, S. Dehn, M. DeBerge *et al.*, "Phagocyte-myocyte interactions and consequences during hypoxic wound healing," *Cellular Immunology*, vol. 291, no. 1–2, pp. 65–73, 2014.

[133] L. A. DiPietro, "Wound healing: the role of the macrophage and other immune cells," *Shock*, vol. 4, no. 4, pp. 233–40, 1995.

[134] C. Fathke, L. Wilson, K. Shah *et al.*, "Wnt signaling induces epithelial differentiation during cutaneous wound healing," *BMC Cell Biology*, vol. 7, pp. 4, 2006.

[135] M.-K. Song, Y.-K. Park, and J.-C. Ryu, "Polycyclic aromatic hydrocarbon (PAH)-mediated upregulation of hepatic microRNA-181 family promotes cancer cell migration by targeting MAPK phosphatase-5, regulating the activation of p38 MAPK," *Toxicology and Applied Pharmacology*, vol. 273, no. 1, pp. 130–9, 2013.

[136] Y. Wang, Y. Zhou, and D. T. Graves, "FOXO transcription factors: their clinical significance and regulation," *BioMed Research International*, vol. 2014, 2014.

[137] C. W. Chow, M. T. Herrera Abreu, T. Suzuki *et al.*, "Oxidative stress and acute lung injury," *American Journal of Respiratory Cell and Molecular Biology*, vol. 29, no. 4, pp. 427–31, 2003.

[138] C. Yang, H. Moriuchi, J. Takase *et al.*, "Oxidative stress in early stage of acute lung injury induced with oleic acid in guinea pigs," *Biological and Pharmaceutical Bulletin*, vol. 26, no. 4, pp. 424–8, 2003.

[139] V. Patel, I. V. Chivukula, S. Roy *et al.*, "Oxygen: from the benefits of inducing VEGF expression to managing the risk of hyperbaric stress," *Antioxidants & Redox Signaling*, vol. 7, no. 9–10, pp. 1377–87, 2005.

[140] A. C. Bulua, A. Simon, R. Maddipati *et al.*, "Mitochondrial reactive oxygen species promote production of proinflammatory cytokines and are elevated in TNFR1-associated periodic syndrome (TRAPS)," *The Journal of Experimental Medicine*, vol. 208, no. 3, pp. 519–33, 2011.

[141] R. J. Aitken, K. T. Jones, and S. A. Robertson, "Reactive oxygen species and sperm function — in sickness and in health," *Journal of Andrology*, vol. 33, no. 6, pp. 1096–1106, 2012.

[142] S. Eligini, I. Arenaz, S. S. Barbieri *et al.*, "Cyclooxygenase-2 mediates hydrogen peroxide-induced wound repair in human endothelial cells," *Free Radical Biology and Medicine*, vol. 46, no. 10, pp. 1428–36, 2009.

[143] M. Iizuka, and S. Konno, "Wound healing of intestinal epithelial cells," *World Journal of Gastroenterology: WJG*, vol. 17, no. 17, pp. 2161, 2011.

[144] D. Maslinska, and M. Gajewski, "Some aspects of the inflammatory process," *Folia Neuropathologica*, vol. 36, no. 4, pp. 199–204, 1998.

[145] P. Libby, P. M. Ridker, and A. Maseri, "Inflammation and atherosclerosis," *Circulation*, vol. 105, no. 9, pp. 1135–43, 2002.

[146] J. M. Rubio-Perez, and J. M. Morillas-Ruiz, "A review: inflammatory process in Alzheimer's disease, role of cytokines," *Scientific World Journal*, 2012.

[147] C. D. Gregory, "Inflammation and cancer revisited: an hypothesis on the oncogenic potential of the apoptotic tumor cell," *Autoimmunity*, vol. 46, no. 5, pp. 312–6, 2013.

[148] B. B. Aggarwal, S. Shishodia, S. K. Sandur *et al.*, "Inflammation and cancer: how hot is the link?," *Biochemical Pharmacology*, vol. 72, no. 11, pp. 1605–21, 2006.

[149] A. K. Muller, M. Meyer, and S. Werner, "The roles of receptor tyrosine kinases and their ligands in the wound repair process," *Seminars in Cell & Developmental Biology*, vol. 23, no. 9, pp. 963–70, 2012.

[150] S. Danckwardt, M. W. Hentze, and A. E. Kulozik, "Pathologies at the nexus of blood coagulation and inflammation: thrombin in hemostasis, cancer, and beyond," *Journal of Molecular Medicine: JMM*, vol. 91, no. 11, pp. 1257–71, 2013.

[151] S. Strukova, "Blood coagulation-dependent inflammation. Coagulation-dependent inflammation and inflammation-dependent thrombosis," *Frontiers in Bioscience*, vol. 11, pp. 59–80, 2006.

[152] T. N. Dugina, E. V. Kiseleva, I. V. Chistov *et al.*, "Receptors of the PAR-family as a link between blood coagulation and inflammation," *Biochemistry (Moscow)*, vol. 67, no. 1, pp. 65–74, 2002.

[153] Y. Nakanishi, M. Nakatsuji, H. Seno *et al.*, "COX-2 inhibition alters the phenotype of tumor-associated macrophages from M2 to M1 in ApcMin/+ mouse polyps," *Carcinogenesis*, vol. 32, pp. 1333–9, 2011.

[154] T. Ikekawa, "Enokitake, *Flammulina velutipes*: host-mediated antitumor polysaccharides," *Food Reviews International*, vol. 11, pp. 203–6, 1995.

[155] T. Ikekawa, N. Uehara, Y. Maeda *et al.*, "Antitumor activity of aqueous extracts of edible mushrooms," *Cancer Research*, vol. 29, pp. 734–5, 1969.

[156] S. P. Wasser, "Medicinal mushrooms as a source of antitumor and immunomodulating polysaccharides," *Applied Microbiology and Biotechnology*, vol. 60, pp. 258–74, 2002.

[157] T. Inomata, G. B. Goodman, C. J. Fryer *et al.*, "Immune reaction induced by X-rays and pions and its stimulation by schizophyllan (SPG)," *The British Journal of Cancer*, vol. 27, pp. 122–5, 1996.

[158] H. Nanba, and K. Kubo, "Effect of Maitake D-fraction on cancer prevention," *Cancer*, vol. 833, pp. 204–7, 1997.

[159] C. Menetrier-Caux, G. Montmain, M. C. Dieu *et al.*, "Inhibition of the differentiation of dendritic cells from CD34+ progenitors by tumor cells: role of interleukin-6 and macrophage colony-stimulating factor," *Blood*, vol. 92, pp. 4778–91, 1998.

[160] E. Y. Lin, V. Gouon-Evans, A. V. Nquyen *et al.*, "The macrophage growth factor CSF-1 in mammary gland development and tumor progression," *Journal of Mammary Gland Biology and Neoplasia*, vol. 7, pp. 147–62, 2002.

[161] C. E. Lewis, and J. W. Pollard, "Distinct role of macrophages in different tumor microenvironment," *Cancer Research*, vol. 66, pp. 605–12, 2006.

[162] E. S. Ch'ng, H. Jaafar, and S. E. Tuan Sharif, "Breast tumor angiogenesis and tumor-associated macrophages: histopathologist's perspective," *Pathology Research International*, vol. 2011, pp. 1–13, 2011.

[163] T. J. Standiford, R. Kuick, U. Bhan *et al.*, "TGF-β-induced IRAK-M expression in tumor-associated macrophages regulates lung tumor growth," *Oncogene*, vol. 30, pp. 2475–84, 2011.

[164] K. Murphy, P. Travers, and M. Walport, *Immunobiology*, 7th ed. Graland Science, 2008.

[165] T. R. Mosmann, H. Cherwinski, M. W. Bond *et al.*, "Two types of murine helper T cell clone. I. Definition according to profiles of lymphokine activities and secreted proteins. 1986," *Journal of Immunology*, vol. 175, no. 1, pp. 5–14, 2005.

[166] T. R. Mosmann, and R. L. Coffman, "TH1 and TH2 cells: different patterns of lympho-kine secretion lead to different functional properties," *Annual Review of Immunology*, vol. 7, pp. 145–73, 1989.

[167] E. Maggi, "The TH1/TH2 paradigm in allergy," *Immunotechnology*, vol. 3, no. 4, pp. 233–44, 1998.

[168] P. Kidd, "Th1/Th2 balance: the hypothesis, its limitations, and implications for health and disease," *Alternative Medicine Review*, vol. 8, no. 3, pp. 223–46, 2003.

[169] M. E. Stern, K. F. Siemasko, and J. Y. Niederkorn, "The Th1/Th2 paradigm in ocular allergy," *Current Opinion in Allergy and Clinical Immunology*, vol. 5, no. 5, pp. 446–50, 2005.

[170] Z. B. Lin, and H. N. Zhang, "Anti-tumor and immunoregulatory activities of Ganoderma lucidum and its possible mechanisms," *Acta Pharmacologica Sinica*, vol. 25, no. 11, pp. 1387–95, 2004.

[171] J. S. Shi, and A. C. Camus, "Hepcidins in amphibians and fishes: antimicrobial peptides or iron-regulatory hormones?" *Developmental and Comparative Immunology*, vol. 30, no. 9, pp. 746–55, 2006.

[172] J. Y. Chen, W. J. Lin, and T. L. Lin, "A fish antimicrobial peptide, tilapia hepcidin TH2-3, shows potent antitumor activity against human fibrosarcoma cells," *Peptides*, vol. 30, no. 9, pp. 1636–42, 2009.

[173] Y. X. Chen, X. M. Xu, S. G. Hong *et al.*, "RGD-tachyplesin inhibits tumor growth," *Cancer Research*, vol. 61, no. 6, pp. 2434–38, 2001.

[174] D. W. Hoskin, and A. Ramamoorthy, "Studies on anticancer activities of antimicrobial peptides," *Biochimica et Biophysica Acta–Biomembranes*, vol. 1778, no. 2, pp. 357–75, 2008.

[175] N. Papo, M. Shahar, L. Eisenbach *et al.*, "A novel lytic peptide composed of DL-amino acids selectively kills cancer cells in culture and in mice," *Journal of Biological Chemistry*, vol. 278, no. 23, pp. 21018–23, 2003.

[176] L. T. Eliassen, G. Berge, A. Leknessund *et al.*, "The antimicrobial peptide, Lactoferricin B, is cytotoxic to neuroblastoma cells in vitro and inhibits xenograft growth in vivo," *International Journal of Cancer*, vol. 119, no. 3, pp. 493–500, 2006.

Permissions

All chapters in this book were first published in WH, by InTech Open; hereby published with permission under the Creative Commons Attribution License or equivalent. Every chapter published in this book has been scrutinized by our experts. Their significance has been extensively debated. The topics covered herein carry significant findings which will fuel the growth of the discipline. They may even be implemented as practical applications or may be referred to as a beginning point for another development.

The contributors of this book come from diverse backgrounds, making this book a truly international effort. This book will bring forth new frontiers with its revolutionizing research information and detailed analysis of the nascent developments around the world.

We would like to thank all the contributing authors for lending their expertise to make the book truly unique. They have played a crucial role in the development of this book. Without their invaluable contributions this book wouldn't have been possible. They have made vital efforts to compile up to date information on the varied aspects of this subject to make this book a valuable addition to the collection of many professionals and students.

This book was conceptualized with the vision of imparting up-to-date information and advanced data in this field. To ensure the same, a matchless editorial board was set up. Every individual on the board went through rigorous rounds of assessment to prove their worth. After which they invested a large part of their time researching and compiling the most relevant data for our readers.

The editorial board has been involved in producing this book since its inception. They have spent rigorous hours researching and exploring the diverse topics which have resulted in the successful publishing of this book. They have passed on their knowledge of decades through this book. To expedite this challenging task, the publisher supported the team at every step. A small team of assistant editors was also appointed to further simplify the editing procedure and attain best results for the readers.

Apart from the editorial board, the designing team has also invested a significant amount of their time in understanding the subject and creating the most relevant covers. They scrutinized every image to scout for the most suitable representation of the subject and create an appropriate cover for the book.

The publishing team has been an ardent support to the editorial, designing and production team. Their endless efforts to recruit the best for this project, has resulted in the accomplishment of this book. They are a veteran in the field of academics and their pool of knowledge is as vast as their experience in printing. Their expertise and guidance has proved useful at every step. Their uncompromising quality standards have made this book an exceptional effort. Their encouragement from time to time has been an inspiration for everyone.

The publisher and the editorial board hope that this book will prove to be a valuable piece of knowledge for researchers, students, practitioners and scholars across the globe.

List of Contributors

Anuradha Majumdar and Prajakta Sangole
Department of Pharmacology, Bombay College of Pharmacy, Kalina, Mumbai, India

Omar Sarheed and Douha Shouqair
RAK College of Pharmaceutical Sciences, RAK Medical and Health Sciences University, Ras Al Khaiamah, United Arab Emirates

Asif Ahmed and Joshua Boateng
Department of Pharmaceutical, Chemical and Environmental Sciences, Faculty of Engineering and Science, University of Greenwich, Kent, UK

Wael Tawfick
Department of Vascular and Endovascular Surgery, Western Vascular Institute, University College Hospital Galway, Galway, Ireland

Edel P Kavanagh and Niamh Hynes
Department of Vascular and Endovascular Surgery, Galway Clinic, Doughiska, Galway, Ireland

Sherif Sultan
Department of Vascular and Endovascular Surgery, Western Vascular Institute, University College Hospital Galway, Galway, Ireland

Department of Vascular and Endovascular Surgery, Galway Clinic, Doughiska, Galway, Ireland

Christian Agyare, Yaw Duah Boakye, Susanna Oteng Dapaah and Theresa Appiah
Department of Pharmaceutics, Faculty of Pharmacy and Pharmaceutical Sciences, Kwame Nkrumah University of Science and Technology, Kumasi, Ghana

Emelia Oppong Bekoe
Department of Pharmaceutics and Pharmaceutical Microbiology, School of Pharmacy, University of Ghana, Legon, Accra, Ghana

Samuel Oppong Bekoe
Department of Pharmaceutical Chemistry, Faculty of Pharmacy and Pharmaceutical Sciences, Kwame Nkrumah University of Science and Technology, Kumasi, Ghana

Jill M. Monfre
University Hospital, University of Wisconsin, Madison, Wisconsin, USA

Eric Boucher, Tatsuya Kato and Craig A. Mandato
Department of Anatomy and Cell Biology, Faculty of Medicine, McGill University, Montreal, Quebec, Canada

Gregorio Castellanos and Antonio Piñero
Surgery Service, Virgen de la Arrixaca University Clinical Hospital, El Palmar, Murcia, Spain

Ángel Bernabé-García and Francisco J. Nicolás
Molecular Oncology and TGFβ, Research Unit, Virgen de la Arrixaca University Hospital, El Palmar, Murcia, Spain

Carmen García Insausti and José M. Moraleda
Cell Therapy Unit, Virgen de la Arrixaca University Clinical Hospital, El Palmar, Murcia, Spain

Peter Mekhail
Aberdeen Royal Infirmary, Aberdeen, UK

Shuchi Chaturvedi
Kings College London, London, UK

Shailesh Chaturvedi
Department of General Surgery, Aberdeen Royal Infirmary, Aberdeen, UK

Fan-Hua Nan
Department of Aquaculture, National Taiwan Ocean University, Keelung, Taiwan

Yu-Sheng Wu, Sherwin Chen and Shiu-Nan Chen
College of Life Science, National Taiwan University, Taipei, Taiwan

Index